POST ANESTHESIA CARE UNIT

Current Practices

POST ANESTHESIA CARE UNIT

Current Practices

Editor

Elizabeth A.M. Frost, M.D.

Professor, Department of Anesthesiology,
Albert Einstein College of Medicine,
Montefiore Medical Center,
Bronx, New York

SECOND EDITION

with 98 illustrations

The C.V. Mosby Company

ST. LOUIS • BALTIMORE • PHILADELPHIA • TORONTO   1990

Editor: Nancy L. Coon
Developmental Editor: Susan R. Epstein
Project Manager: Teri Merchant
Production Editor: Betty Hazelwood
Designer: Kay Kramer

SECOND EDITION

Printed in the United States of America

The C.V. Mosby Company
11830 Westline Industrial Drive, St. Louis, Missouri 63146

Library of Congress Cataloging in Publication Data

Post anesthesia care unit : current practices / editor, Elizabeth A.M.
    Frost. —2nd ed.
        p.   cm.
    Rev. ed. of: Recovery room practice. c1985.
    Includes bibliographical references.
    ISBN 0-8016-0204-1
    1. Postoperative care.   2. Recovery room (Surgery)   I. Frost,
Elizabeth A.M.   II. Recovery room practice.
    [DNLM: 1. Postoperative Care—nurses' instruction.   2. Recovery
Room—nurses' instruction.   3. Surgical Nursing.   WY 154 P8565]
RD51.P64   1990
617′.919—dc20
DNLM/DLC
for Library of Congress   90-5642
                                                                      CIP

GW/MV/MV 9 8 7 6 5 4 3 2 1

CONTRIBUTORS

Jeffrey Askanazi, M.D.

Department of Anesthesiology and Critical Care,
Montefiore Medical Center,
Bronx, New York

Nirmala Balan, M.D.

Loma Linda Anesthesiology Medical Group, Inc.,
Loma Linda, California

Jonathan S. Daitch, M.D.

Captain, USAF, Medical Center,
Wright-Patterson Air Force Base, Ohio

Margaret DeFranco, R.N.

Henrietta, New York

Elizabeth A.M. Frost, M.D.

Department of Anesthesiology,
Albert Einstein College of Medicine,
Bronx, New York

Marilyn (Schneider) Glaser, R.N.

Doctor's Hospital of Prince George's County,
Lanham, Maryland

Paul L. Goldiner, M.D.

Department of Anesthesiology,
Albert Einstein College of Medicine,
Bronx, New York

Ingrid Hollinger, M.D.

Department of Anesthesiology,
Montefiore Medical Center,
Bronx, New York

Laurent Kaleka, M.D.

Rochester, New York

David Myland Kaufman, M.D.

Department of Neurology,
Montefiore Medical Center,
Bronx, New York

Olli Kirvelä, M.D.

Division of Critical Care Medicine,
Montefiore Medical Center,
Bronx, New York

Vladimir Kvetan, M.D.

Division of Critical Care Medicine,
Montefiore Medical Center,
Bronx, New York

Rhoda D. Levine, M.D.

Department of Anesthesiology,
Albert Einstein College of Medicine,
Bronx, New York

Allison D. McIntyre, R.N., C.R.N.A., M.S.

University of Rochester Medical Center,
Rochester, New York

Richard B. Patt, M.D.

Department of Anesthesiology,
University of Rochester Medical Center,
Rochester, New York

Cedric Prys-Roberts, M.A., D.M., Ph. D., F.F.A.R.C.S.

Department of Anaesthetics,
Royal Infirmary,
Bristol, England

Gerald Scheinman, M.D.

Department of Anesthesiology,
Doctor's Hospital of Prince George's County,
Lanham, Maryland

Karen D. Spadaccia, R.N.

Baldwin Place, New York

Ann Marie Terra, R.N.

Thiells, New York

Somasundaram Thiagarajah, M.D.

Department of Anesthesiology,
Beth Israel Medical Center,
New York, New York

Estelle White, R.N.

University of Rochester Medical Center,
Rochester, New York

Dorothy M. Williams, R.N.

Recovery Room,
Sloan Kettering Memorial Hospital,
New York, New York

Marcelle M. Willock, M.D.

Department of Anesthesiology,
Boston University,
University Hospital,
Boston, Massachusetts

To
My Father and Mother

FOREWORD

The past two decades have seen the evolution of PACU practice from an area of mere unskilled, custodial care to an area recognized for managing the problems specific to the postoperative patient. At its meeting in October 1988, the American Society of Anesthesiologists for the first time adopted formal "Standards for Postanesthesia Care." These standards identify which patients shall receive post anesthesia care and mandate the availability of a unit rendering such care. The standard of care for transport to the PACU, as well as the standard of care provided in such a unit, is delineated. A sentence in the opening paragraph of the standards document is appropriate here—"They are subject to revision from time to time as warranted by the evolution of technology and practice." This second edition of *Post Anesthesia Care Unit: Current Practices* is just such a mandate. This text, edited by a leading authority in the field, Elizabeth A.M. Frost, is a comprehensive one, incorporating the most recent advances in technology and pharmacology.

The format of the text is well organized, with Part One devoted to general physiological principles; the treatment of postoperative pain; respiration; the cardiovascular system; fluid management; and the causes of prolonged unconsciousness. Admission and monitoring assessments, as well as discharge criteria, are included in this section.

Part Two deals with patients who have special needs. Included in this section is an excellent chapter on the criteria for establishment of brain death. Both the physiological parameters and the legal implications are completely presented. The chapter on cardiopulmonary arrest is also excellent for its clarity and completeness. The addition of a chapter dealing with the burn patient is important. These unique patients are seen with more regularity in PACUs, with the increasing advances in reconstructive surgery. The increase in ambulatory surgery has created another specialized need that is changing rapidly. The chapter dealing with the ambulatory surgery patient incorporates these changes and presents an up-to-the-minute view of post anesthesia care in this setting.

Part Three of the text covers the administrative aspects of the PACU. The latest ideas on physical structure, nursing requirements, and nursing education are presented here. The final chapter of the text is unique in detailing the liabilities of the risk management and PACU teams, a subject that increasingly concerns everyone providing care in such a unit. A frank discussion of the subject in clear, understandable terms will allow PACU personnel to practice with a better understanding of their risks and responsibilities.

In summary, the second edition of *Post Anesthesia Care Unit: Current Practices* is an excellent work, completely updating this area of practice. It provides a productive review of all the important aspects of post anesthesia care. I congratulate the editor and all the contributors on a very timely, effective, and comprehensive work.

Paul L. Goldiner

PREFACE

Since its publication in 1985, *Recovery Room Practice* has been widely used both in the United States and Europe as a clinical reference book and as a study source. But just as surgical and anesthetic techniques change to meet changing population needs, so must postoperative care be modified. Thus it became apparent that an updating of the material was now appropriate. In accordance with the expanded skill and knowledge required to manage postoperative patients, the term *post anesthesia care unit* provides an appropriate appellation for an area designated for practice of this special expertise. Thus the title of this edition has been changed to *Post Anesthesia Care Unit: Current Practices.*

Although each chapter has been extensively revised and in many instances rewritten, the basic format remains the same. An introduction outlining a short history of postoperative care has been added. Part One deals with basic and specialized nursing in the PACU and current management of acute surgical pain. Part Two considers patients who require special attention, such as children, outpatients, patients with chest or neurosurgical considerations, those operated under regional techniques, and patients with kidney disease. A new chapter has been added that deals with care of the burned patient who has undergone reconstructive surgery.

Part Three on administration is concerned with the physical structure of the PACU, nursing, and educational requirements. The final chapter, which has been rewritten by a nurse and an anesthesiologist and reviewed by lawyers from the University of Rochester, defines the legal considerations involved in nursing care in the PACU.

We believe that open heart procedures are usually managed in an intensive care setting, and we have therefore not included discussion of this group. Obstetrical care has also been excluded, because the trend seems increasingly toward a single labor/delivery/recovery area, bypassing the conventional PACU setting.

Finally, we realize that throughout the nation and indeed the world, there are great differences in patient requirements, staffing, availability of equipment, and standards in post anesthesia care. We trust that by pooling the experience of many physicians and nurses from different types of practices in writing this book, readers will find common information that can be suitably applied in their post anesthesia care units.

Elizabeth A.M. Frost

CONTENTS

INTRODUCTION

A dedicated area for care of postsurgical patients, staffed by specialists, is a fairly recent addition to medical care. Although surgical procedures have been described for thousands of years and general anesthesia has been used for almost 150 years, identification of a specialty of post anesthesia care has evolved slowly. This delay is probably related to the general reluctance of the public before the end of the nineteenth century to go to the hospital at all. All minor operations and many major operations were performed in private houses. Surgical and nursing textbooks provided instruction for the rough and ready preparation of bedrooms and kitchens for surgery. Follow-up care was provided by the surgeon and visiting nurse services. It was not until the 1890s that some prominent surgeons began to limit their practice to the hospital. For example, in 1894 Nicholas Senn, an eminent Chicago surgeon, wrote to the Boston surgeon, Dr. J. Collins Warren, "I enjoy continuous service at St. Joseph's and Presbyterian hospitals. It is here that I earn my daily bread because I have not the time to operate in private houses."

The advances in surgical technique, the understanding of the need for asepsis, and staffing problems made it clear that makeshift domestic operating rooms were not ideal. Also, hospital care became less expensive. In 1909 a middle-class woman wrote the following:

I am going to the New York Hospital at 11 o'clock today. It is the finest hospital in New York and I will be absolutely comfortable there. There is a cheap room vacant that I can get for $25.00 a week. My husband wanted to get a nurse to keep me here. But when we talked the matter over seriously last night, we decided the hospital was the best. Our regular servants are ignorant of medical matters while a nurse is so in the way in this small house. I get absolute rest and freedom from care at the hospital and it doesn't cost quite as much as the nurse.

A nurse at that time cost about 50 cents per hour. In fact, many hospitals relied for much-needed income on sending student nurses out into the community on private duty assignments. Their fees were paid to the hospital. At the Elliot Hospital in Keene, New Hampshire, for example, 22 students gave 330 weeks of private care outside the hospital in 1905. They earned $3176.13 in a year when the hospital's total income was $13,260.96. Of this sum, only $1749 was paid to nurses. Hospital administration reasoned that private duty nursing was an appropriate part of nursing care when it was assumed that most Americans would never enter a hospital, preferring to be treated in their houses.

In 1863 Florence Nightingale suggested the establishment of special areas for recovery of patients from the immediate effects of surgery. The writings on such an idea were largely ignored, coming as they did at a time when surgical procedures, even with anesthesia, were still performed in open wards. The advent of aseptic surgery in the latter half of the nineteenth century added prophylactic to humanitarian reasons for limiting surgery to special operating rooms.

Most postoperative cases were still returned directly to the ward, unless they were considered moribund. The annual report of the Presbyterian Hospital in New York in 1891 noted the following:

Such cases [dying patients], however guarded, are depressing to other patients in the ward as is also the renewal of the body afterward; nor is the ward, however well managed, so fitting a place for the last hour as a room where the patient is separated from all but the necessary attendant or friends.

Clearly, segregation was not to allow closer monitoring of the patient.

The first recovery room as such was opened by Dandy and Firor at the Johns Hopkins Hospital in 1923. They established a three-bed neurosurgical unit close to the operating room. The annual report of the section on anesthesia of the Mayo Clinic mentioned a post anesthesia observation room where 2000 patients had received care. The death of two patients in the immediate postoperative period, during periods of inadequate or no monitoring, spurred the administration at the Hospital of the University of Pennsylvania to designate an area adjacent to the operating room as a recovery room in 1946.

Tremendous impetus was given to the development of postoperative observation areas by the crucial need for critical care of the soldiers wounded in World War II. Several names for such an area were suggested—the recovery room, post anesthesia room, recovery pavilion, special care unit, and postoperative service unit.

Many questions were asked in the early days, such as Who will be responsible for the unit? Is there enough nursing staff at a time stressed by the tumultuous destabilization of the post-war era? Is this a passing fad? Will it be too costly for patients? Should patients be recovered from their surgery and their anesthesia before being returned to their rooms? Does this system mean duplication of beds? Does it mean loss of patient privacy? Will untrained personnel be taking care of unstable patients?

But time and experience quickly proved that a recovery room provided safe, high-quality intensive care to patients who needed it at a critical time in their hospital stay. In 1957 a report from the surgical service of a midwestern hospital stated that the services of three nurses and two students were required to handle the same post anesthesia load that one nurse, a student, and an aide could manage

in a recovery room. Surgeons liked the recovery room because their patients were centralized and not scattered throughout the hospital. As one noted ''with dependable personnel in the recovery room, it helps to conserve the energies of anesthesiologists and surgeons, for they need no longer worry whether their semiconscious patients are being attended.'' Nurses were particularly supportive of the concept of specialized immediate postoperative care. Family members no longer had to be concerned about the necessity of recovering their own relatives because of staff shortages on wards. Nurses on wards were freed to administer bedside care to other patients.

In the intervening 30 years, enormous strides have been made in the development of post anesthesia care. Today hospitals frequently have not one but several recovery areas (for example, a separate ambulatory, cardiac, neurosurgical, or obstetrical unit). The importance of the post anesthesia care unit (PACU) was summarized in a supreme court decision in 1969:

The function of this room is to provide highly specialized care, frequent and careful observation of patients who are under the influence of anesthesia. They remain in this room until they have regained consciousness and their bodies return to their normal functions. The nurses in this room are there for the purpose of promptly recognizing any respiratory problem, cardiovascular problem or hemorrhaging. The patient is more prone to crises after the operation than while in the operating room where the respiration is being controlled. This is the most important room in a hospital and one in which the patient requires the greatest attention, because it is fraught with the greatest potential dangers to the patient. As the dangers or risks are ever-present there should be no relaxing of vigilance.

Nurses, who had been the prime movers in establishing this critical area, began to join together at local, state, and national levels. In October 1980, the groundwork had been completed, legal counsel obtained, and goals and purposes defined. The American Society of Post Anesthesia Nurses (ASPAN) was incorporated. The initial membership of almost 2000 soon grew to more than 4000. In 1981 ASPAN became a member of the National Federation of Specialty Nursing Organizations. Important professional relationships were established with the American Nursing Association and the American Society of Anesthesiologists. From the outset, the publication committee produced a quarterly newsletter, ''Breathline.'' Some 6 years later, a more formal publication, the *Journal of Post Anesthesia Nursing,* appeared, also as a quarterly publication.

ASPAN has continued to provide educational opportunities and has organized National Conferences in major cities throughout the United States. The concept of certification of post anesthesia nurses was developed by a certification committee. By April 1985, an independent organization, the American Board of Post Anesthesia Nursing Certification, was incorporated, and in November 1986, the first 190 post anesthesia nurses fulfilled the requirements for admission to the examination.

At present there are more than 10,000 PACU nurses in the United States. As ambulatory care facilities increase and as the functions of recovery areas expand, so also does the role of these nurses.

In a little over a half century, PACUs have grown from a three-bed experimental area in one hospital, to multiunit facilities with established guidelines and standards in every health care center in the United States that performs surgery.

PART I

GENERAL CARE

CHAPTER 1

Admitting Assessment and Monitoring

Elizabeth A.M. Frost

All patients who receive a general or regional anesthetic should be cared for in the recovery room until the anesthetic effect is sufficiently reversed. The anesthesiologist or physician in charge of the post anesthesia care unit (PACU) determines which patients will be admitted.

Obstetrical units usually have separate recovery areas and generally use the main PACU only under emergency situations or use separate areas of that room.

Occasionally patients may be transferred directly from the operating room to the ward under the following circumstances:

1. Local anesthesia only was used, and the patient's condition is stable.
2. The patient is an infection risk, and no isolation area is available.
3. There is an intensive care unit specially designed for particular care (for example, after cardiac surgery or for premature care.)
4. By agreement with the surgeon and anesthesiologist, the patient makes arrangements for special care on a regular nursing unit.

If the patient is returned directly to his room postoperatively, the standards of nursing care during this period must equal those of the PACU.

The main functions of the PACU nurse are the following (see Appendix 1):

1. To promptly recognize and treat respiratory problems
2. To maintain stability of the cardiovascular system
3. To monitor for hemorrhage
4. To adequately and safely control postoperative pain

ADMISSION ASSESSMENT

The PACU and operating room should be close to one another. Five minutes transfer time is a maximum safe limit. Two individuals must accompany the patient during transfer, one of whom must be part of the anesthesia care team. Availability of adequate monitoring, oxygen, and all resuscitative measures is recommended during transportation of any patient whose consciousness is impaired.

The basic information that the anesthesiologist should give the nurse for admission assessment includes the following:

1. Brief personal history: diagnosis, name, age, sex, native language, physical impairments (for example, deaf, blind)
2. Surgical procedure: operation, surgeon, surgical complications

3. Anesthetic technique: anesthesiologist of record, agents, dosages, drug reversal, complications, estimated time to return of consciousness or reversal of regional block
4. Intraoperative course: vital signs, fluid balance
5. Relevant medical history: maintenance medications, allergies, previous hospitalizations and illnesses
6. Anticipated problems

When the patient is accepted to the PACU, a short form can be inserted or rubber stamped in the medical record (Figure 1-1). PACU orders are either included on a routine form or may be written by the surgeon or anesthesiologist (Figure 1-2).

Assessment of recovery from anesthesia may be made by applying the Aldrete score, which is based on the Apgar score (see Appendix 2). The range is 10 for complete recovery to 0 in comatose patients. The five categories of evaluation in the postanesthetic recovery score (PARS) are as follows:

1. Activity
   Voluntary movement of all limbs
   to command   2
   Voluntary movement of 2 extremities
   to command   1
   Unable to move   0
2. Respiration
   Breathing deeply and coughing   2
   Dyspneic, hypoventilating   1
   Apneic   0
3. Circulation
   Blood pressure ± 20% of
   preanesthetic level   2
   Blood pressure ± 20%-50% of
   preanesthetic level   1
   Blood pressure ± 50% of
   preanesthetic level   0
4. Consciousness
   Fully awake   2
   Arousable   1
   Unresponsive   0
5. Color
   Pink   2
   Pale, blotchy   1
   Cyanotic   0

The score should be recorded on admission and at 15- to 30-minute intervals to document improvement or deterioration. Limitations of the score are apparent when the patient receives a score of 10 but is oliguric, severely nauseated, vomiting, or develops a cardiac dysrhythmia.

The patient's status should be judged by the nurse and anesthesiologist immediately on arrival in the PACU and at a minimum of 15-minute intervals until discharge. Documentation is essential.

MONITORING

The anesthesiologist should review with the nurse the patient functions that have been monitored and should indicate which areas require further observation. Respiratory, cardiovascular, neuromuscular, thermoregulatory, and renal systems, in addition to state of consciousness and fluid and electrolyte balance, are routinely evaluated in the PACU.

Respiratory System

Common measurements of respiratory function are listed in Table 1-1. Good, careful auscultation is irreplaceable in the initial assessment of adequate respiration. Rate should be recorded on admission and at 15-minute intervals. Respiratory pattern, which normally has a regular inspiratory to expiratory ratio of 1:3, should be noted.

Pulse oximetry has been accepted as a simple and accurate means of assessing oxygen saturation and volume status. Routine use is strongly suggested in the early recovery period, especially in patients cared for in the prone position, in those still not recovered from anesthetic effects, and in children with sleep apnea syndromes. In many PACUs, one or two stations are equipped to monitor inspired and expired gases (mass spectroscopy or infrared gas analyses). Continuous measurement of expired CO_2 levels (capnography), especially in the patient whose trachea is still intubated, provides early warning of respiratory depression when a previously stable level begins to decrease.

Abnormalities, such as phasic variations (Cheyne-Stokes respiration), use of accessory mus-

---

PACU Admission

Vital Signs: temperature _____ BP _____ PR _____ RR _____
Anesthesia: regional_____ general_____ other _____
   Regional: level of analgesia _____
   General: unresponsive_____ drowsy _____ awake _____
            airway oral _____ nasal_____ none_____
            endotracheal tube_____ tracheostomy _____

FIGURE 1-1

A short form that the PACU nurse may complete to record patient data at the time of admission. *BP*, Blood pressure; *PR*, Pulse rate; *RR*, Respiratory rate.

Routine PACU Orders

1. O_2 administration: Give O_2 @ _____ L/min _____ mask _____ cannula
2. Vital signs q 15 minutes
3. Endotracheal tube care
   a. Suction prn
   b. Administer O_2 mist/T tube @ _____ %
   c. May be extubated when PACU written scoring criteria are met
   d. Obtain ABGs_____ minutes after admission to unit
4. Continue operating room IV_____ unless otherwise ordered by surgeon
5. Cardiac monitor
6. Pulse oximetry
7. Medications
   a. Atropine 0.5-1 mg IV bolus if cardiac rate is less than _____
   b. Lidocaine 50 mg IV bolus stat for development of PVCs 6 per minute Ventricular tachycardia or bigeminy: call anesthesiologist.
   c. _____ IV for pain
8. Notify anesthesiologist if:
   Blood pressure _____ or _____
   Respiration _____ or _____
   Heart rate _____ or _____

FIGURE 1-2

Postoperative orders to be completed by the anesthesiologist in consultation with the PACU nurse.

TABLE 1-1

Common indicators used to assess respiratory function in the recovery room

Indicator	Normal range
1. Auscultation	bilaterally equal
2. Rate	10-35/min
3. Pattern	regular
4. Pulse oximetry	> 94%
5. Capnography	< 40 mm Hg
6. Tidal volume	4-5 ml/kg
7. Vital capacity	20-40 ml/kg
8. Inspiratory force	-40 cm H_2O
9. Arterial blood gases at 30% O_2	PaO_2 100 mm Hg; $PaCO_2$ 35-45 mm Hg

cles, diaphragmatic breathing, and sternal retraction indicate excess anesthetic effect, neurological complications, or obstruction. Prompt therapy requires reestablishment of an adequate airway, which may mean simply supporting the chin or inserting an oral or nasal airway, or may require reintubation and assisted ventilation. The anesthesiologist and surgeon should be notified.

Tidal volume should be measured if the endotracheal tube is still in place or if any difficulty is suspected. Minute ventilation (normally about 5 to 6 L) is obtained by multiplying respiratory rate by tidal volume. Vital capacity measurement is particularly valuable because it indicates the patient's ability to respond to commands, the adequacy of respiratory drive, and the coordination of the chest wall and lung mechanics.

Inspiratory force is obtained by connecting a manometer through a one-way valve to the endotracheal tube or to a close-fitting mask. The airway is thus temporarily blocked so the force generated is negative. Values of -40 cm H_2O are necessary to cough effectively and prevent atelectasis.

Probably the best measurement of the adequacy of ventilation is obtained from blood gas analyses. Accurate interpretation must take the inspired oxygen concentration into consideration. If an arterial cannula is not in place and monitoring of gases requires repeated arterial puncture, continuous monitoring of oxygen saturation by pulse oximetry

is an acceptable alternative technique. In assessing the adequacy of the circulation, blood pressure, pulse, and heart sounds are monitored. Blood pressure variations up or down of more than 25% of preoperative values should be reported to the physician. The quality of the pulse and heart sounds decreases with myocardial depression.

Continuous electrocardiographic monitoring coupled with a printer to obtain a permanent record as necessary should be routine for all patients. Not only does this monitor afford a visual and auditory indication of rate and rhythm, but it may indicate hypoxia of cardiac muscle if the ST segment is deflected more than 1 mm from baseline. Any dysrhythmia should be noted and reported to the physician. Electrolyte abnormalities (especially potassium) may be apparent by wave changes (for example, T wave) although serum estimations of such changes are more accurate.

Central venous pressure gives an indication of volume status and myocardial function. An upward or downward trend is of far greater significance than single values. Increasingly, pulmonary artery and pulmonary capillary wedge pressures and cardiac output are now measured perioperatively through a flow-directed balloon catheter. Normal values for cardiac measurements appear in Table 1-2.

TABLE 1-2

Approximate range for cardiac measurements obtained in the recovery room

Measure	Normal range
Pulse	55–120/min
Blood pressure	$\frac{90}{50} - \frac{160}{100}$ mm Hg
Central venous pressure	3–8 mm Hg
Right atrial pressure	1–6 mm Hg
Right ventricular pressure	$\frac{20}{0} - \frac{30}{5}$ mm Hg
Pulmonary artery pressure	$\frac{20}{8} - \frac{30}{12}$ mm Hg
Pulmonary capillary pressure	4–12 mm Hg
Cardiac output	4–8 L/min
Cardiac index (cardiac output/ body surface area)	2.5–3.5 L/min/m^2

Neuromuscular Transmission

Two types of neuromuscular blockade can persist into the recovery period. Pattern 1 is phase 1 block or depolarizing block and is produced by succinylcholine. When a nerve stimulator is used, phase 1 block is characterized by sustained tetanus, equal train-of-four responses, and no posttetanic potentiation. Phase 2 block develops after prolonged use of succinylcholine or as a residual effect of nondepolarizing relaxants (for example, *d*-tubocurarine, pancuronium, metocurine). It is associated with tetanic fade, fade of train-of-four responses, and posttetanic potentiation. Although there is no specific antidote for phase 1 block, which usually resolves quickly, phase 2 block may be reversed with anticholinesterase drugs, such as edrophonium, neostigmine, or pyridostigmine.

Tests for residual nondepolarizing block include assessing the patient's ability to lift his head, open his eyes, grasp a hand, and extrude his tongue. Factors that may prolong neuromuscular blockade include acidosis, hypothermia, inhalation anesthetic agents (especially isoflurane), antibiotics (except penicillin G, cephradine, and cephaloridine), hypermagnesemia, hypocalcemia, renal failure (especially with metocurine and pancuronium), and furosemide. After childbirth, patients are particularly sensitive to the effects of succinylcholine. Careful monitoring for inadequate muscle function reversal is especially indicated in patients who have undergone postpartum tubal ligation.

Temperature

Intraoperatively, temperature is altered by administration of cold fluids, exposure of both the interior and exterior of the body to a cool environment, and obtunding of the thermoregulatory center by anesthetic agents. Many anesthetics cause vasodilation with further heat loss, which is particularly problematic in children. Hypothermia of itself may be protective by decreasing oxygen demand. However, if rebound shivering occurs, oxygen consumption may increase by 400%, which may cause a hypoxic state, critical to patients with cardiac or cerebrovascular disease.

Oral recordings are influenced by the temperature of exhaled gases. The rectal temperature is an indicator of core temperature and only changes slowly in relation to other parts of the body. Esophageal temperature, although a good indicator of average body temperature, is usually not feasible in the awake or semiconscious patient. A ceramic bead placed in the tympanic membrane measures the temperature closest to the hypothalamus or thermoregulatory center. Axillary temperature should be used only as a rough indication and is of more value if trends are recorded. Skin temperature is valuable in very small infants and in assessing continued circulation to a limb at risk of vascular occlusion.

Renal Function

Urinary volume is the most commonly recorded estimate of adequate renal function. However, as discussed in Chapter 11, this is only one of many predictors of an intact urinary system. Other measurements include specific gravity, electrolytes, and osmolality.

Level of Consciousness

Cerebral function is estimated postoperatively by the patient's state of awareness. Several scoring systems (Aldrete, Apgar, Carignan, and Glasgow coma scale) developed for different situations depend on estimations from clinical observations (respiration, eye opening, response to command, and motor function).

If coma persists, an overall pattern of cerebral function may be recorded by the electroencephalograph (EEG). Previously, everyday use of EEG monitoring was restricted because interpretation of the analogue signal required certain expertise. With the development of computer facilities, fast transformation allows a spectrum of EEG frequency and amplitude. In one such monitor, the Lifescan® (Diatek), EEG waves are color coded according to frequency and move up a screen with time. A spectral edge, below which a preset percentage of electrical activity occurs, gives a single figure that roughly indicates cerebral activity (edge less than 20 Hz is indicative of low activity or sleep; edge above 20 Hz indicates a more awake patient). Regional changes may indicate abnormal foci. In selected patients, intracranial pressure monitoring and computing of cerebral perfusion pressure (mean systemic arterial pressure minus intracranial pressure) may be indicated.

Pupillary reflexes in response to light should be monitored and the change in each eye recorded for all neurosurgical patients. The absence of clonus in the ankles after spinal operations may be a sign of trauma or surgical injury to the cord. Monitoring of brain and spinal evoked potentials during the recovery phase, although not yet a routine technique, is becoming generally available.

Fluid and Electrolyte Balance

Fluid balance is frequently assessed most accurately first in the PACU. After considerable loss and replacement of fluids, the relative stability of the postoperative period allows time to compute the patient's fluid volume status—a task that often falls to the nurse. It is extremely important to record both input and output in the recovery phase and equate these volumes with the intraoperative fluid shifts.

Electrolyte determination in the postoperative period is generally done by laboratory analysis, although the capability for on-line measurement exists. Indications for early and possibly repeated electrolyte analyses postoperatively include the following:

1. Major physiological fluid loss (diarrhea, vomiting)
2. Administration of large fluid volumes (burns, transurethral resection of the prostate)
3. Bowel surgery (resection of obstructed large bowel)
4. Preoperative electrolyte abnormalities (chronic diuretic administration, hypothalamic disturbances)
5. Neurosurgical procedures, diuresed intraoperatively

Glucose is easily measured at the bedside. Dextrostix determinations are simple and give a qualitative estimate of the need for emergency therapy or more accurate laboratory analysis.

CONCLUSION

The close monitoring afforded the patient in the operating room must be continued into the PACU and individualized according to the needs of the patient.

Noninvasive techniques are preferable because the invasive approach carries the potential for infection. Computers allow an almost limitless ability to assemble data. However, the objective of monitoring—to ensure a safe and smooth postoperative course—must be remembered. It is as important to look at the patient as it is to survey the numbers.

SUGGESTIONS FOR FURTHER READING

Aldrete JA and Kronlik D: A postanesthetic recovery score, Anesth Analg 49:924, 1970.

Carignan G, Keeri-Szanto M, and Lavellie JP: Post anesthetic scoring system. Anesthesiology 25:396, 1964.

Cullen DJ: Recovery room care of the surgical patient. In Hershey SG, editor: Refresher courses in anesthesiology, vol 8, Philadelphia, 1980, JB Lippincott Co.

Fischer TL: Responsibility for care in recovery rooms, Can Med Assoc J 102:78, 1970.

Partridge BL: Use of pulse oximetry as a noninvasive indicator of intravascular volume status, J Clin Monit 3:263, 1987.

Teasdale G and Jennett B: Assessment of coma and impaired consciousness: a practical scale, Lancet 2:81, 1974.

CHAPTER 2

Treatment of Postoperative Pain

Cedric Prys-Roberts

Pain is an almost inevitable consequence of surgery. Pain is a fiction; that is, as a subjective experience it can be described only qualitatively and cannot be quantified. The severity of pain after surgery varies with the perception of the individual and the nature of the injury. Relief of postoperative pain must therefore be directed at the needs of each individual. Traditional approaches to pain relief are inadequate: physicians tend to write inadequate orders, nurses tend to misinterpret these orders, and both underestimate the variety of patient requirements.

Not only does the severity and duration of pain differ from one surgical site to another, the consequences of pain also differ. Pain from the extremities, however severe, does not interfere with breathing, but the pain from upper abdominal and thoracic surgery limits the ability of the patient to breathe deeply and to cough effectively. Both of these limitations contribute to the higher morbidity and mortality associated with major surgery. Adequate and continuous relief of such pain undoubtedly influences the quality and speed of postoperative recovery. By contrast, pain from lower abdominal incisions, especially from transverse rather than vertical incisions, causes less morbidity than that from upper abdominal surgery.

Muscle spasm, which may be considered a protective mechanism to restrict movement of an injured site, also contributes to the severity of postoperative pain. The relief of muscle spasm may in itself improve the comfort of a patient. Most severe postoperative pain is triggered by movement, and if such movement can be restricted without contributing to other causes of morbidity, this too can relieve pain. Positioning of the patient is also important to avoid placing incisions or operated sites under tension or pressure.

ORIGIN AND TRANSMISSION OF PAIN IMPULSES

Three types of receptor are recognized in most tissues: mechanoreceptors, thermoreceptors, and nociceptors. There is also evidence of specific visceral and muscle nociceptors. Action potentials generated in these receptors are transmitted by two classes of nerve fiber to the posterior columns of the spinal cord.

Two types of pain are recognized. The sharp, transient, pricking pain associated with skin trauma is classified as fast pain, as it is transmitted by myelinated Aδ fibers (1 to 5 μm in diameter). The more prolonged and unpleasant burning pain, classified as slow pain, which results from tissue damage, is mediated by unmyelinated C nerve fibers (0.5 to 1.0 μm). Visceral pain and pain from deep somatic structures is also mediated through unmyelinated C nerve fibers and is characteristically difficult to localize and is associated with autonomic disturbances, especially nausea. The Aδ fibers project centrally through the neospinothalmic tracts to the thalamic nuclei that project directly to the cortex. The unmyelinated C fibers, which are predominant in the peripheral nerves, synapse in the substantia gelatinosa of the dorsal horn. The ensuing neurons cross the midline and continue in the paleospinothalmic tract to the thalamus.

Numerous other fibers converge in the substantia gelatinosa, both descending fibers and collateral fibers (Lissauer's tract), all of which can modulate the transmission of impulses in the pain pathway. The general concept of a neuronal gate, as described by Melzak and Wall in their gate-control theory, is relevant to this area of the spinal cord. There are numerous synapses in the various pain pathways, each of which involves at least one chemical transmitter. These transmitters have not been specifically localized to individual synapses, but over the past few years a number of endogenous peptides having opioid characteristics have been identified.

ENDOGENOUS OPIOIDS AND THEIR RECEPTORS

Three types of endogenous peptides have been identified and classified according to the gene sequences that lead to their synthesis (Table 2-1).

TABLE 2-1		
Endogenous opioids, their precursors, and primary receptors		
Origins	Name	Receptors
Proencephalins	met-encephalin leu-encephalin	μ (δ)
Preopiomelanocortins	β-endorphin	μ (δ)
Prodynorphins	dynorphins	κ (μ, δ)

Parentheses indicate secondary receptor sites.

Encephalins are short-chain peptides, based on a five amino acid chain (TYR-GLY-GLY-PHE-LEU, or -MET), which are widely distributed throughout the central nervous system in association with short neurons. β-*endorphins* are long-chain peptides found only in the arcuate nucleus of the hypothalamus and its neuronal projections. *Dynorphins* are the most recently discovered peptides, and although their distribution has not been accurately mapped, they are associated with an opioid pathway descending from the hypothalamus and periaqueductal gray matter to the spinal cord. They are also found in the gastrointestinal tract.

The physiological function of these opioid peptides has yet to be clarified, but they are clearly involved in the endogenous modulation of pain transmission and suppression, possibly as regulators of receptor sensitivity within the brain and spinal cord. They are also probably involved in the regulation of fetal movement. Their mode of action is by increasing potassium conductance in synaptic membranes.

Morphine and other naturally occurring and synthetic opioids bind specifically to certain areas of the brain and spinal cord. These areas are the only sites at which these drugs exert agonist or antagonist activities. In the spinal cord, these opioid receptors are in the substantia gelatinosa of the dorsal horns, specifically in lamina 2 (Rexed) and to a much lesser extent in other parts of the dorsal horn. The association between these localized opioid receptors and the slow pain pathway clearly identifies the pharmacological site of analgesic action. In the central nervous system, opioid receptors are found in the periaqueductal gray matter, the hypothalamus, and throughout the limbic system. Many of the undesirable side effects of opioids are related to actions at these sites, specifically ventilatory depression caused by action on central neurons in the floor of the fourth ventricle, nausea and vomiting caused by action on the chemoreceptor trigger zone in the medulla, and euphoria caused by effects mediated through the limbic system. Identification of different types of opioid receptors at these anatomical sites has been based on the interaction of agonist and antagonist drugs. Analgesic activity is

TABLE 2-2

Characterization of opioid receptors

Name	Associated agonist	Characteristic actions
μ	Morphine	Analgesia, ventilatory depression, **euphoria,** physical dependence with drug seeking
κ	Ketocyclazocine	Analgesia, **apathetic sedation,** physical dependence but little or no drug seeking
σ	SKF 10047	**Dysphoria,** mydriasis, ventilatory stimulation

Two other receptor subtypes (δ, ϵ) have been identified in animal tissues using endogenous (encephalin) and synthetic ligands, but their relevance to the actions of opioids in humans is uncertain.
Typical subjective effects of each class of drugs are highlighted in **boldface.**

TABLE 2-3

Morphinomimetic analgesic drugs (and their antagonists) classified according to opioid receptor activity

Drug	μ	κ	σ
Morphine	A	O	O
Nalorphine	C	P	A
Naloxone	C	C	C
Buprenorphine	P	O	O
Butorphanol	O($\pm$)	A	A
Nalbuphine	C	P	P
Pentazocine	C	A	A

A, agonist; P, partial agonist; C, competitive antagonist; O, no action.

associated with both mu (μ) and kappa (κ) receptors (Table 2-2).

Drugs that produce analgesia (or antagonize it) by morphine-like effects can now be classified according to their spectrum of activities at various receptor types (Table 2-3). In this respect all drugs acting as μ-receptor agonists are represented in this table by morphine. They are diacetyl morphine, codeine, meperidine, fentanyl (and its congeners alfentanil, sufentanil, lofentanil, carfentanil), and methadone. From this table, it can be seen that the effects of morphine (and its congeners) differ from those of buprenorphine and pentazocine and from those of two new analgesics, nalbuphine and butor-

phanol. An understanding of the interrelationships of these drugs is essential when considering interaction between them, for instance, when buprenorphine or pentazocine is given for postoperative pain relief to a patient who has received a μ-agonist, such as morphine or fentanyl, during surgery.

PHARMACOLOGY OF OPIOIDS

The effects of opioid analgesics are determined by their distribution in the body after a specific route of administration. The onset of their action is determined by their lipophilicity, and their duration of action is determined by the interaction of their clearance and their volumes of distribution, both pharmacokinetic parameters.

Morphine is poorly lipophilic; indeed, the two polar hydroxyl groups confer hydrophilicity and limit accessibility of morphine to the opioid receptors locked in the lipoprotenious membranes of the spinal cord. This has importance in understanding why morphine is a most unsuitable drug for use by the epidural or intrathecal route. Morphine has been regarded as a high-clearance drug with an elimination half-life of 3 to 4 hours, but recent studies indicate that it has a slower elimination over a 24-hour period. Its pharmacodynamic and kinetic properties make it suitable for intramuscular or intravenous administration.

Meperidine, having no polar groups, is highly lipophilic and although much less potent than morphine (100 mg meperidine is equipotent to 10 mg morphine), it is still one of the most popular narcotics for postoperative pain relief. It has a longer elimination half-life (5 to 7 hours) than morphine because of lower clearance, but in clinical practice the effects of the two drugs are similar.

Fentanyl was originally considered to be a drug having very short duration of action because small doses (50 to 100 μg) produce ventilatory depression lasting only 20 to 30 minutes. However, the elimination half-life of fentanyl varies from 150 to 180 minutes when given during anesthesia, to 180 to 240 minutes when given to volunteers. Thus the duration of its analgesic and ventilatory depressant effects is determined, as it is for all such drugs, by the actual dose given, the peak concentration of the drug achieved in plasma and other tissues, and the relation of that peak concentration to the concentration required for the desirable (analgesic) and undesirable (ventilatory depression, nausea, and vomiting) effects of the drug. When fentanyl is given in total doses of 10 to 25 μg/kg during anesthesia (1 to 2 hours), the duration of analgesia beyond the anesthetic period may be as long as 4 to 6 hours. When doses of 100 μg/kg or more have been used for cardiac surgery, analgesia and ventilatory depression may last up to 18 to 24 hours.

Alfentanil is a synthetic analogue of fentanyl, having a much lower lipid solubility and a very small initial volume of distribution. Consequently, higher peak plasma levels are easier to reach and the effects of a single dose last a shorter period than the effects of fentanyl. It has been used as a continuous infusion (10 to 20 μg/kg per hour) for postoperative pain relief and as an analgesic in intensive therapy.

Sufentanil has about 5 to 8 times the potency of fentanyl but a shorter duration of action. It has achieved a certain popularity in anesthesia for cardiac surgery but is not yet widely used in general surgery.

Buprenorphine is a derivative of thebaine, a highly lipophilic drug that acts as a partial agonist (agonist-antagonist) at μ-receptors. Its long duration of action reflects a very stable interaction with the receptor even though the pharmacokinetics are similar to those of morphine and meperidine.

Methadone is a synthetic opioid that has a low clearance (100 to 200 ml per minute) and a very long half-life (25 to 45 hours). After the early distribution phase, blood concentration of methadone declines slowly so that a single intravenous dose of 15 to 20 mg can produce adequate analgesia for 12 to 24 hours postoperatively.

Butorphanol is a synthetic morphinan derivative that has strong agonist actions at κ-receptors, but weak antagonist actions at μ-receptors. These characteristics yield a steep dose-response curve with a ceiling effect for ventilatory depression. It has marked sedative properties, a low tendency to induce nausea or vomiting, and a low abuse and dependence potential. Oral (8 mg) or intramuscular (2 mg) doses produce analgesia at plasma concentrations between 0.3 and 1.7 ng/ml. The drug has an elimination half-life of about 3 hours.

Nalbuphine is a synthetic morphinan derivative structurally related to oxymorphone and naloxone. Like naloxone, it is a competitive antagonist at μ-receptors and a partial agonist at κ- and σ-receptors. Nalbuphine (0.15 mg/kg) is almost equipotent with morphine, producing a ceiling ventilatory depression equivalent to that found with morphine 10 mg in a 70 kg subject.

The newer opioids, nalbuphine and butorphanol have little advantage over morphine, meperidine, or fentanyl in the PACU. The main advantages of nalbuphine and butorphanol lie in their low abuse and dependence potential, a property of more relevance to chronic dosing schedules.

Nalbuphine has been used specifically to reverse the μ-receptor–mediated ventilatory depression induced by morphine-like drugs, while retaining analgesia mediated through the κ-agonist effects.

PHARMACOLOGY OF LOCAL ANESTHETICS

The choice of a local anesthetic for postoperative pain relief should be determined largely by its pharmacokinetic profile, which reflects the potential onset and duration of local anesthetic effect and also the propensity of the drug to produce toxic effects. The qualities required for postoperative analgesia are different from those required for a local anesthetic for use during surgery. For instance, the rapid onset of action of lidocaine may be advantageous at the beginning of surgery, whereas its short duration of action, even when combined with epinephrine, makes it less advantageous for postoperative pain relief. Because of its high lipid solubility, bupivacaine is the most suitable local anesthetic currently available for postoperative pain relief.

The chemical structure of a local anesthetic is important in determining its uptake, distribution, and elimination from the body. Amino esters, such as procaine, chloroprocaine, and tetracaine, are hydrolyzed in plasma by cholinesterases; thus their fate after injection into a site for neuronal blockade is largely determined by the vascularity of that area. By contrast, the amino amides, such as lidocaine, etidocaine, mepivacaine, and bupivacaine, are mainly metabolized by microsomal enzymes in the liver. Lipophilicity has a strong influence on the volume of distribution of a drug, which in turn determines the concentration of a drug in the plasma. Bupivacaine is highly lipid soluble and has a strong affinity for the lipoproteinous components of nervous tissue; consequently, it has a large volume of distribution and a slow clearance from the body. Lidocaine and mepivacaine are much less lipophilic than bupivacaine and are more rapidly eliminated from the plasma.

These pharmacokinetic qualities are also important in determining the mode of action of the drug at the site of neural blockade. When lidocaine is injected close to a nerve, little of the drug is absorbed into the lipoprotein structure of the nerve sheath and most of the drug is available for producing the membrane-stabilizing effect at the nodes of Ranvier. When lidocaine is injected into the epidural space, little of the drug is taken up by the fat depots within the space and most of the drug is available at the active site and for uptake into the epidural veins and transport to the liver. Thus the onset of action is rapid and the duration is short, unless epinephrine is used to minimize the uptake of the drug into the bloodstream. By contrast, bupivacaine injected in the epidural space is rapidly taken up into lipid stores, either in the epidural space or in the nerve sheaths, and the onset of neural blockade is delayed and the duration of blockade

extended. Epinephrine as a local vasoconstrictor has little effect on the onset or duration of blockade. To maintain blockade, bupivacaine should be given in a high concentration (0.5% to 0.75%) initially, to saturate the lipid stores of the epidural region, and thereafter as an infusion of lower concentration (0.125%). This approach ensures the most rapid onset of blockade and prevents a waning of the block. The least efficient but, sadly, the most common way of using bupivacaine is to wait until the effect of the initial block has finished before injecting a further dose.

PRACTICAL ASPECTS OF POSTOPERATIVE PAIN RELIEF

Postoperative pain relief should be planned at the preoperative visit and should be carefully adjusted to consider the patient's age and constitution, the site of surgery, and the availability of recovery room and subsequent care. Use of opioids as part of premedication and intraoperative medication influences the subsequent use of these drugs postoperatively. Combinations of opioid with local anesthetic techniques must also be planned. The influence of general anesthetics and benzodiazepines, which also depress ventilation, must be borne in mind when predicting the appropriate dose of opioids postoperatively.

Postoperative Administration of Opioids

The ideal objective in the use of opioids for postoperative pain relief is to produce the highest and most constant concentration at opioid receptors consistent with adequate ventilation. It is adequacy of ventilation that finally determines the safety of any method. By either the intrathecal or epidural approach, *appropriate* opioids can attain the spinal opioid receptors with minimal distribution to other tissues. Parenteral administration of opioids can achieve the appropriate concentration at spinal receptors only by perfusion through the bloodstream. Thus the attainment of a stable plasma concentration is best achieved by giving a continuous infusion of the drug or by frequent injections of small doses.

Routes of Administration
Sublingual

Buprenorphine (0.2 to 0.4 mg) provides adequate analgesia for moderate postoperative pain. Absorption is rapid, and the effect is prolonged because buprenorphine has a strong affinity to opioid receptors.

Intramuscular

Most opioids can be administered intermittently by this route, which allows rapid onset and predictable effects. This route should be avoided in hypovolemic hypotensive patients in whom cardiac output and muscle perfusion may be impaired. For the management of severe postoperative pain, morphine (0.15 mg/kg) or meperidine (1.5 mg/kg) is the most suitable drug for administration by this route. The disadvantage of this route is that the doses normally used are too low to provide adequate pain relief and too intermittent to sustain it.

Subcutaneous

Morphine can be administered by a continuous infusion of 1 to 2 mg per hour together with hyaluronidase to provide excellent relief of pain. The drug can be administered through a 20-gauge teflon cannula placed in a suitable subcutaneous site, such as the lateral aspect of the thigh or the deltopectoral region. Each infusion site can be used for 24 to 36 hours. The drug can be delivered either by an infusion pump or by a burette system. The total drug dose per 24 hours should be comparable with that accumulated by intermittent intramuscular injections.

Intravenous

The main advantage of the intravenous route for administration of opioid drugs is that the distribution phase is relatively short (5 to 10 minutes); thus repeated small doses can be given at 10-minute intervals until either the desired degree of analgesia is achieved or the slowing of breathing (to less than 10 breaths per minute) limits further dosage. Morphine should be given in 1 to 2 mg increments, meperidine in 10 to 15 mg increments.

Intravenous infusion

By using infusion schemes designed to achieve a stable plasma concentration of narcotic analgesic in the shortest possible time, the maximal degree of analgesia consistent with acceptable ventilatory depression can be maintained for long periods. The most suitable agents for intravenous infusion are those that have a rapid clearance (>1000 ml per minute) and a short elimination half-life. Morphine, meperidine, fentanyl and alfentanil have been used in this context, but most clinical reports give little more than dose-infusion rates and indications of the adequacy of pain relief.

Morphine diluted to 0.2 mg/ml can be infused at a rate of 12.5 ml per hour, but the infusion rate could be halved or doubled to meet the requirements of individual patients. This regimen would allow a daily dose of 60 mg, which is equivalent to 10 mg administered regularly at 4-hour intervals. Meperidine diluted to 2 mg/ml can also be infused at the same rate (12.5 ml per hour) to provide a similar degree of analgesia. Infusion of either of these drugs should be preceded by a loading dose equivalent to a 1-hour requirement.

Fentanyl administered as a dose of 5 μg/kg at the commencement of anesthesia and followed by an infusion of 3 μg/kg per hour during and after anesthesia produces consistent plasma concentrations of 2.7 ± 0.3 ng/ml. Such an infusion is compatible with depression of CO_2 responsiveness to about 50% of the patient's preoperative awake value. This is the limit of acceptable ventilatory depression in that $PaCO_2$ levels of 44 to 46 mm Hg are achieved. Such limits must be regarded as the measured upper limits of safety, and in clinical practice an infusion rate of 2 μg/kg per hour may be considered as providing a greater margin of safety.

Alfentanil, a new synthetic analogue of fentanyl, has a much shorter elimination half-life (90 minutes) than morphine or fentanyl. It has been administered as an infusion of 50 or 100 μg/kg per hour during surgery and at 20 μg/kg per hour during the postoperative period. This produces comparable degrees of analgesia and ventilatory depression to those found during fentanyl infusion.

Patient-demand analgesia

Patient-controlled analgesic therapy with intravenous opioids is based on a system that dispenses a preset dose of opioid intravenously from a syringe pump activated by a press button. By administering small doses frequently, with appropriate programming to limit the number of doses in a given period, the patient is able to titrate the drug to control his pain. Although commercial systems have been available for many years, they have not achieved popularity. The sophisticated apparatus that is necessary for such therapy is too expensive to allow this type of approach to be used in all patients, but one patient-demand system per nursing unit can be effectively used for patients with severe pain. The total doses consumed by individual patients are remarkably constant over periods between 6 and 24 hours. Requirements for meperidine have been described as 26 ± 10 mg per hour, and for morphine 2.6 mg per hour.

Epidural

Opioids injected into the epidural space are partly (20% to 40%) absorbed into the plexus of veins contained therein and distributed throughout the rest of the body. This part of the administered dose is distributed and metabolized in the same way as a similar dose administered intramuscularly. Depending on the lipid solubility and molecular size of the opioid, a variable proportion of the remainder will cross the dural membranes to reach the cerebrospinal fluid and, again depending on lipid solubility, will bind to the lipoproteins of the spinal cord and to opioid receptors in the dorsal horn.

Morphine was the first opioid injected (by Behar in 1979) into the epidural space. However, although morphine has been widely used as an epidural analgesic and its effects widely studied, it is perhaps the least suitable drug for this purpose because of its low lipid solubility (oil to water solubility is 1.4). The reports of delayed ventilatory arrest have largely attributed this adverse effect to the longevity of morphine in the cerebrospinal fluid. Unfortunately, diacetyl morphine (heroin), the most suitable opioid for epidural use and widely used in the United Kingdom, is unavailable to anesthesiologists in most countries.

Meperidine, fentanyl, and buprenorphine have been used by the epidural route, but, unfortunately, their analgesic effects are short-lived (1 to 3 hours) when administered intermittently. Table 2-4 summarizes the range of doses of these drugs suitable for epidural or intrathecal analgesia, and the side effects produced.

In patients who come to the PACU with an indwelling epidural catheter in either the lumbar or

---

TABLE 2-4

Opioids suitable for intrathecal (I) or epidural (E) analgesia

Drug	Route	Dose range	Duration (hours)	Pruritus (%)	Nausea and vomiting (%)
Morphine	E*	2.0-7.5 mg	22	22	26
Meperidine	E	25-75 mg	3.5	0	5
Fentanyl	E*	50-200 μg	2.0	0	9
Sufentanil	E	30-50 μg	4.0	?	?
Buprenorphine	E	0.15-0.3 mg	12-24	0	15-20
Diamorphine	E	2.5-5.0 mg	8-18	0	5
Morphine	I	0.5-1.0 mg	18-24	50-70	25

*Duration of action enhanced by epinephrine 1:200,000.

midthoracic region, the appropriate opioid should be dissolved in the same volume of saline that would be used for a segmental local anesthetic block. Nursing staff should realize the importance of recognizing changes of ventilatory frequency and should record these accurately, at 15-minute intervals for the first hour after opioid injection, and at half-hour intervals subsequently. A ventilatory frequency less than 10 breaths per minute is potentially dangerous if the patient is not carefully watched. Below 6 breaths per minute, minute ventilation becomes inadequate and $PaCO_2$ will rise to unacceptable levels.

Intrathecal

At the same time that local anesthetics are injected into the cerebrospinal fluid to produce spinal anesthesia, opioids can be injected to provide prolonged postoperative analgesia. Morphine (0.5 to 1.0 mg) has been more widely used than other opioids. Although it produces profound segmental analgesia, intrathecal morphine has also been associated with undesirable side effects, such as pruritus (50% to 70%), nausea and vomiting, and urinary retention. Pruritus does not respond to antihistamine therapy but can be completely obtunded by small doses of naloxone. More serious have been reports of delayed ventilatory arrest, presumed to occur as a result of diffusion of the hydrophilic morphine from the spinal to the medullary regions of the cerebrospinal fluid. To allow early recognition of such ventilatory depression, nursing staff must record ventilatory frequency at 30- to 60-minute intervals.

TREATMENT OF OPIOID SIDE EFFECTS
Narcotic Overdose

Ventilatory arrest, or profound slowing of breathing (<10 breaths per minute), is the main side effect of opioids. This may be precipitated by simple overdose, or the predicted effect of a given dose may be enhanced by the ventilatory depressant effects of other drugs, such as benzodiazepines, barbiturates, and general anesthetics. Ventilatory arrest may also be enhanced by sleep and antagonized by pain and

wakefulness. Two approaches can be used to reverse ventilatory depression.

Naloxone is a specific antagonist acting at both μ- and κ-receptors, which displaces other agonist opioids from these receptors. Intravenous naloxone (2 to 5 μg/kg) should be given slowly in patients whose ventilatory frequency has dropped below 6 breaths per minute. Its peak effect is reached within 2 minutes, but the duration of its antagonism is much shorter (60 to 90 minutes) than that of many opioids, especially morphine. If ventilatory frequency subsequently decreases to an unacceptable level, a further dose of naloxone must be given.

Doxapram is a nonspecific ventilatory stimulant that may be used either as a single dose (1 mg/kg) to initiate spontaneous breathing, or an infusion of 3 mg/kg per hour. Many patients find the effects of a larger, single dose unpleasant, and an infusion at an initial rate of 30 mg/kg per hour for 10 minutes may be more acceptable. Although doxapram stimulates ventilation, it also increases CO_2 production; thus it may not be very effective in decreasing $PaCO_2$ to normal levels.

Nausea and Vomiting

Nausea and vomiting in the PACU can be the result of a number of factors of which previous administration of opioids is the most common. Patients who have experienced severe nausea or vomiting after anesthetics are more likely to suffer the same problems on subsequent occasions, irrespective of the type of anesthesia administered. The best prophylaxis is to use a powerful butyrophenone antiemetic as part of the anesthetic technique. Droperidol (5 to 7.5 mg) is a much more potent and dependable antiemetic than the others that will be mentioned, and is more effective when given at the beginning of the anesthetic rather than in the PACU. Its antiemetic action lasts about 12 to 18 hours.

Many patients feel nauseated and retch within the first 5 to 10 minutes after waking, especially after a nitrous oxide anesthetic administered by mask. This is because of retention of nitrous oxide in the stomach cavity. Other than turning the patient on the side to protect the airway, no specific therapy is required.

Persistent nausea and vomiting of clear or bile-stained material is best treated in the PACU by the intravenous administration of one of the following drugs (mentioned in order of cost).

Metoclopramide

Metoclopramide is an effective antiemetic with a spectrum of activity similar to the phenothiazines, but it also increases propulsive activity in the stomach and closes the lower esophageal sphincter. It has little anticholinergic effect. It may cause severe extrapyramidal reactions, including oculogyric crisis, especially in children. The normal dose is 5 mg intravenously in young adults (up to 21 years of age), but more may be given to older patients.

Prochlorperazine

This phenothiazine is a potent antiemetic that acts primarily on the chemoreceptor trigger zone and is therefore particularly useful to inhibit opioid-induced nausea and vomiting. It is most effective when given as an intravenous injection of 6.25 mg, but its effect is more prolonged when given as an intramuscular injection of 12.5 mg. Dystonic reactions may occur in patients who have been taking other phenothiazines.

Perphenazine

The least expensive but as effective antiemetic as those mentioned, perphenazine is given either by intravenous injection of 2.5 to 5.0 mg, or by intramuscular injection of 5 to 10 mg. As with all phenothiazines, dystonic reactions may occur in response to overdosage.

REGIONAL AND LOCAL ANESTHETICS

Supplementation of regional anesthetic techniques used during surgery to provide postoperative pain relief can be more effective than the use of opioids, especially after intraabdominal or thoracic surgery. For many purposes the intraoperative dose provides adequate initial pain relief in the PACU, and further injection techniques are inappropriate.

Caudal Analgesia

Children having prolonged genitourinary procedures, such as plastic surgery for hypospadias or epispadias, can be given excellent postoperative pain relief by a further injection of bupivacaine (0.25%) into the caudal space at the end of surgery, while the child is still anesthetized. This will provide many hours of excellent analgesia.

Intercostal Block

Intercostal nerve blockade can be established by the surgeon, under direct vision, before closing a thoracotomy wound. Three milliliters of 0.5% bupivacaine can be accurately placed alongside each of the two intercostal nerves above and below, and at the level of the interspace used for the thoracotomy.

For unilateral operations, such as cholecystectomy, intercostal block can be achieved by placing a fine catheter through a Tuohy needle, or a teflon intravenous cannula (18-gauge) into one intercostal space (T8) posteriorly (at the rib angle). An initial injection of 12 to 15 ml of 0.5% bupivacaine followed by a slow continuous infusion of 0.125% bupivacaine will provide blockade of the intercostal nerve at the site of injection and allow spread to adjacent intercostal nerves by diffusion through the paravertebral space.

Move recently, diffuse blockade of intercostal nerves has been achieved by intrapleural injection of local anesthetics.

Epidural Blockade

Lumbar epidural blockade is highly suitable for postoperative pain relief after surgery of the lower abdomen, the pelvis, and the legs. The main disadvantage of sustained analgesia by continuous infusions into the lumbar epidural space is the arterial hypotension consequent on sympathetic nervous blockade. Provided the block does not extend above the T10 level, the degree of hypotension can be minimized. This is rarely sufficient to provide adequate pain relief after major intraabdominal procedures when local anesthetics are used. The principle of injecting a single dose of 0.5% bupivacaine followed by intermittent repeat doses of 0.25% bupivacaine or an infusion of 0.125% bupivacaine should be followed.

Thoracic segmental epidural blockade can be achieved by placing a catheter in the seventh or eighth thoracic interspace by the paraspinous approach. In the midthoracic region the spinous processes of the vertebrae are steeply inclined in a caudad direction, making the midline approach difficult and uncertain. A Tuohy needle can be inserted about one finger's breadth lateral to the lower margin of the spinous process of T7 and advanced perpendicular to the skin until the tip encounters the lamina of T8. The needle is then angulated toward the midline and the tip walked along the lamina until one can feel the tip of the needle slipping over the edge. The tip is then in the ligamentum flavum, and entry into the epidural space can be identified with standard loss of resistance techniques. A catheter placed at this the T7-T8 interspace and advanced only about 2 cm can be used to provide segmental blockade limited to the range T4-T12, thus providing excellent pain relief after intraabdominal or thoracic surgery. Bupivacaine (0.5%) should be injected slowly, in a volume of 1 ml per segment (5 to 8 ml) and supplemented by a slow infusion of bupivacaine (0.125%) at a rate of 6 to 7 ml per hour. Alternatively, appropriate opioids can be dissolved in a similar volume of saline to provide analgesia over the same segmental distribution.

For patients with severe respiratory disease who require total analgesia after intraabdominal surgery, combined opioid and local analgesia through a thoracic epidural catheter is most effective.

SUGGESTIONS FOR FURTHER READING

Bromage P: The price of intraspinal narcotic analgesia: basic constraints. Anesth Analg 60:461, 1981.

Bullingham RES editor: Opiate analgesia, Clinics in anaesthesiology 1(1), London, 1983, WB Saunders Co.

Frost EAM and Andrews IC, editors: Recovery room care. Int Anesthesiol Clin 21(1), Boston, 1983, Little, Brown & Co, Inc.

Kitahata LM and Collins JG, editors: Narcotic analgesics in anesthesiology, Baltimore, 1982, Williams & Wilkins.

Mankikian B et al: Improvement of diaphragmatic function by a thoracic extradural block after upper abdominal surgery, Anesthesiology 68:379, 1988.

Prys-Roberts C and Hug CC Jr, editors: Pharmacokinetics of anaesthesia. Oxford, 1984, Blackwell Scientific Publications, Inc.

Raj P: Postoperative pain. Curr Opin Anaesthesiol 1(3):392, 1988.

CHAPTER 3

Respiration: Mechanical Ventilation and Oxygen Therapy

Allison D. McIntyre

Postoperative respiratory insufficiency is one of the most commonly encountered complications in the post anesthesia care unit (PACU), and healthy patients are not immune. Anesthetic techniques, which include narcotics and muscle relaxants, can alter an individual's ability to control his airway and ventilatory exchange. In the patient with preoperative respiratory disease or dysfunction, the effects can be even more pronounced. Common treatable causes of early dysfunction are shown in Figure 3-1. Essentials of monitoring are outlined in Figure 3-2.

The respiratory complications seen in the PACU may be caused by arterial hypoxemia, alveolar hypoventilation, and upper and lower airway obstruction.

ARTERIAL HYPOXEMIA

Postoperative arterial hypoxemia has multiple etiological factors. The most common cause is atelectasis, which results in ventilation to perfusion mismatching in the lung. Whenever poorly ventilated areas of the lung are well perfused and well-ventilated areas of the lung are poorly perfused, there will be ventilation to perfusion mismatching. Other causes of ventilation to perfusion mismatching include intrapulmonary shunts, increased oxygen consumption (as with shivering and hyperthermia), low cardiac output, effects of intraoperative positioning, abdominal distention, abdominal pain, residual effects of anesthetics, and a decrease in functional residual capacity (FRC). FRC is the volume of gas remaining in the lungs after a normal expiration. It is reduced in obese patients, in patients with abdominal distention or ascites, and in pregnant patients. It is reduced also in patients with circumferential chest or abdominal dressings that are too restrictive.

Aspiration of acidic gastric fluid can cause profound hypoxemia, as can a pulmonary embolus. The signs and symptoms of aspiration include tachypnea, tachycardia, rales, rhonchi, and eventually chest x-ray examination changes in the majority of patients. The earliest and most reliable sign of aspiration is arterial hypoxemia. The signs and symptoms of pulmonary embolism include acute dyspnea and tachypnea.

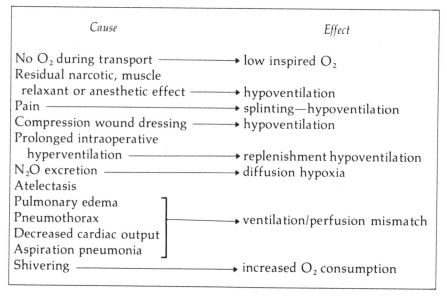

FIGURE 3-1

Common treatable causes of early postoperative respiratory dysfunction.

Diffusion hypoxia is a problem more frequently seen in the operating room than in the PACU. When nitrous oxide is discontinued at the end of an anesthetic, large quantities of nitrous enter the alveoli from the blood, which dilutes the oxygen and other gases in the alveoli. The patient usually becomes hypoxic if allowed to breathe room air at this point. Diffusion hypoxia can be prevented if 100% oxygen is administered to the patient for 5 to 10 minutes after the discontinuation of nitrous oxide.

Posthypoventilation hypoxia is a complication that can occur when patients are hyperventilated intraoperatively. The patient will hypoventilate postoperatively in an attempt to increase $PaCO_2$ stores, and hypoxia can result. Treatment is to give 100% oxygen until the patient exhibits a normal ventilatory pattern.

Pneumothorax can occur postoperatively after insertion of central monitoring cannulae and after neck surgery, mastectomy, nephrectomy, and regional anesthesia. Arterial hypoxemia caused by atelectasis and intrapulmonary shunts (ventilation to perfusion mismatching) result. A pneumothorax of more than 20% in a spontaneously breathing patient or any pneumothorax in a mechanically ventilated person should be treated by insertion of a chest tube.

Pulmonary edema can cause hypoxemia and may result from noncardiogenic or cardiogenic sources. Noncardiogenic pulmonary edema can occur postoperatively as a result of aspiration of acidic gastric contents, upper airway obstruction, massive transfusion, sepsis, and anaphylaxis. Cardiogenic pulmonary edema is usually the result of left ventricular failure and high pulmonary vascular pressures.

Definitive diagnosis of arterial hypoxemia requires arterial blood gas analyses and is considered to be present when the PaO_2 is less than 60 mm Hg at any inspired oxygen concentration. Early clinical signs of hypoxemia are nonspecific, and the effects of residual anesthetics attenuate circulatory and ventilatory responses to arterial hypoxemia. Transcutaneous pulse oximetry offers a fast, easy, noninvasive means of measuring oxyhemoglobin saturation in the blood. Accuracy depends on skin perfusion. It offers the advantage of continuous monitoring immediately postoperatively and can alert PACU staff to adverse trends in oxygenation.

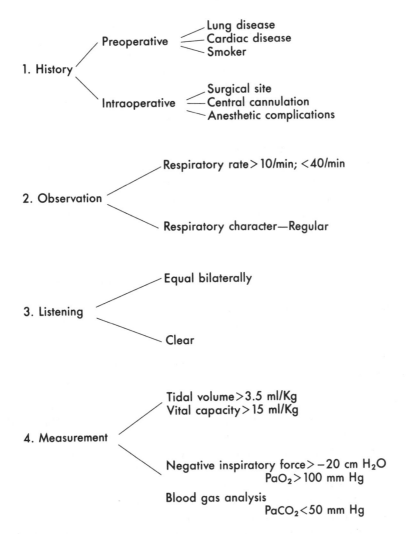

FIGURE 3-2

Essentials of monitoring ventilation. Deviation from the values listed means therapeutic intervention is necessary.

Initial treatment of arterial hypoxemia includes increasing the inspired oxygen concentration and encouraging the patient to cough and deep breathe to decrease atelectasis and improve ventilation to perfusion mismatching. If arterial hypoxemia persists despite a 100% inhaled oxygen concentration and the above measures, tracheal intubation and mechanical ventilation are indicated. Positive end-expiratory pressure (PEEP) increases the FRC, de-creases ventilation to perfusion mismatching, and increases the PaO_2.

ALVEOLAR HYPOVENTILATION

Hypoventilation is defined as decreased alveolar ventilation resulting in an arterial carbon dioxide tension ($PaCO_2$) of greater than 44 mm Hg. Alveolar hypoventilation can occur postoperatively as a result of central respiratory depression, poor respiratory muscle function, and acute or chronic lung disease.

Inhaled and intravenous anesthetics can depress the central respiratory center and desensitize the patient to the stimulating effects of CO_2. Narcotics can produce a biphasic respiratory depression. The first phase occurs intraoperatively and is temporarily reversed by the stimulating effects of extubation and transfer to the PACU. After the patient is admitted and settled in the PACU, external stimulation decreases and respiratory depression can again occur. Narcotic-induced alveolar hypoventilation can be effectively reversed by the narcotic antagonist naloxone (Narcan). When naloxone is titrated in small doses, respiratory depression can be reversed while the analgesic effects of the narcotic are maintained. The effects of naloxone are often of shorter duration than the respiratory depressant effects of the narcotic, and a second dose may be required. Narcotic agonist/antagonist drugs, such as butorphanol (Stadol) and nalbuphine (Nubain), are occasionally used to reverse narcotic-induced respiratory depression.

Poor respiratory muscle function can be caused by residual neuromuscular blockade that results in alveolar hypoventilation. Residual neuromuscular blockade may be the result of inadequate pharmacological reversal, potentiation of the neuromuscular blocker by aminoglycoside antibiotics, respiratory acidosis, hypokalemia, hypermagnesemia, and hypothermia. Adequate recovery of neuromuscular blockade can be reasonably assured if the patient can sustain head lift for 5 seconds, has a vigorous hand grasp, can protrude the tongue for several seconds, and has an inspiratory force of -20 cm H_2O or greater and/or a vital capacity of 10 to 15 ml/kg. Pharmacological reversal of the nondepolarizing muscle relaxants (pancuronium, curare, metocurine, gallamine, atracurium, and vecuronium) is achieved with either edrophonium, neostigmine, or pyridostigmine with atropine or glycopyrrolate.

Alveolar hypoventilation can occur also in obese patients, patients with abdominal and gastric distention, and patients with preoperative respiratory disease or dysfunction. The site of surgical incision can also affect the ability to deep breathe. After upper abdominal surgery patients experience the greatest decrease in vital capacity.

Evaluation of arterial blood gases is the best method of diagnosing alveolar hypoventilation. Occasionally an increase in blood pressure and tachycardia are seen with hypercarbia, but may not occur in postanesthetized patients and patients with an attenuated response to increased levels of CO_2.

Vital capacity and inspiratory force also indicate the effectiveness of ventilation. If the minimal acceptable volumes cannot be attained (10 to 15 ml/kg and -20 cm H_2O respectively) and if the $PaCO_2$ is greater than 44 mm Hg, mechanical ventilation should be instituted.

RESPIRATORY DYSFUNCTION

Several causes of respiratory difficulties in the PACU have been identified.

Upper and Lower Airway Obstruction

Upper airway obstruction is usually caused by the tongue and pharyngeal soft tissues falling back and occluding the airway. This results in inadequate ventilation. The classic signs of upper airway obstruction are intercostal and suprasternal retractions and lack of air movement on auscultation. The most effective method of relieving obstruction is to extend the head and displace the mandible anteriorly if necessary. If this fails to relieve the obstruction, an oropharyngeal or nasopharyngeal airway should be inserted. A nasopharyngeal airway is usually better tolerated by the patient emerging from general anesthesia, and an oropharyngeal airway can cause vomiting and laryngospasm. The patient with an upper airway obstruction should be placed in the lateral position to facilitate drainage of oral secretions and prevent aspiration. If these measures are unsuccessful in relieving the obstruction, an endotracheal or nasotracheal tube should be inserted.

Laryngospasm

Spasm of the laryngeal muscles causes narrowing or closure of the larynx. Laryngospasm can occur during emergence from general anesthesia or just after extubation. It is usually caused by secretions, blood, or upper airway manipulation that irritates the glottis. If the laryngospasm is incomplete, ventilation may be possible by extending the head, anteriorly displacing the mandible, and manually assisting ventilation with 100% oxygen and positive airway pressure. If ventilation cannot be achieved with these methods or if the laryngospasm is complete, 0.15 to 0.3 mg/kg succinylcholine should be given to relax and open the vocal cords. Ventilation should be assisted until the effects of the succinylcholine have worn off and ventilation is adequate.

Laryngeal edema

Stridulous respirations may result from laryngeal edema or vocal cord paralysis. Laryngeal edema is usually a result of irritation to the larynx either from surgical manipulation, traumatic or repeated intubations, use of a larger than needed endotracheal tube in children, or excessive coughing while intubated. Treatment of laryngeal edema includes administration of warmed, humidified oxygen and inhalation of an aerosolized topical mucosal vasoconstrictor, such as racemic epinephrine. Intravenous steroids are occasionally used to minimize soft tissue swelling, particularly when extensive and marked airway edema is anticipated. The effectiveness of steroids remains controversial.

Bronchospasm

Bronchospasm is treated in the PACU by inhaled or intravenous bronchodilators (Table 3-1). The newer β-agonist bronchodilators have predominantly greater β-2 (bronchodilating) effects than β-1 (tachycardia, dysrhythmias) side effects. These drugs include metaproterenol (Alupent or Metaprel)

TABLE 3-1

Inhalation drugs used as bronchodilators

Generic name	Trade name	Inhalation by IPPB	Inhalation from metered nebulizer	Peak response (minutes)	Duration of action (minutes)
Isoproterenol preparations	Isuprel Hydrochloride Solution; Isuprel Mistometer (metered dose)	0.5 ml (0.5%) in 1.5 ml N saline	2-3 doses; 125 μg/dose	10-15	60-90
Racepinephrine	Vaponefrin	0.5 ml (2.25%) in 1.5 ml N saline		5-10	120-180
Isoetharine HCI	Bronkosol	0.5 ml (1%) in 1.5 ml N saline	1-2 doses; 340 μg/dose	10-15	90-120
Metaproterenol sulfate	Alupent	0.5 ml (5%) in 1.5 ml N saline	2-3 doses; 0.65 mg/dose	10-15	180-240
Atropine sulfate		2 mg in 1 ml N saline; 0.05-0.1 mg/kg; no more than t.i.d.		5-10	240-360
Albuterol	Ventolin; Salbutamol		2 doses; 90 μg/dose	10-15	240-360

Reprinted with permission from Int Anesthesiol Clin, 21:1, 1983.
IPPB, Intermittent positive-pressure breathing; *N*, Normal; *t.i.d.*, Three times daily.

and salbutamol/albuterol (Proventil or Ventolin). Albuterol has the least amount of β-1 activity. Isoetharine (Bronkosol) has more β-1 activity than the previously mentioned agents, and cardiovascular side effects occur more often. Overall, when bronchodilators are inhaled, there is a lower incidence of β-1 side effects than when they are received systemically.

Aminophylline given with inhaled bronchodilators acts synergistically. A loading dose of aminophylline is usually given intravenously, followed by a continuous infusion.

Steroids are occasionally used for treatment of bronchospasm. Beclomethasone (Vanceril) can be inhaled, and methylprednisolone (Solu-Medrol) is given intravenously.

Frequent auscultation of the chest should be done to assess effectiveness of therapies.

OXYGEN THERAPY

Supplemental oxygen is routinely given to nonintubated patients postoperatively. There are many available devices. The inhaled oxygen concentration, level of humidification, and degree of patient comfort vary with the different modes of oxygen therapy. Table 3-2 delineates flow rates and resultant FiO_2 values for the different devices.

Nasal Cannulae

Nasal cannulae are usually well tolerated by patients postoperatively. Oxygen is delivered via two short prongs that are inserted into the nares (Figure 3-3). The inhaled oxygen concentration (FiO_2) delivered to the patient depends on the flow rate of oxygen (L/min) and the patient's minute ventilation (tidal volume × respiratory rate). The inhaled oxygen concentration is lower if the minute ventilation is high (hyperventilation) because the inspiratory flow rate exceeds the oxygen flow rate. This causes room air to be entrained by the patient. Conversely, the inhaled oxygen concentration is increased by hypoventilation.

Increasing oxygen flow rates from 1 to 6 L/min increases the inhaled oxygen concentration. Flow rates greater than 6 L/min should be avoided, however, because there is no further increase in FiO_2. Minimal humidification is provided with nasal cannulae, and higher flow rates may dry the nasal mucosa.

Face Masks

Face masks used for supplemental oxygen therapy include simple, partial rebreathing, nonrebreathing, and venturi. They deliver a higher FiO_2 than nasal cannulae.

TABLE 3-2		
Oxygen delivery devices for nonintubated patients		
Equipment	**O$_2$ Flow (L/min)**	**FiO$_2$**
Nasal cannulae	1-6	0.25-0.55
Open face mask	6-12	0.35-0.65
Face mask/nasal cannula combination	6-12 (mask); 6 (cannulae)	0.44-0.85
Face tent	8-10	0.21-0.55
Nonrebreathing mask (mask with reservoir)	Any rate that prevents the reservoir from collapsing	0.60-0.80
Venturi mask	4-12	0.24, 0.28, 0,31, 0.35, 0.40

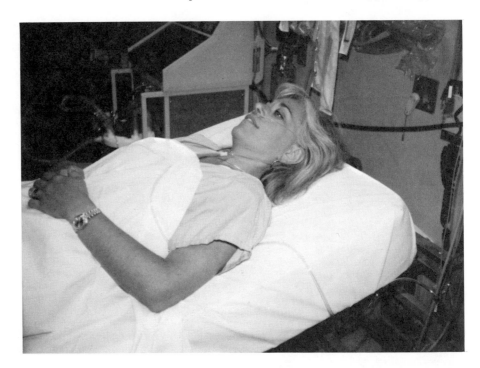

FIGURE 3-3
Nasal cannula.

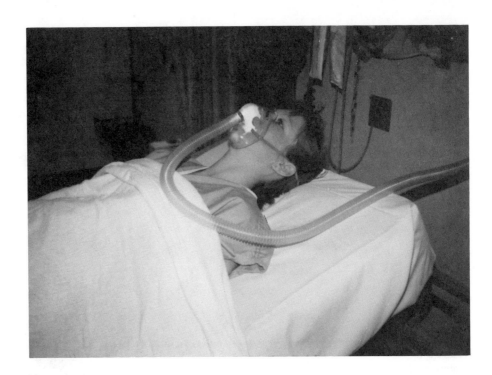

FIGURE 3-4
Simple face mask.

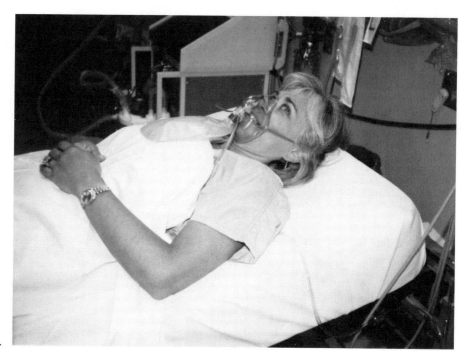

FIGURE 3-5
Partial rebreathing mask.

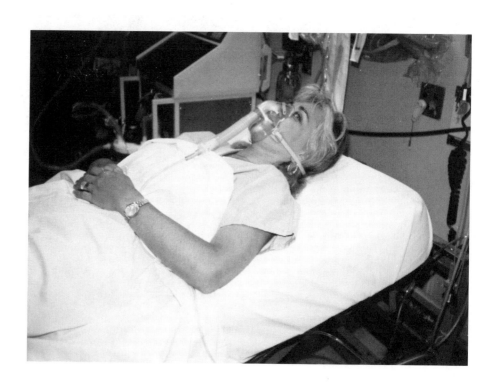

FIGURE 3-6
Venturi mask.

Simple face mask

A simple face mask (Figure 3-4) delivers a high level of humidity as a result of the wider bore of its tubing. Oxygen flows into the mask through this tubing, and exhaled gases leave through the holes in the side of the mask. The inspired oxygen concentration depends on the flow rate of oxygen and the minute ventilation of the patient as a result of room air entrainment. A snug-fitting mask gives a more consistent FiO_2 than an improperly positioned mask.

Partial rebreathing mask

A partial rebreathing mask (Figure 3-5) combines a face mask with an oxygen reservoir bag. The initial portion of the patient's exhaled gas (which contains little or no CO_2) mixes with the oxygen in the reservoir bag and is inspired with the next inhalation. As the reservoir bag fills and the pressure increases, the last portion of the patient's exhaled gas (which contains CO_2) is forced out through the holes on the side of the mask.

Nonrebreathing mask

A nonrebreathing mask combines a simple face mask with an oxygen reservoir bag. A unidirectional valve prevents rebreathing of exhaled gases. Exhaled gases exit through the holes at the side of the mask. An inhaled oxygen concentration of 100% can be achieved if the flow rates are high enough to maintain an inflated reservoir bag.

Venturi mask

A venturi mask (Figure 3-6) delivers precise inhaled concentrations of oxygen that are not affected by the patient's minute ventilation. Various concentrations of inhaled oxygen are available either through interchangeable air injectors (different color = different preset percentage) or dialable controls on a single air injector. The design of this mask prevents CO_2 rebreathing by the patient.

Tracheostomy Masks

Tracheostomy masks (Figure 3-7) are designed to deliver humidified oxygen to the patient with a tra-

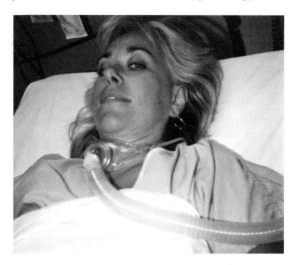

FIGURE 3-7
Tracheostomy mask.

cheostomy. They are available in adult and pediatric sizes.

Face Tents

Face tents (Figure 3-8) can be used with or without oxygen, and the large bore tubing allows delivery at a high humidity.

Oxygen Tents (Croup Tents)

Oxygen tents are usually used for children and provide an oxygenated, temperature- and humidity-controlled environment. The maximum attainable inspired oxygen concentration is usually 50%.

HUMIDIFICATION SYSTEMS

Humidification and warming of inhaled gases normally occur in the nose and upper respiratory tract. The relative humidity of alveolar gases at 37° C is 100%. When dry gases are inhaled or the upper airways are bypassed by a tracheal tube, water is vaporized from the airway mucosa to maintain the 100% relative humidity of gas in the alveolus. Dehydration of the airway mucosa and increased

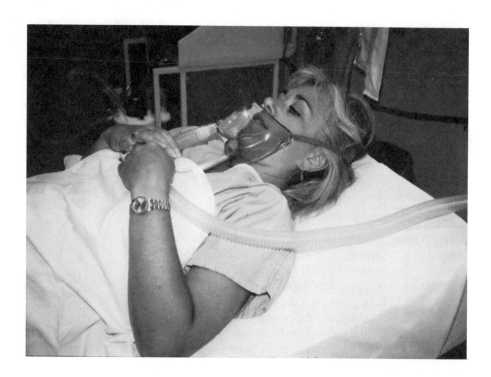

FIGURE 3-8
Face tent.

viscosity of mucous secretions result. Ciliary and surfactant activity is reduced, and the removal of secretions is inhibited. Retention of mucous secretions produces atelectasis, inflamed airway mucosa, and a decrease in ventilation to perfused areas of lung (ventilation/perfusion mismatch). It is therefore desirable and beneficial to humidify dry inhaled gases by use of a humidifier or nebulizer.

Humidifiers

The two types of humidifiers are the pass over and the cascade (bubble through). The principle involved with pass over humidifiers is evaporation of the warmed water that gases "pass over." This increases the water vapor content of the gas. Cascade (bubble through) humidifiers are frequently used in mechanical ventilators. Gases are bubbled through heated water to saturate the gas with as much water vapor as possible. The warmer a gas is, the more water is carried. Conversely, as saturated gas travels through ventilator tubing, it cools and

causes the water vapor to condense. To deliver humidified gas at body temperature, the water in the humidifier must be 38° to 40° C. Temperature of the inhaled gases should be monitored at the closest possible point to the patient to prevent tracheal "burn."

Nebulizers

Nebulizers suspend particles of liquid (water or medication) in a gas. Two types are available: jet and ultrasonic.

Jet nebulizers

High-pressure gas is forced through a restricted orifice that produces a high-velocity jet stream in the nebulizer chamber. This high-velocity gas stream is directed over the end of a small capillary tube that is immersed in the liquid to be nebulized. When the liquid exits the top of the small tube, it is aerosolized by the jet of gas and very small (30μm) particles are formed and carried to the patient.

Ultrasonic nebulizers

An ultrasonic nebulizer creates ultrahigh-frequency oscillations that are transmitted to a transducer. These high-frequency vibrations produce fragmentation of a liquid into very small particles. The aerosolized particles are then carried to the patient by air or oxygen. Nebulizers are used as humidifiers and also to deliver bronchodilating drugs to airways.

Complications of humidifying gases are bacterial contamination (which can cause infection), water intoxication, hyperthermia, and tracheal mucosal burn if the temperature of inhaled gases is too high.

MECHANICAL VENTILATION

Several types of ventilators are encountered in the PACU.

Pressure-cycled Ventilators

Pressure-cycled ventilators deliver gas to the patient at a predetermined flow rate until a certain airway pressure is reached, regardless of the tidal volume delivered. The tidal volume and inspiratory time are directly related to pulmonary compliance and may vary considerably. The FiO_2 delivered is not constant, and the use of a pressure-cycled ventilator is usually limited to intermittent positive-pressure breathing (IPPB) therapy. An example of this type of ventilator is the Bird.

Volume-cycled Ventilators

A volume-cycled ventilator delivers a preset tidal volume over a preset inspiratory time, regardless of the peak inspiratory pressure required. A pressure limit is often set to prevent excessive pressure from being generated within the system. The delivered tidal volume and the FiO_2 are relatively constant. There are five ventilation modes on volume-cycled ventilators:

1. **Control** The ventilator initiates and delivers a preset tidal volume that is unaffected by the patient's respiratory efforts.

2. **Assist** The ventilator delivers a mechanical breath of a preset tidal volume when it senses a drop in airway pressure as the patient initiates a spontaneous breath.

3. **Assist/Control** The patient receives a minimum number of preset breaths of a preset tidal volume but can receive additional mechanical breaths of the same tidal volume by initiating a spontaneous breath.

4. **Intermittent Mandatory Ventilation (IMV)** A preset tidal volume at a preset rate is delivered by the ventilator, but the patient can breathe spontaneously between mechanical breaths.

5. **Synchronous IMV (SIMV)** This is similar to IMV in that a preset tidal volume at a preset rate is delivered mechanically by the ventilator when the ventilator senses an inspiratory effort by the patient. This limits the number of times a mechanical breath is given during exhalation.

Ventilator Settings

Ventilator settings for a patient in the PACU are usually similar to the ventilator settings that were used for that patient in the OR. Respiratory rates are usually 8 to 12 breaths/min, tidal volumes are 10 to 15 ml/kg, and inhaled oxygen concentrations are 30% to 50%. Adjustments of these settings should be based on evaluation of the patient's arterial blood gases. Normal arterial blood gas values are: pH, 7.35 to 7.45; $PaCO_2$, 35 to 45 mm Hg; and PaO_2, 80 to 100 mm Hg.

PEEP and CPAP

Positive end-expiratory pressure (PEEP) is produced by applying positive pressure to the airway at the conclusion of exhalation. It is initially set at 3 to 5 cm H_2O pressure and increased in 2.5 to 5.0 cm H_2O increments, depending on the patient's arterial PaO_2, cardiac output, and blood pressure. PEEP (1) prevents expiratory alveolar collapse, (2) increases functional residual capacity (FRC), (3) increases pulmonary compliance, and (4) improves arterial oxygenation. It improves ventilation/perfusion matching as previously collapsed but perfused alveoli are expanded and is of particular value in patients with adult respiratory distress syndrome (ARDS) when the PaO_2 cannot be maintained above 60 mm Hg despite inhaled oxygen concentrations in excess of 50%. Hemodynamically, PEEP may decrease venous return and cardiac output. PEEP may also cause pulmonary barotrauma as a result of overdistention of alveoli, increased extravascular lung water, and redistribution of pulmonary blood flow.

Continuous positive airway pressure (CPAP) is positive expiratory pressure generated to a spontaneously breathing patient via a tracheal tube or mask.

High-frequency Ventilation

High-frequency ventilation is a type of controlled ventilation that is characterized by very small tidal volumes and rapid ventilatory rates. It has traditionally been used to ventilate patients with ARDS and bronchopleural fistulae. The mechanism underlying its efficacy is unknown. There are three types of high-frequency ventilation:

High-frequency, positive-pressure ventilation (HFPPV)	50-150 breaths/min
High-frequency jet ventilation (HFJV)	60-660 breaths/min
High-frequency oscillation	60 Hz or 3600 cycles/min

HFPPV is not affected by airway resistance and pulmonary compliance. During inspiration of the low tidal volumes, there is a low mean positive airway pressure, resulting in minimal effects on cardiac output and a decreased incidence of barotrauma. HFPPV provides continuous positive pressure throughout the ventilator cycle. HFJV delivers a small tidal volume at high flow rates through a narrow orifice. Because jet flow is delivered through a small lumen tube, gas is entrained, which makes it difficult to determine the actual oxygen concentration and tidal volume delivered. Exhalation occurs either around the tube or through another lumen and is passive.

EXTUBATION CRITERIA

The following criteria are usually associated with uncomplicated extubations:

1. Vital capacity greater than 10 to 15 ml/kg
2. Inspiratory force numerically greater than -20 cm H_2O
3. A $PaO_2 > 80$ mm Hg at an FiO_2 greater than .4 and an acceptable pH
4. Cardiovascular and metabolic stability (extubation should be postponed until the patient is hemodynamically stable)
5. No residual neuromuscular blockade
6. Intact airway reflexes (coughing, gagging) sufficient to protect the airway and clear secretions; patients who should be extubated only when fully awake (synonymous with intact airway reflexes) include those with a full stomach before anesthesia, those with mandibular wiring or banding, those with difficult airways, and children with sleep apnea syndromes

SUMMARY

A knowledge of the physiology and principles of airway management and oxygen therapies is essential to effectively care for the postanesthetic patient. This knowledge combined with diligence and timely intervention enables PACU nurses to expertly manage respiratory complications. A summary of abbreviations and tables of normal values of respiratory measurements are found in Appendix 3.

SUGGESTIONS FOR FURTHER READING

Bowe EA and Klein EF Jr: Postoperative respiratory care, Int Anesthesiol Clin 21(1):77, 1983.

Feeley TW: The recovery room. In Miller RD, editor: Anesthesia, ed 2, New York, 1986, Churchill Livingstone, Inc.

Hornbein, TF: Drugs and postoperative recovery of ventilation, Amer Soc Anesth Refresher Course Lecture, San Francisco, 1988.

Mickler TA and Hoellerich VL: Respiratory intensive care. In Firestone LL, Lebowitz PW, and Cook CE, editors: Clinical anesthesia procedures of the Massachusetts General Hospital, Boston, 1988, Little, Brown & Co, Inc.

Stoelting RK and Miller RD: Basics of anesthesia, New York, 1984, Churchill Livingstone, Inc.

Stone DJ: Recovery room. In Firestone LL, Lebowitz PW, and Cook CE, editors: Clinical anesthesia procedures of the Massachusetts General Hospital, Boston, 1988, Little, Brown and Co, Inc.

CHAPTER 4

Cardiovascular Action: Too Much, Too Little, or Irregular

Cedric Prys-Roberts

Recovery from anesthesia can be associated with marked instability of the cardiovascular system. Extremes of arterial hypotension or hypertension, bradycardia or tachycardia, and dysrhythmia are by no means uncommon and require a high degree of vigilance for detection and correction. Although these abnormalities may be well tolerated by younger patients, they frequently herald the onset of serious consequences in the older patient, such as myocardial infarction, cerebral hemorrhage or infarction, renal failure, and acute cardiac arrest. Recognition, decision making, and action must follow in short succession.

MONITORING

The key to success in recognizing disturbances of cardiovascular function lies in continuous monitoring of as many variables as are consistent with the patient's preexisting medical state and the nature of the surgery. The more unpredictable the condition of the patient in the PACU, the more variety of monitoring techniques and the greater emphasis on continuity of monitoring are required.

Arterial Pressure

Monitoring of arterial pressure can be considered under three headings: (1) continuation of direct intraarterial pressure recording used during surgery, (2) automatic, discontinuous, noninvasive measurements, and (3) intermittent, manual recordings.

Direct intraarterial pressure measurement

This provides the most continuous and potentially the most accurate information. The observer derives a number of subsidiary indices of performance. Figure 4-1 shows how the arterial pressure pulse may be interpreted and how abnormal conditions may be identified. These patterns can be clearly and accurately identified only if certain simple principles are adhered to in the measurement process: (1) air bubbles should be avoided in the transducer domes, stop-cock systems, and catheters connecting to the patient's artery; and (2) the catheter with connecting tubing is kept as short and stiff as possible.

For a more detailed discussion of measurement techniques, the reader should consult the literature.

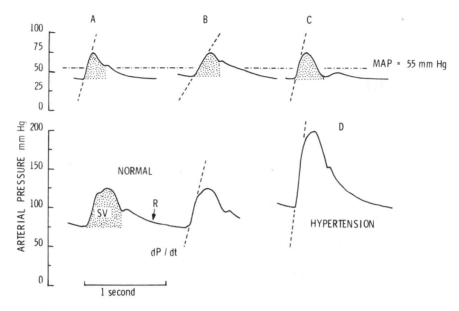

FIGURE 4-1

Arterial pressure waveforms as seen on a monitor screen or oscillograph tracing. The normal tracing shows that over and above the systolic and diastolic arterial pressure values, three additional pieces of information can be derived: (1) the area *(shaded)* under the systolic ejection curve is proportional to the stroke volume; (2) the rate of change of arterial pressure (dP/dt) is proportional to the contractile performance of the left ventricular muscle; and (3) the diastolic decay of pressure is an exponential, whose time constant is the product of resistance and compliance of the systemic vasculature. Hence the steepness of the diastolic pressure decay is proportional to the systemic vascular resistance. **A,** Arterial pressure waveform during hypovolemia. **B,** Arterial pressure waveform during myocardial depression by halothane anesthesia. **C,** Arterial pressure waveform during an infusion of sodium nitroprusside. **D,** Arterial pressure waveform in hypertension.

Systolic and diastolic pressures should be recorded from whatever display or recording system is used, because these alone are the measurements common to all three categories. A wide pulse pressure (systolic/diastolic pressure) is usually indicative of a high stroke volume, and vice-versa. A high diastolic pressure and a steep diastolic pressure run-off indicate a high vascular resistance (Figure 4-1, *D*). Low systolic and diastolic pressures could indicate either direct myocardial depression (Figure 4-1, *B*), inadequate cardiac filling caused by hypovolemia (Figure 4-1, *A*), or persistence of drug effects from the anesthetic period causing marked arterial dilation with consequent low vascular resistance (Figure 4-1, *C*). Mean arterial pressure may be useful as a means of recording a trend but has little physiological significance. In each of these three circumstances (Figure 4-1, *A, B,* and *C*), mean arterial pressure would have been the same and would have given *no indication of the cause* of the low arterial pressure. Steepness of the upstroke of the arterial pressure wave (dP/dt) indicates good contractility, whereas a sluggish upstroke may indicate poor contractility (Figure 4-1, *B*). Beware of making the latter interpretation if there is any doubt about damping of the waveform caused by air bubbles in the connecting tubing.

Dysrhythmias, which cause a shortening of the

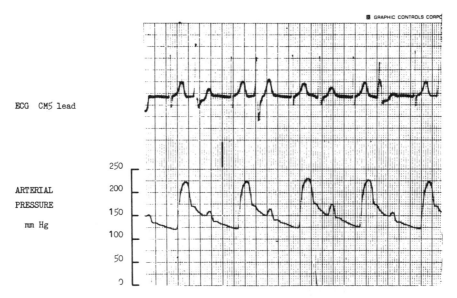

FIGURE 4-2

Influence of ventricular and junctional extrasystoles on the left ventricular output as manifest in the arterial pressure trace. Note that because extrasystolic beats come too early and do not allow adequate time for ventricular filling and for the atrial kick, the arterial pressure generated for these beats is almost nonexistent.

interbeat interval, may cause marked diminution of stroke volume and thus arterial pressure on occasional or alternate beats (Figure 4-2).

Automatic noninvasive measurements

During the past few years, a number of devices have become available that automatically inflate a standard sphygmomanometer cuff on the arm and, using the oscillometry principle, detect separately the systolic, mean, and diastolic pressures, and determine the heart rate. A typical machine of this type is the Dinamap. Its accuracy and reproducibility in clinical practice have been described. It can measure both systolic and diastolic pressures from 50 to 250 mm Hg with a reproducibility of $\pm$ 15 mm Hg (95% confidence limits for a single measurement). This and other automatic systems are valuable for repeated measurements at frequent preset intervals in the PACU. They have two disadvantages: (1) they are relatively poor at accurately measuring pressures during a sudden increase or

decrease of pressure; and (2) they can produce bruising and nerve damage if set to inflate too frequently for long periods.

Intermittent manual recordings

The standard method of sphygmomanometry has been the mainstay of PACU blood pressure measurement and is perfectly satisfactory for routine postoperative management. Detection of the onset of Korotkoff sounds for measurement of systolic pressure gives poor absolute accuracy and reproducibility (95% confidence limits: $\pm$21 mm Hg) compared with the Dinamap, but better reproducibility for diastolic pressures ($\pm$16 mm Hg) when determined as phase 5 limits (disappearance of Korotkoff sounds).

Electrocardiogram (ECG)

The ECG is essential to monitor cardiac dysrhythmias, disturbances of cardiac conduction, and is-

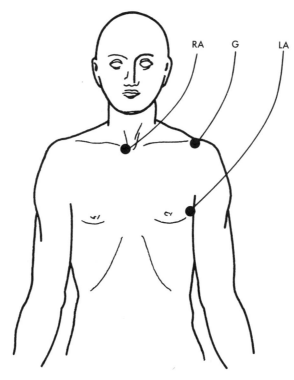

CM5 LEAD CONFIGURATION

FIGURE 4-3

Lead placement for CM_5 configuration. When using this with a three-lead display (Lead I), the R arm lead should be placed just below the sternal notch, the L arm lead in the anterior axillary line at the fifth intercostal space (as for Lead V), and the indifference lead on the left shoulder.

chemia of the myocardium. Any of the standard 12 leads can be used to detect dysrhythmias or a prolonged P-R interval characteristic of first-degree heart block. To detect myocardial ischemia, which is commonly of left ventricular origin, either a standard V_5 unipolar lead or preferably the CM_5 bipolar lead (Figure 4-3) should be used. The CM_5 lead consistently gives a positive R wave of good amplitude and has the highest probability, for any single lead, of detecting ST segment elevation characteristic of transmural ischemia or more commonly ST segment depression characteristic of subendocardial ischemia. Continuous monitoring of heart rate is usually obtained from the ECG waveform.

Central Venous Pressure (CVP)

Catheters may be advanced to the superior vena cava or right atrium from the internal or external jugular veins, the subclavian vein, or a peripheral vein at the elbow. Measurement of CVP by transducer or a simple saline manometer yields a mean value of pressure over the cardiac cycle. In the PACU, the finding of a low CVP (<1 mm Hg) in combination with a low arterial pressure is strongly suggestive of hypovolemia. By contrast, a low arterial pressure associated with elevated CVP (>10 mm Hg) is more likely to represent impaired cardiac function.

Pulmonary Artery Balloon-tipped Catheters

Measurement of pulmonary artery (PA) pressures (systolic and diastolic) is normally used only in patients with severe pulmonary hypertension or right ventricular failure and is of little value in monitoring the normal patient. In the early 1960s PA catheters were floated without balloon control through the central veins and right ventricle but could not be wedged. In 1969 Swan and his colleagues described a balloon-tipped catheter that could be placed in a distal branch of the pulmonary artery to yield an estimate of left atrial pressure when the balloon was inflated and phasic PA pressures with the balloon deflated. A thermistor placed at the tip of the catheter behind the balloon allows measurement of cardiac output by the thermodilution method. Such measurements are usually of value only in patients with severely compromised myocardial function or severe ventricular hypertrophy and those who have undergone cardiac surgery.

Pulse Oximetry

The pulse oximeter gives an indication of peripheral tissue oxygenation by measuring simultaneously the pulse volume (usually in a finger) and the oxyhemoglobin saturation (SaO_2). The latter is measured by transmission spectrophotometry, at two wavelengths in the red and infrared light spectrum, during the pulsatile phase of tissue perfusion. The pulse volume waveform is usually displayed on a screen and is used to determine the heart rate.

Pulse oximetry can detect detrimental changes of tissue oxygen delivery arising either from (1) a decrease of SaO_2 (induced by decreased inspired oxygen concentration, obstruction of the airways, or defects in pulmonary gas exchange) or a decrease of cardiac output or (2) arteriolar constriction—both of which will decrease pulse volume. Pulse oximetry has a rather slow response to accidental failure of oxygen delivery to the patient than do other methods of detecting a decrease of airway PO_2, such as a paramagnetic O_2 analyzer or a fuel cell analyzer. It has proved to be a valuable tool in identifying potential and occasionally real oxyhemoglobin desaturation occurring during the transfer of a patient from the operating room to the recovery area or during the postoperative course of the elderly patients who are recovering after hip surgery. Although it is sometimes claimed to be the ''ultimate'' monitor of oxygenation, it should be recognized that pulse oximetry is subject to a number of artifactual problems and that it is only one of a number of methods, each of which has advantages and disadvantages, for measuring oxygenation. Its place in PACU monitoring remains to be validated by good quality studies, although recent reports indicate that pulse oximetry may indeed become a standard monitor in the immediate postanesthetic period.

CARDIOVASCULAR DISTURBANCES AND THEIR MANAGEMENT

This section is organized on a problem-oriented basis. Two main problems, arterial hypotension and hypertension, their recognition, causation, and management, are considered under three associated states of heart rate: normal heart rate (55 to 100 per minute), bradycardia (<55 per minute), and tachycardia (>100 per minute). Dysrhythmias and their management are considered within the context of hypotension and hypertension, as well as separately.

Problem: Arterial Pressure Too Low

Low arterial pressure can be defined only arbitrarily, depending on the preoperative arterial pressure of each patient. In the PACU predetermined limits should be set with the anesthesiologist as to what constitutes important hypotension or hypertension. For a normotensive patient a systolic blood pressure 25% below the preoperative value (<100 mm Hg in normotensive patients, <130 mm Hg in hypertensive patients) would be considered a clinically important change requiring urgent attention. When systolic pressures fall to levels 40% below preoperative values, aggressive therapy is required. The nature of therapy depends on the cause of the hypotensive episode.

Causes: decreased cardiac output

Normal heart rate: stroke volume decreased

- Direct myocardial depression by anesthetics. This represents a continuation of depressant effects of inhalational or intravenous anesthetics on the myocardium. Poor myocardial contractility is evident as small pulse pressure and low dP/dt of arterial pressure trace.

To treat these patients (1) encourage deep breathing to wash out any remaining inhalational anesthetics; (2) stimulate myocardial activity by infusion of isoproterenol (0.02 µg/kg per minute) or dopamine (1 to 2 µg/kg per minute).

- Low output failure: cardiogenic shock. The most florid clinical sign of acute left ventricular failure is pulmonary (alveolar) edema, which is the third stage of a process that starts with pulmonary congestion and proceeds through interstitial edema. Early pulmonary congestion is recognized by a history of tachypnea, orthopnea, and paroxysmal nocturnal dyspnea. Interstitial edema may be recognized by the signs of basal crepitations and rales and by the appearance of Kerley B lines on the chest x-ray examination. Florid pulmonary edema may occur in the PACU when acute left ventricular failure is precipitated by sudden hypertension.

The management of low output failure is shown in Figure 4-4, in which the signs of pulmonary edema and congestion are linked to measurements of cardiac output and pulmonary artery wedge pressures.

For pulmonary congestion, the general principle is to give a diuretic and a vasodilator that exerts a venodilating effect, for example, a nitrate: (1) furosemide 40 to 80 mg intravenous; (2) nitroglycerin (NTG) 0.6 mg sublingual; or (3) isosorbide dinitrate 5 to 15 mg sublingual; (4) intravenous infusion of NTG 0.5 to 5 µg/kg per minute.

For low cardiac output syndrome—cardiogenic shock—give (1) combined therapy with infusions of inotropic and vasodilator drugs (dopamine 5 to 10 µg/kg per minute, with sodium nitroprusside 0.5

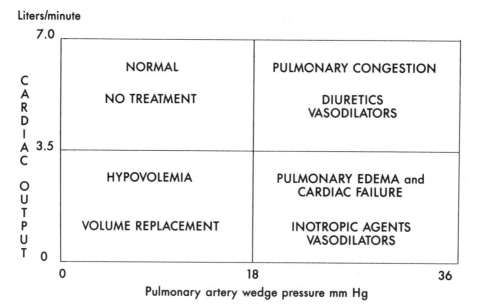

FIGURE 4-4

Management of low-output failure.

to 5.0 μg/kg per minute, (2) epinephrine infusion 2 to 10 μg/kg per minute, and (3) aortic balloon-pump counterpulsation.

New drugs available for inotropic management are the phosphodiesterase III inhibitors, such as amrinone.

- Myocardial ischemia. When arterial hypotension is caused by myocardial ischemia, it is usually secondary to some other cause of hypotension that has resulted in inadequate coronary perfusion caused by a low diastolic arterial pressure. Myocardial ischemia occurs in two forms: subendocardial ischemia, which is recognized by the appearance of deep ST segment depression (Figure 4-5, *A*) or transmural ischemia, characterized by ST segment elevation (Figure 4-5, *B*). The latter may occur after acute myocardial infarction or, more rarely, as a manifestation of coronary artery spasm (Prinzmetal's variant angina).

To treat myocardial ischemia, prevent further deterioration of coronary blood flow by maintaining diastolic pressure above the critical value for that patient (usually > 80 to 100 mm Hg). Dopamine infusion (1 to 3 μg/kg per minute) can be effective,

but take care to avoid a heart rate increase, which will also increase the myocardial oxygen requirements. Phenylephrine infusion can be used also, but avoid an excessive increase of systolic arterial pressure. At all times, ensure the patient is adequately oxygenated by increasing inspired O_2 concentration to at least 40%.

- Impaired cardiac filling. Hypovolemia without baroreflex response is the result of impaired cardiac filling. Recognition of minor degrees of hypovolemia is difficult, because many other factors combined with minor blood loss can cause marked hypotension. Tachycardia in association with arterial hypotension, especially when the pulse pressure is small, is traditionally described as the cardinal sign of blood loss. One must remember that when heart rate increases in response to a decreasing arterial pressure, the response is mediated through the carotid sinus baroreceptors. It has been established that anesthesia suppresses this barostatic response, but there is little evidence available to indicate how long such depression lasts after termination of anesthesia. Certainly for 30 to 60 minutes after the end of anesthesia, one

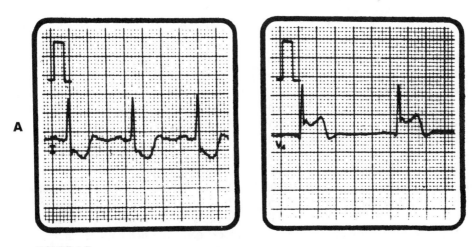

FIGURE 4-5
ST segment depression. **A,** Indicative of subendocardial ischemia and ST segment elevation. **B,** Indicative of transmural ischemia.

should anticipate that modest degrees of blood loss (< 10% of the predicted blood volume) would not provoke a significant tachycardia. Other signs of sympathetic nervous activity in response to hemorrhage, such as sweating and pallor, may also be diminished in the first hour after anesthesia. Central venous pressure will almost always be decreased when hemorrhage exceeds 5% of the blood volume. In this respect, accurate setting of the reference point (midaxillary line in the supine position) is most important. Obviously, if the reference point is set even 2 cm too high, it will give the impression that the CVP is 2 cm too low. If a CVP measurement is available, it is an easy task to test the hypothesis of hypovolemia by rapidly infusing about 200 ml of crystalloid solution, observing the response (it is hoped, a rapid increase) of both arterial pressure and CVP. Even in the absence of CVP measurements, an acceptable increase of arterial pressure (>10 mm Hg) in response to such a fluid load is ample evidence.

Treatment is as follows: (1) Raise legs or tip bed head down. (2) Give 250 to 500 ml lactated Ringer's solution, giving the first 250 ml rapidly and watching the response of both arterial pressure and CVP. (3) If there is a marked increase of arterial pressure in response to this amount of fluid, consider expanding the patient's blood volume with 250 to 500 ml whole blood or an alternative colloid solution, such as plasma protein factor (PPF), salt-poor albumin, dextran, or gelatin.

Cardiac tamponade. This is evident as hypotension with decreased pulse pressure, paradoxical effect of breathing on arterial pressure (decrease of arterial pulse during inspiration), and distention of neck veins. Causes are pericardial effusion or hemopericardium, for instance, knife wounds to the chest or upper abdomen. Initial pericardial drainage is performed by insertion of an 18-gauge needle in the midline behind the xiphisternum, toward the base of the heart.

Bradycardia

- Sinus bradycardia. This is usually a residual effect of neostigmine given at the end of anes-

thesia to reverse muscle relaxation and may be very marked in patients receiving β-receptor blockers. This is also a common finding after spinal anesthesia or thoracic epidrual blockage and is common in patients with body temperatures below 32°C. To treat, give atropine 0.6 mg or glycopyrrolate 0.2 mg, repeated at 5 minutes if heart rate is still below 50 per minute. Glycopyrrolate has a slower onset of action than atropine, but the duration of cholinergic blockade is about twice as long as atropine.

- Junctional bradycardia. No P waves are visible on ECG (Figure 4-6). This is usually caused by interaction of volatile anesthetics and their effect on cardiac conduction, with the effect of neostigmine. To treat, give (1) atropine 0.6 mg intravenously; (2) calcium chloride 5 ml of a 10 % solution, to aid and improve cardiac conduction; (3) isoproterenol infusion (0.02 μg/kg per minute) if the use of atropine and calcium chloride has been ineffective.

- Heart block (Figure 4-7). In first-degree heart block, the ECG P-R interval is greater than 0.12 seconds. In Möbitz Type I (Wenckebach) second-degree heart block, the ECG P-R interval lengthens with successive beats until one QRS complex is then dropped. In Möbitz Type II second-degree heart block, the P-R interval is constantly long, but occasional beats are dropped. There is also 2:1 or 3:1 block with an atrial rate 2 or 3 times that of the ventricular rate. In third-degree heart block, there is complete dissociation of P and QRS waves, usually with a slow heart rate.

To treat, give isoproterenol infusion (0.02 μg/kg per minute). Do not increase the infusion rate above 10 μg per minute in the absence of a reversal of heart block, because this may increase ventricular irritability and precipitate ventricular fibrillation. In all cases of severe refractory bradycardia or heart block, call a physician immediately, with a view to inserting a transvenous pacemaker catheter.

Tachycardia

- Sinus tachycardia. The commonest cause of sinus tachycardia is increased sympathetic ner-

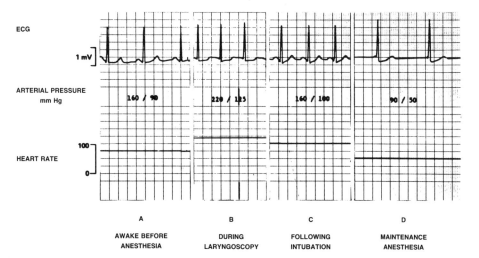

ECG

1 mV

ARTERIAL PRESSURE
mm Hg

160 / 90   220 / 125   160 / 100   90 / 50

HEART RATE

100

0

A
AWAKE BEFORE
ANESTHESIA

B
DURING
LARYNGOSCOPY

C
FOLLOWING
INTUBATION

D
MAINTENANCE
ANESTHESIA

FIGURE 4-6
Episodes of junctional tachycardia (B) and bradycardia (D) occurring during anesthesia.
Compare with the normal ECG awake (A), and note that ST segment has occurred on both
occasions.

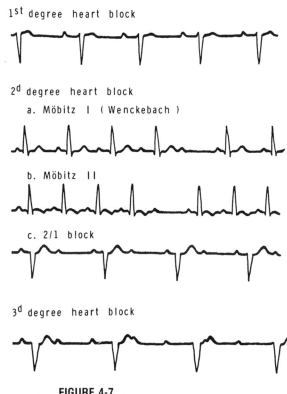

1st degree heart block

2d degree heart block
    a. Möbitz I (Wenckebach)

    b. Möbitz II

    c. 2/1 block

3d degree heart block

FIGURE 4-7
Heart block: different ECG patterns.

vous activity stimulated by pain, bladder distention, or apprehension. If heart rate is greater than 150 per minute, cardiac filling may be inadequate and may cause myocardial ischemia in susceptible patients. To treat, give propranolol 1 to 2 mg or metroprolol 2 to 5 mg intravenously if heart rate is greater than 120 per minute. Esmolol is a new β-adrenoceptor antagonist having a very short duration of action (5 to 10 minutes) and may have a place in PACU practice. It can be given as an infusion of 500 μg/kg per minute for 1 minute, followed by 300 μg/kg per minute.

- Junctional tachycardia. This is commonly caused by increased sympathetic nervous activity in patients with depressed cardiac conduction, caused by either the effects of anesthetics or digitalis toxicity. If the patient has not been receiving digitalis, give propranolol 1 to 2 mg intravenously or verapamil 5 mg intravenously to control the heart rate. When junctional tachycardia is a complication of digitalis overactivity, many authorities advise the use of DC countershock.

- Atrial fibrillation. When this is associated with a ventricular rate more than 120 per minute, cardiac output falls markedly because of poor filling. This may occur because of inadequate treatment with cardiac glycosides.

If the heart rate is greater than 120 per minute, propranolol (0.2 mg intravenously) may be given every minute until the rate can be decreased to about 100 to 110 per minute. DC countershock may also be used in these circumstances if a β-blocker is in any way contraindicated. Digoxin may be given to patients with rapid atrial fibrillation, but the peak effect is slow in onset and a satisfactory decrease of heart rate may take a few hours to achieve. Digoxin 0.25 to 0.5 mg may be given intravenously.

- Wolff-Parkinson-White Syndrome. Recurrent atrial tachycardia associated with this condition may cause impaired ventricular filling. Heart rate should be controlled with small intravenous doses of propranolol (0.5 to 1 mg) or verapamil (2 to 5 mg).

Causes: decreased systemic vascular resistance (SVR)

Normal heart rate: no baroreflex response to low blood pressure

- After spinal or epidural anesthesia. When there is evidence that somatic blockade is still effective, low arterial pressure is usually the result of arteriolar dilation coupled with expansion of the venous capacitance vessels. Treatment is as follows: (1) Raise patient's legs or tip bed head down. (2) Give 250 to 500 ml lactated Ringer's solution intravenously. (3) Give methoxamine 1 to 2 mg intravenously, repeated at 5-minute intervals if necessary. Do not give methoxamine to patients with heart rates less than 55 per minute. (4) Give ephedrine 5 to 10 mg intravenously followed by another 5 mg intramuscularly. Avoid giving ephedrine to patients with coronary artery disease, especially if they are not receiving β-adrenoceptor antagonists.

- Persistent effects of vasodilator drugs given during the course of anesthesia. Drugs such as trimetaphan, hydralazine, or sodium nitroprusside may produce delayed and protracted arteriolar dilation after the end of anesthesia. To treat, give methoxamine 1 to 2 mg intravenously, repeated at 5 minutes if necessary.

Tachycardia. Low arterial pressure associated with tachycardia may imply a normal baroreflex activity, in which case, treatment of the hypotension should follow the pattern described for hypovolemia.

- Septicemia (endotoxic shock). In patients who have undergone elective or emergency gall bladder or colonic surgery, the possibility of endotoxic shock should be considered when hypotension and tachycardia are present in a patient in the PACU. Characteristic features are arterial pressure wave with little or no diastolic run-off, a warm, dry skin (in the early stages), a high cardiac output, and low CVP.

Treatment is as follows: (1) Infuse colloid solutions (salt-poor albumin or fresh frozen plasma) to counteract the loss of protein from the extracellular blood. (2) Give methylprednisolone 1 mg/kg, dexamethasone 8 mg, or hydrocortisone hemisuccinate 500 to 800 mg. (3) Give antibiotic therapy effective against *Escherichia coli* and other gram-negative organisms: gentamycin 1 mg/kg and metronidazole 500 mg intravenously.

- Hemodilution. Inadequate red cell replacement despite an adequate volume replacement with crystalloid or colloid solutions can lead to excessive hemodilution, especially in patients who start with mild to moderate anemia. To treat, transfuse whole blood or red cell concentrates.

Problem: Arterial Pressure Too High

The definition of hypertension is arbitrary. For the purposes of patient care in the PACU we can define hypertension as systolic pressure greater than 180 mm Hg with diastolic pressure greater than 90 mm Hg in previously normotensive patients, and systolic pressure greater than 220 mm Hg with diastolic pressure greater than 110 mm Hg in previously hypertensive patients.

Causes: cardiac output increased

The common finding is of a patient with a high pulse pressure, resulting in systolic hypertension with normal or low diastolic pressure. These conditions are commonly found in patients with arteriosclerosis (rigid arterial disease) in whom a small change of the stroke volume ejected into the rigid arterial system results in large changes of pulse pressure. Pain or bladder distention are the most frequent causes of such systolic hypertension.

Normal heart rate: no baroreflex response to hypertension

- Arteriosclerotic patients. Treatment is as follows: (1) Give morphine sulfate 5 to 10 mg intravenously slowly to relieve pain. (2) Catheterize patient if the urinary bladder is distended and the patient cannot void. (3) Give labetalol 5 to 10 mg intravenously if systolic pressure is greater than 250 mm Hg.
- Hypertensive patients. Awakening after anes-

thesia and surgery may be associated with sudden and severe hypertension in patients with preexisting hypertension, both treated and untreated. Because of the adaptive hypertrophy in the arterioles of hypertensive patients, their arterial pressures show exaggerated responses to stimuli that generate vasoconstriction. These patients may develop systolic arterial pressures between 200 and 300 mm Hg and diastolic pressures between 130 and 160 mm Hg during the first 30 to 60 minutes after the end of anesthesia. Such pressures pose a serious threat to the well-being of the patient and can cause (1) cerebral hemorrhage, (2) acute left ventricular failure with pulmonary edema, (3) acute myocardial ischemia, and (4) disruption of recently grafted arteries.

Treatment is as follows: (1) Infuse sodium nitroprusside 0.5 to 5.0 μg/kg per minute to reduce arterial pressure to 160/100 mm Hg. (2) To maintain this pressure, give labetalol 5 to 10 mg intravenously, repeated at 10 minutes if heart rate is greater than 100 per minute or the rate-pressure product stays above 18,000. Hydralazine 5 to 10 mg intravenously, repeated at 20-minute intervals can be given as a treatment of moderate hypertension (diastolic pressure 100 to 110 mm Hg).

- Carotid endarterectomy patients. Carotid surgery is often performed in arteriosclerotic patients. Excessive hypertension in the postoperative period may be associated with transient or permanent neurological deficit, myocardial ischemia, or acute pulmonary edema. This requires aggressive therapy to bring systolic arterial pressure into a range (150 to 170 mm Hg) compatible with adequate cerebral perfusion but with diminished risk of a local hematoma, intracranial hemorrhage, cerebral edema, and other problems created by hypertension.

For treatment of hypertension, see above, but select labetalol or a combination of propranolol and hydralazine as the first lines of treatment rather than sodium nitroprusside. If sodium nitroprusside is used, beware of suddenly reducing the arterial pressure too much. Sodium nitroprusside increases intracranial pressure, and thus cerebral perfusion may become inadequate.

Tachycardia. Hypertension combined with tachycardia is a manifestation of increased sympathetic nervous activity, usually in response to noxious stimuli, of which pain is the most important to recognize. Distension of the urinary bladder is also a common cause in patients who have undergone genitourinary surgery. Misplacement of urinary catheters, so that the balloon is inflated in the prostatic bed or the urethra of the male, is also an uncommon but important cause of postoperative hypertension. Sympathetic storms are uncommon, but some unusual causes should be borne in mind: thyrotoxicosis, tetanus, and the Landry-Guillain-Barré syndrome.

The combination of hypertension and tachycardia increases the work of the heart dramatically. Rate-pressure product (RPP) was introduced to highlight this combination effect. RPP is the product of systolic arterial pressure (SAP and heart rate (HR). Normal values are in the range 7200 (SAP 120 × HR 60) to 12,000 (SAP 120 × HR 100, or SAP 150 × HR 80). Values in excess of 24,000 (SAP 240 × HR 100, or SAP 200 × HR 120) clearly represent a very high myocardial oxygen requirement to fulfill the required work. Such a demand can easily be met for the normal heart by increased coronary blood flow; for instance, exercise may increase the RPP to at least the same extent. For the patient with coronary artery disease, such a requirement may precipitate acute subendocardial ischemia, manifest as depressed ST segments in the ECG (see Figure 4-5, *A*) or, more rarely, elevated ST segments indicating transmural ischemia (Figure 4-5, *B*). Aggressive therapy to reduce both systolic arterial pressure and heart rate must begin as soon as possible to avoid the consequences of prolonged ischemia—acute myocardial infarction.

Treatment is as follows:

(1) Ensure adequate analgesia (see Chapter 2).
(2) Give propranolol 1 to 2 mg, or metoprolol 2 to 5 mg, intravenously, at 10-minute intervals until heart rate is less than 100 per minute, or administer esmolol infusion of 500 µg/kg per minute for 1 minute, followed by 300 µg/kg per minute until heart rate is less than 100 per minute.
(3) Give hydralazine 10 to 20 mg intravenously in patients with a known history of treated or untreated hypertension; hydralazine may cause tachycardia and require propranolol therapy.
(4) If the patient has a history of chronic clonidine therapy, adopt a more aggressive regimen for controlling arterial pressure using sodium nitroprusside.

Bradycardia. The combination of hypertension (blood pressure greater than 220/110 mm Hg) and bradycardia (HR less than 50 per minute) is unusual and requires less aggressive therapy provided the patient is in sinus rhythm. It implies active baroreflexes. The commonest cause is a hangover effect of neostigmine in a previously untreated or poorly treated hypertensive patient. Such a large pulse pressure indicates an adequate stroke volume, which, despite the bradycardia, should meet the patient's requirements.

- Elevated intracranial pressure (ICP). Hypertension at slow heart rates may represent the attempt of the vascular control system to maintain cerebral perfusion in the presence of elevated ICP. Management is considered in Chapter 9.
- Hypertensive patients. The commonest cause of systolic or diastolic hypertension with bradycardia is unrelieved pain.

Problem: Dysrhythmia without Hypotension or Hypertension

Many dysrhythmias occur during the patient's recovery from anesthesia that are not associated with hypotension or hypertension (as defined at the beginning of this chapter). Provided these occur at heart rates between 50 and 90 per minute, they are unlikely to require treatment. Examples are unifocal ventricular extrasystoles occurring less than five times per minute (especially in patients known to have such a dysrhythmia preoperatively) or atrial fibrillation that is clearly well controlled either with or without digitalis therapy.

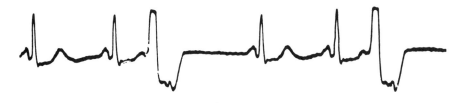

Lead I

FIGURE 4-8
Ventricular extrasystoles: R on T phenomenon.

However, there are some dysrhythmias that precede one of four life-threatening conditions: complete heart block with syncope, asystole (cardiac standstill), ventricular tachycardia, and ventricular fibrillation.

Ventricular extrasystoles.   If these occur with every other beat, the cardiac rhythm is said to be coupled (synonymous with *bigeminy*). Coupled ventricular extrasystoles are not dangerous in themselves and occur commonly in association with hypercapnia (Figure 4-2 is a good example of a coupled rhythm). Check arterial blood gases, and if $PaCO_2$ is higher than 55 mm Hg, take steps to improve the patient's ventilation or to establish artificial ventilation. If there is no apparent cause, adopt the decision process outlined below.

Multifocal ventricular extrasystoles.   When there is more than one aberrant pacemaker, there is a danger of precipitating either ventricular tachycardia or fibrillation. Another serious precursor of these conditions is the existence of an R on T phenomenon (Figure 4-8) when the R wave occurs during the T wave (a time when part but not all of the ventricular muscle is no longer refractory).

To treat, give lidocaine 1 mg/kg intravenously followed by an infusion at 2 to 4 mg per minute, or a repeat dose in 15 to 20 minutes. Ventricular tachycardia should be managed in exactly the same way as multifocal ventricular extrasystoles. Ventricular asystole or fibrillation constitutes cardiac arrest, and the general process of cardiopulmonary resuscitation (CPR) should be set in motion (see Chapter 14).

SUGGESTIONS FOR FURTHER READING

Davis RF: Acute postoperative hypertension, Amer Soc Anes Refresher Course Lecture no 245, San Francisco, 1988.

Frost EAM and Andrews IC, editors: Recovery room care. Int Anesthesiol Clin 21(1):59, 1983.

Kaplan JA, editor: Cardiac anesthesia, vol 2, Cardiovascular pharmacology. New York, 1983, Grune & Stratton, Inc.

Mason DT, editor: Cardiac emergencies. Baltimore, 1978, Williams & Wilkins.

Prys-Roberts C, editor: The circulation in anaesthesia. Oxford, 1980, Blackwell Scientific Publications, Inc.

Prys-Roberts C, editor: Hypertension, ischemic heart disease and anesthesia. Int Anesthesiol Clin 18(4):1, 137, 1980.

Prys-Roberts C, editor: Vascular disease and anaesthesia (Postgraduate Educational Symposium). Br J Anaesth 53(7):673, 1981.

Saidman LJ and Smith NT, editors: Monitoring in anesthesia, ed 2, Woburn, 1983, Butterworth, Publishers.

Thys DM and Kaplan JA: The ECG in anesthesia and critical care, pp. 1, 77, 155, New York, 1987, Churchill Livingstone, Inc.

CHAPTER 5

Postanesthetic Fluid Management

Olli Kirvelä
Vladimir Kvetan
Jeffrey Askanazi

The evolution of fluid therapy for surgical patients to a large degree reflects changing attitudes toward the handling of sodium in injury. Attention has shifted from plasma and renal handling of salt and water to the extracellular space and the overall behavior of sodium. This change in attitude has resulted in marked changes in fluid therapy for acute surgical patients. Isotonic saline, which once was contraindicated in the immediate postoperative period, is now regarded as essential. However, it is clear that excesses can result in complications.

Essential to proper fluid therapy is an understanding of body composition and of the changes that occur in injury. The abnormal body composition of the injured patient after resuscitation is the result of the therapy superimposed on the body's response to the injury. The daily fluid and electrolyte therapy for such a patient is the sum of normal requirements and the additional needs of the specific stage of convalescence after injury.

NORMAL BODY COMPOSITION

The adult body is composed of three functional components: fat, cell mass, and extracellular structures. The amount of each varies as a function of age, sex, and body size.

Total body water (TBW) is the largest single component of body weight, being greatest in the young, muscular man (more than 60%) and least in the elderly, obese woman (less then 45%). In general, total body water is considered to be distributed into two major fluid spaces: intracellular fluid (ICF), which makes up 25% to 30% of average body weight, and extracellular fluid (ECF), which makes up 20% to 25% of normal body weight.

The body content of electrolytes is discussed in terms of their exchangable components as measured with an isotope dilution technique. Body stores of potassium can be measured by whole body counting of the naturally occurring isotope. Neutron activation has recently been used to measure many tissue components. Minerals that are incorporated into bone, collagen, and connective tissue exchange very slowly with plasma and generally are not considered in determining the composition of parenteral fluid therapy needed to achieve daily balance.

The total exchangeable potassium can be considered as equivalent to the body stores of potassium for clinical purposes. A healthy man (70 kg) has a pool of exchangeable potassium of 2700 to 3400 mmol; a woman, 2100 to 2300 mmol. The major fraction of this pool is intracellular, the small extracellular portion approximating 1% to 2% of the total.

In contrast to potassium, exchangeable sodium is only 65% of total body sodium. Men (70 kg) contain approximately 2800 mmol; women, approximately 2600 mmol. The fraction of sodium in the skeleton is only slowly exchangeable. In a normal 70 kg man there is approximately 2100 mmol of chloride.

NORMAL DAILY BALANCE
Water

The daily amount of water and dilute liquids required by the normal individual varies widely with habit and climate, but in temperate climates the average adult exchanges 2500 to 4500 ml of water daily with a body pool of 25 to 45 L. Fluid intake averages 1000 to 2500 ml per day. Water in foods averages 1000 to 1500 ml. Water of oxidation adds 200 to 400 ml per day.

Losses occur by three routes: evaporation from the respiratory tract and skin, urinary output, and the water content of stool. The first two are termed *insensible losses*. In the normal individual, water intake and losses balance each other very closely. Daily body weight usually fluctuates by less than 2%, and often by less than 1% if measured at the same time of the day. Insensible losses depend on body size, physical exertion, environmental temperature, and humidity. Surface evaporation and sweat together average 600 to 800 ml per day. Total insensible water loss is between 300 and 500 ml per meter of body surface area per day, with minimal activity in a temperate environment. Sweat volume is small in a temperate climate except with vigorous activity but may reach several liters a day, with serious losses of both water and sodium chloride, in warm, humid environments with exposure to the sun. Markedly obese patients have an increased water loss, largely because of sweat. Such patients show marked changes in daily weight consistent with unusually large fluctuations in ECF.

Electrolytes

The daily sodium intake of the normal individual varies between 50 and 100 mmol. Maintenance of normal body composition is primarily the result of renal excretion of any excess intake. When there is a low intake or extrarenal losses, the kidney can reduce sodium excretion to as low as 1 mmol per day. As renal function is lost in disease, the capability to extremely reduce sodium excretion may be lost, and certain renal disorders have a wasting of sodium considerably in excess of the daily intake.

The daily intake of potassium varies from 40 to 80 mmol per day. However, potassium metabolism is strongly influenced by acid-base balance, and the normal kidney does not respond to a reduction in intake by prompt conservation of potassium in the way that it does for sodium.

SERUM ELECTROLYTE CONCENTRATIONS

Several studies have reviewed the electrolyte composition of body fluids. A definite relationship exists between the serum concentration of sodium and potassium and the total exchangeable sodium and potassium. There is poor correlation between serum sodium and total body sodium.

$$\text{Serum sodium} = \frac{(\text{Total exchangeable Na}^+) + (\text{Total exchangeable K}^+)}{(\text{Total body water})} - 26$$

Thus serum sodium can be increased by additional potassium or sodium or restriction of free water. Retention of water in excess of sodium can lead to hyponatremia even with an excess of total body sodium. Administration of potassium can raise the serum sodium concentration in hyponatremia patients.

Most potassium is contained in the ICF, leaving only a small fraction of body potassium in plasma. Thus the absolute reduction of serum potassium that occurs with depletion can be expected to reflect a very large total body potassium deficit. However, a change in acid-base status may alter the serum potassium levels quite markedly as H^+ is exchanged for K^+. Thus alkalosis may lower serum

K^+ markedly, particularly if there is a preexisting total body deficit.

To maintain electroneutrality:

$Serum(Na^+) + (Ca^{++}) + (Mg^{++}) + (K^+) = (Cl^-) + (HCO_3^-)$
$+ (Protein) + (Sulphate) + (Phosphate) + (Organic acids)$

Thus:

$$(Na^+) + (K^+) = (HCO_3^-) + (Cl^-) + 14$$

The factor of *14* is commonly termed the *anion gap*. If (sodium + potassium) − (bicarbonate + chloride) exceeds 18, the substantial addition of an anion must be suspected.

These are (1) $HPO_4^=$ and $SO_4^=$, as in renal failure; (2) lactic acid, as in hypoxia, shock states, and salicylate intoxication; and (3) keto acids, as in diabetic ketoacidosis. If the anion gap is less than 5, hypoproteinemia is the most likely cause.

GASTROINTESTINAL TRACT LOSSES

The normal daily volume of secretion into the gastrointestinal tract is not exactly known but is estimated to be 8000 to 10,000 ml per day, of which saliva constitutes 1 to 2 L; gastric juice (including body acid and mucoid secretions), about 500 to 750 ml; and pancreatic juice, approximately 100 ml. In addition, secretion of the upper small bowel mucosa contributes between 2000 to 3000 ml. However, all but 100 to 200 ml of the secretions are normally reabsorbed by the small bowel and the colon.

Abnormal losses from the gastrointestinal tract include water and electrolytes and varying amounts of protein. The electrolyte content of fluid from the gastrointestinal tract varies significantly with the level from which most of the fluid is derived. Table 5-1 shows the average value and the range of variation of sodium, potassium, chloride, and bicarbonate in fluids from different levels of the intestine. It is important to note that, of all the secretions, only bile and pancreatic juice are approximately isotonic in their electrolyte content. The average calculated osmolality of saliva is about 160 mOsm; of upper small bowel content, 220 mOsm; and of fluid from the distal ileum, about 240 mOsm. Other substances, including mucoproteins, other polysaccha-

TABLE 5-1

Electrolyte content of gastrointestinal secretions (mmol/L)

Source of fluid	Na⁺	K⁺	Cl⁻	HCO₃⁻
Saliva	60	20	16	50
Gastric	30-90	4-12	50-155	0
Upper small bowel	70-120	3-7	70-120	10
Ileum	90-140	3-8	80-125	15-20
Bile	145	4-7	80-110	50
Pancreas	120-140	5-8	60-80	70

From Randall HT: Fluid, electrolyte, and acid-base balance, Surg Clin North Am 56:1019, 1976.

rides, urea, calcium, and phosphate, add to these approximations of the total osmolality.

The values shown in Table 5-1 may be used for semiquantitative replacement of gastrointestinal tract losses. When volumes of these losses exceed 2000 ml in 24 hours or when substantial losses (1 l or more per day) continue for more than a few days, it is wise to send an aliquot of the 24-hour drainage to the laboratory for measurement of electrolytes and protein and to determine the pH of a fresh specimen. More precise replacement can be made with this information. It is important to note that replacement of abnormal losses should be provided in addition to baseline requirements.

The data listed in Table 5-2 are intended only as approximate guidelines in fluid replacement. Fluid therapy should be individualized for a given patient. In general, urinary output serves as a useful guide to fluid therapy and should be maintained at levels of 600 ml per day or more. If output decreases below 600 ml per day in association with a decreasing central venous pressure or a decrease in body weight, an increase in fluid requirements is indicated. A decrease in urinary output, associated with a rising central venous pressure and weight gain, may indicate the onset of interstitial pulmonary edema, and diuretic therapy should be instituted.

The common use of the term *dehydration* can lead to confusion, since there are two different clin-

TABLE 5-2

Baseline fluid requirements

	Age (years)	Fluid (ml/kg per day)
Average adults	25-55	35
Young active adults	16-30	40
Older patients	55-65	30
Elderly	>65	25

Modified from Randall HT: Fluid, electrolyte, and acid base balance, Surg Clin North Am 56:1019, 1976.
Adult values are based on ideal weight for height and age.

ical syndromes that may be referred to as dehydration. One syndrome is caused by the loss of sodium and chloride with contraction of the extracellular volume, resulting in decreased skin turgor, a rapid pulse, and a lowered blood pressure. Laboratory findings are related to increased hemoglobin and hematocrit with lower sodium and chloride values in the plasma, although urine volume and concentration are not remarkable. Another syndrome is associated with the primary loss of water without loss of electrolytes. Skin turgor, together with circulatory signs and symptoms, is usually normal even though thirst becomes intense. Oliguria with maximal urine concentration is associated with elevated plasma sodium and chloride. When referring to dehydration, sufficient description should be provided to clarify which of these two syndromes is under discussion.

FLUID AND ELECTROLYTE CHANGES IN INJURY

Normal individuals usually tolerate large amounts of intravenously administered sodium chloride. In the immediate postoperative period, these same individuals will tend to retain some of the administered fluid and may even develop respiratory symptoms from relatively modest excesses of sodium chloride. This observation of postoperative salt intolerance was recognized as early as 1911. As complications caused by salt loss were increasingly observed, an era of postoperative saline administration ensued. The studies that emphasized the dangers of salt deprivation led to a period when many surgeons administered saline whether losses had occurred or not, and the manifestations of fluid overload sometimes became evident. Reports soon followed cautioning against excessive salt administration. In 1944 Coller retracted his previously published formula for fluid administration and stated that no salt solution should be given for the first 2 postoperative days.

Wiggers noted that animals that did not survive hemorrhagic shock demonstrated hemoconcentration even though the shed blood was returned. Gilman demonstrated that animals that were deficient in ECF were sensitive to relatively small degrees of hemorrhage. Reynolds demonstrated that dogs in hemorrhagic shock treated with saline alone could survive with a return of cardiac output.

A series of studies by Shires et al. emphasized the disparate reduction of functional ECF volume induced by hemorrhagic shock. This deficit is not alleviated by return of the shed blood alone or by moderate overexpansion of the intravascular volume with plasma. Rather, the reduction in ECF could be alleviated by use of a balanced salt solution as an adjunct to shed blood replacement. It must be emphasized that these measurements of a reduced function ECF were made either during or soon after the injury or shock.

The changes in the ECF after injury or shock vary with time. During shock there is a reduction in the ECF, whereas after resuscitation the ECF is expanded.

Pluth et al. and Moore et al. demonstrated an expansion of the extracellular space after injury and resuscitation that did not appear to be the result of excessive fluid administration. Roth et al. also reported an increase in ECF after injury and suggested moderation in the use of lactated Ringer's solution for resuscitation. Elwyn and Shoemaker reported an expansion of the extracellular space in postoperative patients that was similar to that seen in nutritional depletion. The changes seen in nutritional depletion resolved with adequate nutrition.

The weight gain caused by fluid administration as immediate treatement for operation or injury is variable and a function of the severity of the injury, as well as the preexisting clinical state of the patient. Elective operations, such as total hip replacement or colon resection, are commonly associated with a 3% to 5% weight gain, whereas major trauma may be associated with a 10% to 15% gain in body weight after fluid resuscitation. In our view, such acute weight gains are difficult to avoid. Fluid administration should be guided by parameters such as blood pressure, central venous pressure, and urinary output. It is important to note that from the third to the sixth day after injury, a diuresis will ordinarily develop. Failure to return to initial weight by the tenth day after operation or injury should be regarded as a warning of an impending complication (such as congestive heart failure, sepsis, or renal failure).

It has been suggested by Flear et al. that the post-injury changes in ECF and ICF probably are reflective of a change in permeability of cell membranes and a disturbance in ionic exchange. Thus injury is thought to lead to an increased escape of nondiffusible solutes into the ECF. This causes a decrease in the osmolality of cell fluids and at the same time increases the osmolality and resultant volume of the ECF.

Skeletal muscle represents the major component of lean body tissue and can be safely sampled by needle biopsy. Studies performed by Bergstrom et al. and Askanazi et al. using the needle biopsy technique have evaluated the role of nutrition and activity level in muscle fluid sequestration. Patients undergoing total hip replacement were assigned to receive a daily intravenous infusion of either 5% dextrose solution or 5.5% amino acid solution (with appropriate electrolytes and vitamins) for the first 4 postoperative days. Muscle biopsies were performed in the nonoperated thigh preoperatively and on the fourth day postoperatively. These studies demonstrated that an increase in muscle sodium and chloride occurs in noninjured portions of the body. These changes are not affected by the form of nutritional support administered. There was an increase in muscle ECF in these patients, which was unaffected by the nutritional support system administered. In normal subjects on bedrest, receiving either a regular diet or a 5% dextrose solution, there

were no comparable changes in muscle composition.

With increasing severity of injury and injury complicated by sepsis, there is a progressive increase in muscle ECF, sodium, and chloride, while the intracellular space is decreased. Muscle potassium and magnesium tend to decrease with increasing degrees of injury.

These studies suggest that there is an obligatory expansion of the ECF after injury. This is associated with characteristic changes in muscle membrane potential. This expansion requires fluid and sodium administration above maintenance levels and results in an increase in body weight. The physiological effect of this weight gain is variable and depends on the underlying clinical state of the patient. In a young, healthy individual, a 10% to 12% weight gain (7 L positive fluid balance) may be well tolerated, whereas a much smaller weight gain may be poorly tolerated by the elderly patient who has decreased cardiopulmonary system reserve.

Hypertensive patients receiving chronic diuretic therapy are somewhat vasoconstricted and often salt depleted. These patients often are dehydrated and require additional fluid. Fluid restriction can result in severe dehydration and possible irreversible renal failure and is contraindicated. These patients may be hypokalemic and should be given potassium with their intravenous fluids.

Urological Concerns

The transurethral resection of the prostate (TURP) is known to have a risk of causing the "TURP" syndrome. This is a vascular overload caused by the rapid absorption of irrigating fluid and associated with the length of operative time. Hypotension, bradycardia, an elevated central venous pressure, and seizures may accompany the hyponatremia. The first set of postoperative electrolytes obtained in the PACU may provide a clue to the diagnosis. If absorption is suspected, ethanol in low concentrations can be put into the irrigation solution and diagnosis can be made simply by using a breath analyzer. Treatment varies with the severity of the hyponatremia and water intoxication. If hyponatremia with an associated volume deficit is present, isotonic sodium chloride or lactated Ringer's solution may be used. When the hyponatremia is severe (Na^+ 90 mEq in the hypoosmotic patient), hypertonic saline (3%) can be used to correct the serum sodium.

Type of Anesthetic

There is an association between the type of anesthetic given and the amount of fluid and blood given. With regional anesthesia, the area anesthetized and agent used generally will guide fluid requirement. For example, an epidural block for orthopedic surgery necessitates administration of large amounts of fluid. With resolution of the anesthetic, the affected area may vasoconstrict and lead to fluid overload. Therefore in certain patient groups, the use of vasoconstricting agents (for example, phenylephrine hydrochloride) should be considered instead of large volumes of fluid to control blood pressure to avoid post anesthesia problems.

Burns

Care of the burn patient is complex. Some general guidelines are noted below. The rule of nines is a relatively easy way to calculate the percentage of the burn. Basically the surface area of each upper extremity is 9% of body surface area. The rest of the body is broken down as follows: head, 9%; lower extremity front, 9%; lower extremity back, 9%; front and back torso, 18% each. There are several formulas for fluid replacement in burn patients, and they are generally calculated from the percentage of the burn. The Parkland formula is as follows (per 24 hours):

$$\text{Colloid amount} = \frac{\% \text{ burn} \times \text{weight in kg} \times 0.5 \text{ ml}}{24 \text{ hours}}$$

$$\text{Lactated Ringer's solution} = \frac{\% \text{ burn} \times \text{weight in kg} \times 1.5 \text{ ml}}{24 \text{ hours}}$$

$$D_5W \text{ (detrose 5\% in water)} = \frac{2000 \text{ ml}}{24 \text{ hours}}$$

USE OF COLLOID IN FLUID RESUSCITATION

The use of albumin, dextran, or hydroxyethylstarch solution in resuscitation of injured patients is a controversial issue. The proponents of the use of colloid as part of fluid therapy argue that resuscitation with crystalloid alone dilutes plasma proteins, thereby reducing plasma oncotic pressure. Reduced oncotic pressure favors fluid movement from the intravascular to the interstitial compartment and thereby predisposes the patient to the development of interstitial pulmonary edema. In contrast to these findings, Lowe et al., Moss et al., and Virgilio et al. found no advantage to the administration of colloid solutions. Lucas et al. demonstrated that patients receiving large quantities of albumin had a greater dependency on ventilator support, which compromised renal function.

Our own policy is to use a balanced salt solution together with whole blood for resuscitation of postoperative and injured patients. Albumin infusions are generally confined to patients whose serum albumin is below 2.5 g/dl and who are also receiving nutritional repletion. In the absence of infection, the capillary bed is considered to be intact; therefore a rise in serum albumin level may be expected with albumin infusion.

FLUID AND ELECTROLYTE REQUIREMENTS IN CONVALESCENCE

The purpose of administering parenteral fluids and electrolytes is to prevent deficiencies that otherwise result from the inability of the patient's gastrointestinal tract and kidneys to fulfill their normal function. Also, in acute trauma or when there has been a substantial loss of water, electrolytes, or both from the body without adequate replacement, parenteral fluid therapy is required to restore a normal distribution of body fluids.

The requirements for parenteral therapy can be considered in three categories:

1. **Normal requirements.** What does the patient require in water, electrolytes, basic calories, and micronutrients to minimize the effects of dehydration and of starvation caused by cessation or reduction of oral intake? The calculation of baseline requirements disregards any

preexisting losses, but baseline volumes may require modification in patients with ECF expansion associated with delusional hyponatremia.

2. **Preexisting deficits or excesses.** What deficits (or excesses) does the patient have in water, electrolytes, blood volume, plasma proteins, and micronutrients? What should be done to correct these abnormalities?

3. **Abnormal losses.** What does the patient require to replace ongoing abnormal fluid and electrolyte losses resulting from the disease or its treatment? This includes ECF sequestration.

A part of the fluid and electrolyte requirement will be obtained through metabolism of body tissue in a semistarving state. Endogenous water is derived from the shrinkage or breakdown of protoplasm, which is roughly 75% water, as well as the water of oxidation that results from fuel oxidation. Other endogenous water derived from muscle breakdown approximates 800 to 850 ml/kg of body cell mass lost. This water is almost completely sodium-free but is rich in potassium, magnesium, phosphate, and sulphate.

Oxidation of fat provides approximately 1 ml of water per gram of fat oxidized. Moore estimated that about 100 ml of water is available for each 100 kcal derived from the burning of body tissues, part of which is fat and part body cells. The daily caloric requirement of the surgical patient depends in part on sex and age but much more on the extent and type of trauma, the presence of infection, the degree of immobilization, and the amount of energy required to maintain body temperature in the presence of abnormal evaporative water losses, either from hyperventilation or from evaporative cooling that occurs as the result of extensive thermal injury.

The daily caloric requirement of the afebrile patient of average size, at bed rest, will vary from 1300 to 1900 kcal, 400 to 500 kcal of which is often provided by the administration of isotonic glucose into a peripheral vein. The baseline production of endogenous water or oxidation in this situation will be 150 to 200 ml, or about 10% of the total daily requirement. However, fever, trauma, and infection will increase endogenous water production, along with the increased oxidation of tissue fuel. The use of glycerol instead of dextrose as an energy substrate after surgery may help to control blood glucose levels in diabetic patients. It can be infused into peripheral lines in low concentrations, and its protein-sparing effect in hypocaloric amounts equals that of glucose.

CLINICAL EVALUATION OF THE PATIENT

External abnormal loss may be in the form of excessive loss of water and electrolytes by normal routes of excretion or secretion, or losses that may occur from intraluminal tubes, drains, fistulas, or wounds. The most common source of abnormal external loss in surgical patients is the gastrointestinal tract; next in frequency are losses from surgical wounds, increased evaporation from the skin and respiratory tract, and losses from direct injury to the skin. Sequestration of ECF into areas of traumatized or infected tissue produces a decrease in the usual distribution of ECF without external loss or change in body weight.

Body Weight

Daily changes in body weight present the most practical index of the changing state of hydration. The daily weight of a patient on conventional fluid therapy by peripheral vein should reveal a loss of approximately .2% to .4% of body weight per day until adequate oral nutrition is instituted. Exceptions occur with blood transfusions or deliberate changes in hydration, as well as during the first 48 hours after trauma or operation when local sequestration of fluid occurs and parenteral fluid is given to compensate for it. The patient who gains weight in other circumstances while on routine fluid therapy is usually being overhydrated or may have developed some complication, most often sepsis. The patient who loses weight at a faster rate, except during a temporary posttraumatic diuresis, is in need of more aggressive fluid therapy. Frequent measurements of body weight are probably the single most important method of recognizing changes in water balance.

Factors That Modify Fluid Requirements

Factors that increase baseline requirements for fluid intake are essentially those that increase the insensible water loss. Fever increases the water requirements to a variable degree. Hyperventilation results in increased water loss by evaporation and cutaneous losses. A patient with a temperature of 103° F (39.4° C) will require an average of an additional 500 ml of water per day. The endogenous water production associated with the hypermetabolism of fever is also increased, but not enough to offset the increased losses.

Sweating will increase the average adult water requirements by 500 ml per day for each degree Fahrenheit of ambient temperature above 85° F (29.5° C), depending on the humidity. Sweat is about one-half normal sodium chloride, so that additional salt must be provided in the therapy. The potassium content of sweat is negligible. When the environmental temperature rises above 90° F (32° C), the seriously ill, febrile patient should be cooled, preferably by air conditioning, because the insensible loss of water from evaporative cooling becomes very large.

Increased Metabolism

Hyperthyroidism substantially increases the turnover of water in parallel with increases in caloric requirements. Hyperthyroid patients in the semi-starving state tend to consume massive amounts of lean tissue and fat, producing unusual amounts of endogenous water, and simultaneously losing water by respiratory evaporation, skin sublimation, and sweating.

Use of Blood and Blood Products

Indications for the use of the various available blood products are listed in Appendix 4.

SUGGESTIONS FOR FURTHER READING

Askanazi J et at: Effect of immediate postoperative nutritional support on length of hospitalization, Ann Surg 203:236, 1986.

Bergstrom J et al: Influence of injury and nutrition on muscle water and electrolytes: effects of elective operation, Ann Surg 193:134, 1981.

Bomberger RA, McGregor B, and DePalma RG: Optimal fluid management after aortic reconstruction: a prospective study of two crystalloid solutions, J Vasc Surg 4:164, 1986.

Coller FA, Campbell KNV, and Vaughan HH: Postoperative salt intolerance, Ann Surg 119:533, 1944.

Demling RH: Fluid replacement in burned patients, Surg Clin North Am 67:15, 1987.

Flear CTG, Bhattacharya SS, and Singh CM: Solute and water exchanges between cells and extracellular fluids in health and disturbances after trauma, JPEN 4:98, 1980.

Gilman A: Experimental sodium loss analogous to adrenal insufficiency: the resulting water shift and sensitivity to hemorrhage, Am J Physiol 108:662, 1934.

Graves TA et al: Fluid resuscitation of infants and children with massive thermal injury, J Trauma 28:1656, 1988.

Gump FE: Fluid and electrolyte management. In Kinney JM, Bendixen HH, and Powers SR, editors: Manual of surgical intensive care, Philadelphia, 1977, WB Saunders Co.

Hagerdal M and Lundberg D, editors: Intravenous fluid therapy, Acta Anaesthesiol Scand Suppl 82 v:29, 1985.

Kaperonis AA et al: Effects of total hip replacement and bed rest on blood rheology and red cell metabolism, J Trauma 28:453, 1988.

Karanko MS, Klossner JA, and Laaksonen VO: Restoration of volume by crystolloid versus colloid after coronary artery bypass: hemodynamics, lung water, oxygenation, and outcome. Crit Care Med 15:559, 1987.

Kruskall MS et al: Transfusion therapy in emergency medicine, Ann Emerg Med 17:327, 1988.

Lev-Ran A et al: Double-blind study of glycerol vs glucose in parenteral nutrition of postsurgical insulin-treated diabetic patients, JPEN 11:271, 1987.

Lowe RJ et al: Crystalloid vs colloid in the etiology of pulmonary failure after trauma: a randomized trial in man, Surgery 81:676, 1977.

Moore FD: Common patterns of water and electrolyte change in injury, surgery, and disease, N Engl J Med 258:277, 377, 427, 1958.

Moore FD et al: Body cell mass and its supporting environment: body composition in health and disease, Philadelphia, 1963, WB Saunders Co.

Moss GS et al: Effects of saline and colloid solutions on pulmonary function in hemorrhagic shock, Surg Gynecol Obstet 133:53, 1971.

Pluth JR et al: Effect of surgery on the volume of distribution of extracellular fluid determined by the sulfate and bromide methods. In Berguer PE and Lushbough EE, editors: Medical Physiology, Springfield, IL: USAEC, 1967, pp. 217-239.

Randall HT: Fluid, electrolyte, and acid-base balance, Surg Clin North Am 56:1019, 1976.

Reynolds M: Cardiovascular effects of large volumes of isotonic saline infused intravenously in dogs following severe hemorrhage, Am J Physiol 158:418, 1949.

Roth E, Lax LC, and Maloney JV Jr: Changes in extracellular fluid volume during shock and surgical trauma in animals and man, Surg Forum 18:43, 1967.

Shackford SR et al: Serum osmolar and electrolyte changes associated with large infusions of hypertonic sodium lactate for intravascular volume expansion of patients undergoing aortic reconstruction, Surg Gynecol Obstet 164:127, 1987.

Shackford SR et al: The effect of hemorrhage and resuscitation on serum levels of immunoreactive atrial natriuretic factor, Ann Surg 207:195, 1988.

Shires T, Williams J, and Brown F: Simultaneous measurement of plasma volume, extracellular fluid volume, and red blood cell mass in man using ^{131}I, $^{35}SO_4$ and ^{51}Cr, J Lab Clin Med 55:776, 1960.

Shires T et al: Fluid therapy in hemorrhagic shock, Arch Surg 88:688, 1964.

Shires T, Carrico CJ, and Cohn D: Role of the extracellular fluid in shock, Int Anesthesiol Clin 2:435, 1964.

Shires T: The role of sodium-containing solutions in the treatment of oligemic shock, Surg Clin North Am 45:365, 1969.

Shires GT: Fluid and electrolyte therapy. In Inney JM, Egdahl RH, and Zuidema GD, editors: Manual of preoperative and postoperative care, ed 2, Philadelphia, 1971, WB Saunders Co.

Virgilio RW Smith DE and Zarins CK: Balanced electrolyte solutions: experimental and clinical studies, Crit Care Med 7:98, 1979.

Wiggars MD and Ingraham RC: Hemorrhagic shock: definition of criteria for its diagnosis, J Clin Invest 25:30, 1946.

CHAPTER 6

Why Is the Patient Not Awake Yet?

Elizabeth A.M. Frost

After general anesthesia, most patients are admitted to the PACU at least drowsy if not unconscious. By far the majority regain consciousness within a few minutes to an hour. However, a small percentage remain somnolent for longer periods. An understanding of the possible underlying causes of such unresponsiveness is essential to the correct management and successful outcome of the postoperative period. The commonest reasons why the patient is not awake shortly after the end of surgery are as follows:

Prolonged anesthetic action or overdose
Drug interaction
Respiratory insufficiency
Cardiovascular instability
Thermoregulatory dysfunction
Fluid and electrolyte imbalance
Allergic or atypical drug reaction
Intraoperative catastrophe
Preoperative state

PROLONGED ANESTHETIC EFFECT

If patients are admitted comatose to the PACU, the most usual reason is anesthetic effect. Table 6-1 outlines the stages of anesthetic management where

drug administration may give rise to difficulties postoperatively.

It is important to review premedication orders because many tranquilizer drugs, such as diazepam, have half-lives of 12 hours or more, which means that their effect often extends well into the postoperative period. Midazolam, once thought to have a much shorter half-life, has marked individual variation and, especially in older patients, may exert long-lasting effects.

The commonly used inhalation agents—enflurane, isoflurane, and halothane—are usually associated with rapid awakening when they are discontinued (that is, within 15 minutes). Studies have indicated that recovery should not be delayed even in markedly obese patients if anesthetic time was less than 3 hours. However, the anesthetic effect may persist because administration lasted more than 3 hours or because of interactions with other drugs. Delayed awakening is most marked after the very fat-soluble agents methoxyflurane and ether, both seldom used today.

Intravenous techniques involve the administration of several drugs (barbiturates, narcotics, tranquilizers, muscle relaxants). Several factors can combine to prolong the action of these agents. Sodi-

TABLE 6-1		
Unresponsiveness because of prolonged effects or overdose of anesthetic drugs		
Anesthetic drugs	**Diagnosis**	**Treatment**
Premedication	Order sheet in chart	Supportive (assist ventilation, maintain cardiovascular stability, maintain normothermia)
Inhalation agents	Anesthetic record	Supportive
Barbiturates	Anesthetic record	Supportive
Narcotics	Anesthetic record	Naloxone (Narcan)
Muscle relaxants	Peripheral nerve stimulator	Correct acid-base imbalance; give neostigmine and atropine

um thiopental has a very short duration of action when it is used only as a single bolus for induction. However, it is extremely fat soluble and, if it is used as a continuous infusion over several hours or during emergence, return to consciousness may be considerably delayed as the drug is slowly released from the tissues. Moreover, it is reabsorbed by the renal tubules and recirculated in the body.

After administration, barbiturates bind to protein. Only free barbiturate is effective. Thus in patients with decreased protein levels (for example, liver disease), more drug is available to exert a hypnotic effect. Other factors that increase the hypnotic effect of barbiturates are as follows:

Cardiac output
Blood volume
Fat solubility
Renal excretion
Microsomal enzyme induction

Also, if other drugs are present to competitively bind the protein sites, a greater effect is seen with average barbiturate doses (for example, x-ray contrast material). Biotransformation of barbiturates by microsomal enzyme systems reduces the effect of these drugs. This is seen in patients who are addicted to barbiturates and in chronic alcoholics. The result is that these patients require a higher dose for the same effect. The opposite effect, that is, a decrease in microsomal enzyme activity and delayed awakening, is seen after acute alcoholic intoxication.

Small doses of narcotics, such as fentanyl (3 to 15 μg/kg), usually do not contribute to postoperative somnolence, especially if they have been administered over 3 to 4 hours. However, if doubt exists, naloxone hydrochloride 0.4 mg may be titrated intravenously. This drug acts very quickly to reverse any analgesia, and the patient may wake suddenly in severe pain. Some techniques, such as those used in cardiac surgery or to reduce stress responses, may employ much larger doses (for example, 50 to 150 μg/kg fentanyl). These patients may be markedly depressed postoperatively, requiring several hours or even days of respiratory support despite administration of narcotic antagonists.

Neuromuscular paralysis persisting into the postoperative period may be caused by several factors, as follows:

Atypical cholinesterase
Puerperium
Acid-base imbalance
Hypothermia $\rightarrow$ normothermia
Drug interactions
Overdose

If the action of muscle relaxant drugs has not been reversed at the end of surgery, the patient may appear unresponsive although he is actually paralyzed and not anesthetized. The patient's condition (for example, severe intracranial disease with elevated intracranial pressure or respiratory impairment) may require continued ventilatory support postoperatively, which is often best achieved by sedation and the use of neuromuscular blocking agents. Under these circumstances, the anesthesiologist may have elected not to give specific relaxant antagonists. Inadequate reversal may also be the result of metabolic acidosis. Any acid-base imbalance should be corrected before withdrawing ventilatory support. A low body temperature decreases the effectiveness of *d*-tubocurarine but not of pancuronium. As the patient becomes warmer during recovery, neuromuscular paralysis may become more intense.

Rarely (1:2500 individuals possess a homozygous genotype) prolonged paralysis follows average doses of succinylcholine (0.5 to 1 mg/kg) because of the presence of atypical pseudocholinesterase, which metabolizes the drug very slowly or not at all. Increased effect of muscle relaxants is usually the result of drug interaction (see discussion) or decreased calcium or potassium levels. The effect of succinylcholine is also increased in the puerperium because serum cholinesterase activity is decreased. A diagnosis may be made by reviewing the anesthetic record and using a nerve stimulator to measure the twitch response in the ulnar nerve. In patients with prolonged paralysis, improvement of muscle power may be followed more comfortably in the awake patient by using the train-of-four response, which is a series of four supramaximal single shocks delivered to the ulnar nerve at 2 Hz for 2 seconds. A decreased response from the first to the fourth response (ratio of 4 to 1 twitch of up to 50% indicates marked nondepolarizing block. Edrophonium chloride 20 mg and atropine 0.5 mg may be used as a clinical test and as an indicator of the effectiveness of neostigmine (a longer-acting drug). A train-of-four value of 75% to 80% indicates adequate neuromuscular function. Some clinicians believe that because assessment of train-of-four ratio is inaccurate, it is difficult to identify complete reversal of neuromuscular blockade. Moreover, the relationship between return of train-of-four and adequate ventilation is unknown for atracurium and vecuronium. Thus it has been suggested that nondepolarizing blockade should be routinely antagonized. Others, pointing to the adverse cardiovascular effects caused by these antagonists, maintain that adequate ventilation exists if the patient can sustain a head lift for 5 seconds, open his eyes, and squeeze the anesthesiologist's hand.

DRUG INTERACTION

During hospitalization, the average patient receives 8 drugs. An additional 5 to 10 agents are used during anesthesia. Many are multicomponent preparations. The relationship between the number of drugs administered and the incidence of reactions is not linear, as one might suppose. If less than 6 drugs are used, the reaction rate approximates 4%. However, if more than 11 drugs are given, the complication rate increases disproportionate to the number of drugs consumed (for example, 20 drugs have a 45% reaction rate). Some of the commonly used drugs that interact with anesthetic agents to cause increased sedation are listed in Table 6-2.

Maintenance Medications
Cardiovascular drugs

Methyldopa (Aldomet) and reserpine reduce the effective dose of halothane. Propranolol, which is

---

TABLE 6-2

Drugs that interact with anesthetics

Maintenance medications

Cardiovascular: antihypertensive drugs, antidysrhythmic agents, digitalis glycosides
Antibiotics
Psychotrophic drugs: lithium, monoamine oxide inhibitors, phenothiazine derivatives, street drugs
Cimetidine

Intravenous agents

Narcotics, barbiturates, benzodiazepines, ketamine, trimethaphan

Inhalation agents

Nitrous oxide, isoflurane, halothane, enflurane

Muscle relaxants

compatible with isoflurane and halothane, may cause cardiovascular collapse in the presence of cyclopropane or ether. In combination with morphine, effectiveness of histamine is increased and severe bronchospasm may occur in the asthmatic patients. Propranolol and other adrenergic blockers acutely potentiate neuromuscular blockade caused by nondepolarizing agents. In patients maintained on moderate doses of propranolol, neostigmine may cause severe bradycardia associated with somnolence, which may persist for several hours. Neuromuscular blockade is also prolonged by chronic administration of diuretics (reduced potassium levels), quinidine, procaine hydrochloride, and lidocaine. There is a narrow safety range with digitalis preparations. Hyperventilation causes alkalosis, which decreases serum potassium levels and increases the effect of digitalis. During halothane administration, on the other hand, more digitalis is required, which may result in an overdose as the patient wakes up, causing cardiac dysrhythmias and heart failure.

Antibiotics

Neuromuscular blockade is increased by streptomycin sulfate, neomycin, kanamycin sulfate, gentamycin sulfate, tobramycin sulfate, tetracyclines, polymyxin, colistin sulfate, lincomycin, clindamycin, and erythromycin. This interaction is usually seen when antibiotics are given intravenously or intraperitoneally during surgery, but the margin of safety of neuromuscular transmission may be reduced for many hours postoperatively. Administration of antibiotics in the early postoperative period may be particularly dangerous when respiratory assistance has been withdrawn and the effect of other depressant drugs is still evidenced. Antibiotics that do not interfere with neuromuscular transmission include penicillin G, cephradine, and cephaloridine.

Psychotropic drugs

Lithium increases the effect of all muscle relaxants except *d*-tubocurarine and gallamine and increases the reversal time of pancuronium by neostigmine. It also increases the hypnotic effect of pentobarbital.

The monoamine oxidase inhibitors (pargyline hydrochloride, tranylcypromine, phenelzine sulfate, isocarboxazid) increase the effect of narcotics, barbiturates, and succinylcholine. Tricyclic antidepressants (imipramine, amitriptyline, desipramine, doxepin) increase respiratory depression and analgesia with narcotics and hypnosis with barbiturates. A similar effect occurs with the phenothiazine derivatives (promethazine, chlorpromazine, perphenazine) and butyrophenones (droperidol).

Intravenous Agents

Narcotics cause respiratory depression, which decreases the rate at which inhalation agents can be excreted through the lungs. Morphine can potentiate acute alcohol intoxication (for example, injured drunk driver). All the narcotics have a synergistic central nervous system depressant effect with inhalation agents. Morphine-induced respiratory depression is potentiated by the H_2 antagonist cimetidine. Ventilatory response to CO_2 is depressed for as long as 24 hours.

Barbiturates and benzodiazepines reduce the intraoperative inhalation requirements, prolonging the hypnotic effect that may be particularly evidenced after short procedures. Barbiturates can acutely inhibit the metabolism of ketamine and increase its action. Barbiturates can be readily displaced from protein-binding sites by other drugs, such as dyes used during intraoperative radiological studies, thus increasing their hypnotic effect.

Drugs such as phenothiazine derivatives, barbiturates, hydroxyzine, and droperidol, which have been used to control the adverse central nervous system effects of ketamine, all delay return to consciousness. Ketamine reduces the effective dose of inhalation agents for hours and enhances *d*-tubocurarine blockade.

The action of trimethaphan, a ganglionic blocking agent that also releases histamine, is potentiated by general and spinal anesthesia, diuretics, and antihypertensive medications. Profound hypotension, prolonged coma, and respiratory depression may occur. Therapy includes respiratory support, fluid administration, and phenylephrine hydrochloride infusion.

Inhalation Agents

Effective inhalation anesthetic concentration is significantly reduced by the addition of nitrous oxide. Appropriate intraoperative decrease in administration must be made to avoid postoperative depression. There is marked synergism between all the inhalation agents (especially isoflurane) and nondepolarizing muscle relaxants.

RESPIRATORY INSUFFICIENCY

Respiratory depression commonly occurs in the immediate postoperative period. All degrees of ventilatory inadequacy, from mild depression to overt failure, may occur and lead to prolonged unconsciousness. The diagnosis is made if one or more of the criteria listed in Table 6-3 are met. Table 6-4 lists common causes of postoperative respiratory insufficiency.

Intraoperative Hyperventilation

Intraoperative hyperventilation causes alkalosis and decreases $PaCO_2$. Postoperatively the patient hypoventilates as CO_2 is restored. However, there are no oxygen stores, and unless supplemental oxygen is given, hypoxia develops.

TABLE 6-3	
Criteria used in diagnosis of respiratory insufficiency	
Respiratory pattern	irregular
Respiratory rate	<10/min >40/min
Tidal volume	<3.5 ml/kg
Vital capacity	<15 ml/kg
Inspiratory pressure	>−20 cm H_2O
$PaCO_2$	>50 mm Hg
PaO_2	<70 mm Hg

TABLE 6-4		
Causes of inadequate respiration in the postoperative period		
Cause	**Diagnosis**	**Therapy**
Intraoperative hyperventilation	Observation Anesthetic record	O_2 mask
Anesthetic agents	History Anesthetic record	Supportive (ventilation; cardio-vascular stability)
Fluid overload	Chest x-ray Central venous pressure Input/Output discrepancy in anesthetic record	Diuretics Intubation Positive-pressure ventilation
Operative site	Observation Patient complains of pain	Narcotics Regional block
Intraoperative complication	Anesthetist's and surgeon's reports Chest x-ray	Fluid replacement Assisted ventilation Chest tube inserted if necessary
Aspiration	Observation Chest x-ray Blood gases Anesthetist's report	Assisted or controlled ventilation Suction Antibiotics; steroids Bronchoscopy Bronchodilators
Preexisting disease	History	Ventilatory support Bronchodilators Antibiotics

Adapted from Frost E: Postoperative coma in recovery room care, Int Anesthesiol Clin 21(1):22, 1983.

Anesthetic Agents

All anesthetic agents, especially narcotics, cause respiratory depression. Therapy is supportive until the drug effect has been reversed or worn off. Small doses of narcotics (for example, Demerol 25 mg) may cause marked respiratory depression in the PACU if the patient is still under the influence of other anesthetic agents.

Fluid Overload

Excess intraoperative fluid administration or use of hyperosmolar solutions, such as mannitol, may cause congestive cardiac failure in the elderly, in small babies, or in patients with a history of cardiac disease. Central venous pressure is elevated, sputum is pink and frothy, there is obvious respiratory distress, and a fluffy picture is seen on the chest x-ray film. Reintubation and positive-pressure ventilation, furosemide (40 mg intravenously), and morphine sulfate (2 to 5 mg intravenously) are required.

Operative Site

Thoracic and upper abdominal surgical procedures are associated with considerable pain and splinting of the diaphragm. Appropriate therapy includes regional epidural blockade, intercostal nerve block, and small doses of narcotics.

Special attention must be paid to patients who have undergone anterior cervical spinal surgery. Ventilation may have been marginal preoperatively because of cord injury and spasm. Edema caused by surgical trauma and decreased function of auxiliary muscles of respiration may cause ventilatory failure postoperatively. If in doubt, ventilatory support should be continued for several days if necessary.

Intraoperative Complications

Intraoperative complications that can cause postoperative respiratory problems (pneumothorax, endobronchial intubation, hemothorax, asthmatic attack, pulmonary collapse) are uncommon but should have been included in the anesthesiologist's or surgeon's report.

Aspiration

Pulmonary aspiration of stomach contents is rare after extubation but may occur during transfer of the comatose patient. It is more likely to occur if a nasogastric tube is present. Diagnosis is usually made by observation. Arterial blood gas analyses are a much more sensitive indicator of lung damage than a chest x-ray examination, which may not show changes for 24 hours. If the amount aspirated is more than a few milliliters or if the pH of the secretions obtained immediately is less than 5, the patient should be reintubated and given ventilation support. Bronchoscopy may be indicated to reexpand collapsed lung segments and to remove particulate matter.

Shivering

Reduced body temperature and infusion of cold fluids may cause postoperative shivering, which can increase oxygen use by 400% and reduce PaO_2, especially if there is ventilatory difficulty already or a fixed low cardiac output. Therapy involves oxygen administration, careful warming, sedation, and, if available, small doses of methylphenidate (Ritalin).

Preexisting Disease

Appropriate evaluation of postoperative respiratory difficulties must include a review of preoperative lung function. Additive effects of anesthetic drug depression and chronic obstructive pulmonary disease may precipitate respiratory failure.

CARDIOVASCULAR INSTABILITY

As with the respiratory system, instability of the cardiovascular system is not uncommon in the PACU. Both hypotension and dysrhythmias may cause coma. Hypotension may be caused by inadequate volume replacement, drug overdose, intraoperative catastrophe, or acute cardiopulmonary disease. Cardiac dysrhythmias may be precipitated by myocardial ischemia, hypoxia, or drugs. Diagnosis requires a careful review of the chart and examination of the patient. Therapy is determined by the underlying cause.

THERMOREGULATORY DYSFUNCTION

Regulation of body temperature is impaired during anesthesia (poikilothermic state). Core temperatures may decrease by 6° C or more, especially in children if the ambient temperature is low. At this level, the depressant effects of all anesthetic agents are exaggerated. Diagnosis is made immediately when the temperature is checked on admission to the PACU. Rewarming should be done gradually to prevent burns in areas of low perfusion. Continuous electrocardiographic monitoring for ventricular dysrhythmias is essential. Sudden body movements (especially of the extremities) should be avoided because this may push large volumes of relatively cold peripheral blood into the heart. Close attention must be paid to respiratory status if *d*-tubocurarine was used because neuromuscular paralysis may become more intense during rewarming.

Postoperative hyperthermia may be the result of preexisting disease, an infective process, drug reaction, or malignant hyperthermia. This last syndrome may be triggered by pain or stress and is associated with persistent coma, high fever, supraventricular tachycardia, hyperventilation, unstable blood pressure, acute pulmonary and cerebral edema, and acute renal failure. Therapy requires cardioventilatory support, sodium bicarbonate, external and internal cooling, dantrolene sodium, procaine hydrochloride, steroids, diuretics, and insulin in glucose.

FLUID AND ELECTROLYTE IMBALANCE

Complications of fluid and electrolyte imbalance are most likely to occur in elderly or debilitated patients (especially after major intestinal surgery) or in severe hypertensive patients maintained on diuretics and in diabetic and neurosurgical patients who have received large doses of mannitol or who have disturbances involving the thalamohypophyseal pathways.

Serum electrolyte estimation should be performed shortly after admission to the PACU and the results correlated with vital signs. Any abnormalities, particularly of sodium, potassium, or glucose levels, should be corrected. Two situations deserve special attention.

Diabetes Mellitus

Patients with severe diabetes are usually stabilized for 1 to 2 days preoperatively on a regimen of a sliding regular insulin dosage determined according to urinalysis (that is, 1+ sugar in urine—no insulin; 2+, 5 units; 3+, 10 units; 4+, 15 units). However, preoperative fasting, stress, infection, steroids, and intraoperative glucose administration may cause either a hypoglycemic or hyperglycemic state postoperatively. Urinalysis should be performed immediately on admission to the PACU. At least a small amount of sugar should be detected. Bedside glucose determination with Dextrostix provides a rough guide to sugar levels ($\pm$ 50 mg/dl) and is no substitute for laboratory determinations in these patients. Insulin, which has a half-life of about 10 minutes, is rapidly cleared by metabolism and renal excretion. Intravenous bolus injections are short acting, and small amounts given continuously are probably more effective (for example, 100 units in 100 ml saline over 1 to 2 hours). Potassium 20 mEq should be added to the infusion. Insulin decreases blood sugar levels at approximately 100 to 200 mg/dl per hour as opposed to rehydration, which by dilutional effect can cause a fall of as much as 700 mg/dl per hour. Ketosis is best treated postoperatively by small doses of insulin (5 units).

Patients in hypoglycemic coma usually respond to a rapid injection of 50 ml 50% dextrose in water within 5 minutes. The clinical features of hypoglycemia and hyperglycemia are contrasted in Table 6-5. Hypoglycemia is most likely to occur (1) in patients maintained on oral agents (the effects of chlorpropamide last for 2 days), (2) if there is coexistent renal failure, which delays insulin excretion, or (3) in patients fasted (for example, nonfunctioning intravenous lines) or vomiting. Hyperglycemia occurs in association with sepsis, stress, or if the

TABLE 6-5

Clinical features of hypoglycemia and hyperglycemia

Hypoglycemia	Hyperglycemia
Coma	Dehydration
Seizures	Hypokalemia
Tachycardia	Metabolic acidosis
Low blood pressure	Hyperventilation (air hunger)
	Coma
Blood sugar <70 mg/dl	Blood sugar >300 mg/dl

TABLE 6-6

Abnormalities caused by changes in antidiuretic hormone (ADH) production

Overproduction of ADH (SIADH)	Underproduction of ADH (Diabetes insipidus)
Causes	
CNS pathology	Head trauma
Pneumonia	Intracranial surgery
Pulmonary Tb	(hypophysectomy)
Bronchogenic Ca	
Diagnosis	
Oliguria	Polyuria (300 ml/hr)
Hyponatremia	Hypernatremia
UO ↑, PO ↓	UO ↓, PO ↑
Normal renal and adrenal function	Urine specific gravity ↓
Normotension	Hypotension
No dehydration	Dehydration
Confusion, delirium, coma	Seizures, coma

UO, urine osmolality; PO, Plasma osmolality.

patient has not received insulin or has been hydrated with dextrose solutions.

Hyperosmolar, nonketotic coma is a rare cause of hyperglycemia that occurs in elderly, debilitated patients or associated with major trauma and is caused by disturbance of thirst mechanisms. Blood glucose levels are more than 1000 mg/dl. Patients are severely dehydrated, and coma and seizures are common. However, these patients respond promptly to small doses of insulin (10 to 20 units) and to rehydration.

Abnormalities of Antidiuretic Hormone Secretion

Oversecretion or undersecretion of antidiuretic hormone (ADH) from the pituitary can cause fluid and electrolyte complications postoperatively. Table 6-6 compares the causes and diagnostic features of overproduction (syndrome of inappropriate antidiuretic secretion, SIADH) and underproduction of ADH (diabetes insipidus).

Treatment of SIADH involves administration of sodium as a 3% to 5% saline solution preceded by furosemide 20 mg to promote diuresis. Fluid restriction is necessary. Diabetes insipidus should be treated over a 24-hour period with hypotonic solutions (for example, 5% dextrose in 0.25% saline solution) with potassium chloride supplementation as necessary. Too rapid correction of hypernatremia can cause water intoxication and cerebral edema. Vasopressin tannate 5 units subcutaneously is specific therapy. 1-Desamino-8-*D*-arginine vasopres-

sin (DDAVP) is rapidly effective by nasal insufflation. Its use is restricted to cooperative patients. An intravenous preparation is available. ECG monitoring is required during administration because signs of myocardial ischemia may develop.

ALLERGIC OR ATYPICAL DRUG REACTION

Individual response to drug action is the rule. Occasionally an allergic or atypical reaction may occur that interferes with early return to consciousness. Some of the drugs that may prove problematic are listed in Table 6-7.

INTRAOPERATIVE CATASTROPHE

Rarely complications in the operating room may be the cause of prolonged postoperative coma. Some of the causes and the differential diagnoses are listed in Table 6-8. Early and close communication among all the medical personnel involved in the patient's care is essential.

TABLE 6-7

Allergic or atypical drug response

Cause	Diagnosis	Treatment
Penicillin	Skin reactions Bronchospasm Tachycardia Hypotension	Antihistamines Epinephrine
Droperidol	Anesthetic record Decreased ventilation Positive Babinski sign	Ventilatory support
Phenothiazines (Valium, Versed)	Hypoventilation Hypotension Anesthetic record	Ventilatory support Fluid replacement
Muscle relaxants	Hypoventilation Peripheral nerve stimulator	Assisted ventilation Neostigmine and atropine
Narcotics	Hypoventilation Hypotension	Naloxone
Ketamine	Hallucinations	Diazepam
Barbiturates	Hypoventilation	Assisted ventilation

Adapted from Frost E: Postoperative coma in recovery room care, Int Anesthesiol Clin 21(1):29, 1983.

TABLE 6-8

Some intraoperative factors that can result in prolonged coma

Cause	Diagnosis	Treatment

Shock
  Hemorrhagic
  Septic
	Vital signs
	  BP $\downarrow$
	  Pulse $\uparrow$
	  Temperature $\uparrow$ or $\downarrow$
	  CVP $\downarrow$
	Physician's report
		Fluid replacement
		Steroids
		Antibiotics
		Ventilatory assistance

Myocardial infarction	ECG Enzyme studies	Cardiovascular support (vasopressors, anti- dysrhythmic agents) O_2 mask

Intracranial lesion
  Blood shift
  Herniation
	Vital signs
	  BP $\uparrow$
	  Pulse $\uparrow$ or $\downarrow$
	Neurologic exam; unequal pupils
	Radiologic studies
		Support ventilation
		Diuretics
		Steroids
		Barbiturates

Hypoxia	Physician's report PaO_2 $\downarrow$	Support ventilation

Adapted from Frost E: Postoperative coma recovery room care, Int Anesthesiol Clin 21(1):24, 1983.

Shock

Sudden loss of volume (fluid or blood) may cause shock. Multiunit transfusions are often associated with pulmonary and renal problems after a few hours. Careful monitoring is essential. Septic shock may develop rapidly after manipulation of a large abscess, infarcted bowel, or gangrenous area. The clinical picture is one of severe hypotension, tachycardia, and hypothermia, without obvious bleeding. Treatment requires cardiopulmonary support, steroids, and antibiotics.

Myocardial Infarction

All degrees of cardiac ischemia may be caused by hypotensive or hypertensive episodes or by stress. Typical ECG changes develop. Diagnostic serum enzyme levels may be masked by surgical trauma. Technetium 99 pyrophosphate infarct scintigrams that become positive in 12 to 24 hours may help in making a positive diagnosis.

Intracranial Lesion

Rupture of an intracranial aneurysm before clipping carries a poor prognosis. If major vessels have been occluded to control bleeding or if there has been deep or extensive tumor dissection requiring prolonged brain tissue retraction, cerebral edema may cause increased intracranial pressure and coma.

Another problem that may become obvious in the PACU is that of intracranial air. Intraoperatively, the brain size is decreased by diuretic administration and hyperventilation. Air becomes trapped within the skull. As the brain reexpands, this air may be put under pressure, resulting in a tension pneumocephalus and coma.

In any patient with altered intracranial dynamics, small increases in $PaCO_2$ may cause marked deterioration in the level of consciousness. Should hypertension or respiratory or cardiac abnormalities associated with decrease in sensorium occur in any neurosurgical patient, prompt therapy must include neurosurgical consultation and immediate attempts to control intracranial pressure at less than 20 mm Hg (reintubation, hyperventilation, diuretics, head-up position). A CT scan should be performed as soon as possible.

Patients who have undergone bilateral carotid endarterectomy either as one procedure or during two operations spaced several months apart are very sensitive to the respiratory depressant effects of small doses of narcotics. As hypoxemia develops, without normal carotid body function, there is no increase in ventilation.

Preoperative State

Finally, accurate assessment of the cause of postoperative somnolence must include a review of the patient's preoperative mental status. A patient comatose before surgery will most likely remain so for some time postoperatively. As in all the several situations that contribute to delayed awakening, close communication, including a verbal report, is essential between the PACU nurse, anesthesiologist, and surgeon.

SUGGESTIONS FOR FURTHER READING

Ammon JR: Perioperative management of the diabetic patient, Am Soc Anes, Refresher Course, lecture no. 215, San Francisco, 1988.

Cullen BF and Miller MG: Drug interactions and anesthesia: a review, Anesth Analg 58:413, 1979.

Frost E: Differential diagnosis of postoperative coma. In Recovery room care. Frost EAM and Andrews IC, editors: Internat Anesth Clin, Boston, 1983, Little, Brown & Co, Inc.

Halsey MJ: Drug interactions in anaesthesia, Br J Anaesth. 59:111, 1987.

May FE, Stewart RB, and Cluff LE: Drug use in the hospital: evaluation of determinants, Clin Pharmacol Ther 16:834, 1974.

Meyers EF, Alberts D, and Gordon MO: Perioperative control of blood glucose in diabetic patients: a two-step protocol, Diabetes Care 9:40, 1986.

Miller R: Monitoring of neuromuscular blockade, Am Soc Anes, Refresher Course, lecture no. 255, San Francisco, 1988.

Smith JW, Seidl LG, and Cluff LE: Studies on the epidemiology of adverse drug reactions. V. Clinical factors influencing susceptibility, Ann Intern Med 65:629, 1966.

Waud BE: Interaction of muscle relaxants and other drugs. In ASA refresher courses in anesthesiology, vol 9, Hershey SG, editor, Philadelphia, 1981, JB Lippincott Co.

CHAPTER 7

Criteria for Discharge

Marilyn (Schneider) Glaser

Assessing the patient's readiness for discharge from the PACU (post anesthesia care unit) is a significant responsibility of the PAN (post anesthesia nurse). Determining the criteria to be applied in this assessment is a joint responsibility of the department of anesthesiology, the PACU nurse-manager, the department of surgery, and any designated others. Together, these individuals identify the criteria to be used by the nursing and anesthesiology staffs for evaluating the patient's response to anesthesia and surgery. These criteria should be written as departmental policy to serve as the standards against which the nurse and anesthesiologist evaluate the patient for discharge and the PACU.

Several national agencies have addressed the issue of determining the patient's readiness for discharge from PACU. These include the Joint Commission on Accreditation of Healthcare Organizations (JCAHO), the American Society of Anesthesiologists (ASA), and the American Society of Post anesthesia Nurses (ASPAN).

JCAHO

The JCAHO Accreditation Manual for Hospitals 1988, states:

A licensed independent practitioner who has appropriate clinical privileges and who is familiar with the patient is responsible for the decision to discharge a patient from a post anesthesia recovery area or, when the surgical or anesthesia services are provided on an ambulatory basis, from the hospital. When the responsible licensed independent practitioner is not personally present to make the decision to discharge or does not sign the discharge order, the name of the licensed independent practitioner responsible for the discharge is recorded in the patient's medical record; and the relevant discharge criteria are rigorously applied to determine the readiness of the patient for discharge. The discharge criteria are approved by the medical staff.

Therefore JCAHO guidelines require discharge criteria as a standard against which to assess the patient's readiness for discharge. The areas of assessment required by the JCAHO are the following:

Vital signs and level of consciousness

Intravenous fluids administered, including blood and blood products

All drugs administered

Post anesthesia visits

Any unusual events or postoperative complications and the management of those events

If the decision of the individual hospital is that the licensed independent practitioner does not need to be physically present to sign the discharge order, discharge criteria must be clearly defined in departmental policy and all applicable criteria assessed and documented on the PACU nursing record.

ASA

The ASA suggests (1977) that an anesthesiologist evaluate the "status of the patient on admission and discharge from the postoperative recovery suite," and that the "anesthesiologist shall determine and document when the period of postoperative surveillance has terminated." In its *Practice Advisory* (1978) ASA said, "Patients may be discharged [from PACU] only after vital signs are stable and after an evaluation of the patient's condition by a responsible physician or designee."

The ASA is in the process of developing discharge standards for anesthesiologists.

ASPAN

ASPAN, in its Standards of Nursing Practice (1986), states that evaluation of the following parameters are necessary before discharge of a patient in phase One (hospitalized patients):

1. Airway patency and respiratory function
2. Stability of vital signs, including temperature
3. Level of consciousness and muscular strength
4. Mobility
5. Patency of tubes, catheters, drains, intravenous lines
6. Skin color and condition
7. Condition of dressing and/or surgical site
8. Fluid intake and output
9. Comfort

Another aspect of discharge criteria and planning recommended by ASPAN includes communicating with the patient's family or significant others, and with the patient's care unit.
Standards for the nurse, according to ASPAN, are the following:

The postanesthesia nurse shall discharge the patient in accordance with written policies set forth by the department of anesthesia and also in accordance with the circeria and data collected through the use of the nursing process. A final nursing assessment and evaluation of the patient's condition will be performed and documented. If a numerical scoring system is used, the discharge score will be recorded to reflect the patient's status. The PAN arranges for the safe transport of the patient from the PACU.

Discharge standards are dynamic. Additional standards will emerge, such as the use of pulse oximetry and minimum O_2 saturation.

NUMERICAL SCORING SYSTEMS

The use of a numerical scoring system for assessment of the patient's recovery from anesthesia has been investigated, and widely used for the past 15 years. The first anesthesia and surgery scoring system was developed by Gaston Carignan et al. in 1964. This evaluated long-term recovery from anesthesia, measuring five physiological system parameters at the second, fifth, and fifteenth postoperative days (Figure 7-1). The Apgar scoring system was introduced for evaluation of newborns in 1958 and formed the basis for subsequent scoring systems. Carignan's scoring system was developed because of the need for "observing, tubulating, and presenting in condensed form, the postanesthetic course of a large number of patients."

A postanesthetic recovery score (PAS) analogous to the Apgar score and applicable to the postanesthetic period was introduced by Aldrete and Kroulik in 1970. Physical signs, which could be easily observed and commonly seen, were selected for evaluation. To simplify assessment, a numerical score of 0, 1, or 2 is assigned in each of five selected areas: activity, respirations, circulation, consciousness, and color. A maximum score of 10 indicates a patient in optimum postanesthetic condition to return to the nursing unit. It was recommended that scoring assessment be performed on admission to PACU and hourly thereafter until discharge from PACU. This has been modified with usage over the years, and many PACUs have added a 15-minute postadmission assessment. Figure 7-2 shows the PAS introduced by Aldrete and Kroulik. It should be noted that PACUs have adapted, modified, and condensed the graph. Figure 7-3 is an example of a PAS currently in use. The scoring system is employed with the following considerations:

Activity. Muscular activity may be spontaneous or on command. This assists in evaluating recovery from the effects of regional and local anesthetic techniques, as well as general anesthesia.

	0	1	2	3	4	5
Circ.	BP stable. Pulse always under 100	BP-change less than 30%. Pulse 100–120	Vasopressors OR Digitalis	BP under 100 in spite of treatment	Decompensated	Severe shock
Resp.	Rate under 15, Breath-holding more than 25 sec.	Rate 15–20. Productive cough	Rate over 20, rales OR temp. up to 100°	Temp. over 100°, partial atelectasis	Major atelectasis	Pneumonia
C.N.S.	Amnesic, satisfied	Confused OR recalls induction	Dissatisfied with anesthesia for any reason	Extrapyramidal signs	Major neurological complications	Coma
G.I.	Nothing	No more than 3 episodes of nausea	Nausea, vomited once only	Vomiting	Ileus	Evisceration OR perforation
Renal	Voids over 800 cc.	Over 800 cc. per catheter	Voids 500–800 cc.	500–800 cc. per catheter	Under 500 cc.	Anuria

FIGURE 7-1

Carignan scoring system
(Hospital of Notre Dame, Montreal, Canada).

POST ANESTHESIA SCORE SYSTEM

	SCORE	AT ARRIVAL	HOUR 1	2	3

ACTIVITY
Able to move 4 extremities _____ 2 ___ _____ ___ ___ ___
Able to move 2 extremities _____ 1 ___ _____ ___ ___ ___
Able to move 0 extremities _____ 0 ___ _____ ___ ___ ___

RESPIRATION
Able to deep breathe and cough freely __ 2 ___ _____ ___ ___ ___
Dyspnea or limited breathing_____ 1 ___ _____ ___ ___ ___
Apneic _____ 0 ___ _____ ___ ___ ___

CIRCULATION
BP ± 20%
    of preanesthetic level _____ 2 ___ _____ ___ ___ ___
BP ± 20% to 50%
    of preanesthetic level _____ 1 ___ _____ ___ ___ ___
BP ± 50%
    or more of preanesthetic level _____ 0 ___ _____ ___ ___ ___

CONSCIOUSNESS
Fully awake_____ 2 ___ _____ ___ ___ ___
Arousable on calling_____ 1 ___ _____ ___ ___ ___
Not responding_____ 0 ___ _____ ___ ___ ___

COLOR
Pink_____ 2 ___ _____ ___ ___ ___
Pale, dusky, blotchy, jaundiced, other____ 1 ___ _____ ___ ___ ___
Cyanotic_____ 0 ___ _____ ___ ___ ___

                    TOTALS   _____ ___ ___ ____

FIGURE 7-2

A post anesthesia score system.

SCORE	CRITERIA	ADM	15 MIN	DIS
Activity				
2	Able To Move 4 Extremities			
1	Able To Move 2 Extremities			
0	Able To Move 0 Extremities			
Resp.				
2	Able To Breathe Deeply & Cough			
1	Dyspnea or Limited Breathing			
0	Apnea			
Circ.	Preanesthetic Level			
2	BP is ± 20 mm Hg of preanesthetic level			
1	BP is ± 20-50 mm Hg of preanesthetic level			
0	BP is ± 50 mm Hg of preanesthetic level			
Awareness				
2	Fully Awake			
1	Arousable on Calling			
0	Not Responding			
Color				
2	Pink			
1	Pale, Dusky, Blotchy, Jaundiced			
0	Cyanotic			
TOTAL SCORE				

FIGURE 7-3

Post anesthesia score
(AMI Doctors Hospital of Prince Georges County).

Respirations. The ability to breathe deeply and cough is the maximum achievable; apnea is the other extreme. Limited respiratory efforts (for example, splinting, airway adjuncts, dyspnea) rate the median value.

Circulation. Blood pressure is rated in relation to its preanesthetic level, and circulatory function is evaluated. A percentage of the preanesthetic systolic arterial blood pressure is determined and rated. (Some PACUs have modified this and consider the pressure difference in mm HG, which is simpler and faster to calculate, instead of percentage).

Consciousness. Full alertness, orientation to person, place, and time, and the ability to answer questions and summon assistance receives the maximum value. Response to calling the patient by name is assigned the median value. If no response is elicited by oral communication, the 0 value is assigned. Painful stimulation is not employed to elicit a response.

Color. A normal skin and mucous membrane color receives the highest score; obvious cyanosis rates the lowest score. Assessments between these two—pallor, duskiness, blotchy discoloration, flushed appearance, and jaundice—receive the median value. Even if alterations in color existed preoperatively, the postoperative assessment is rated objectively.

Many PACUs use the PAS as one criterion for discharge. Department policy may state, ''Patient may be discharged from PACU when PAS reaches 9,'' but a PAS constitutes only minimal criteria for discharge and other parameters also must be considered.

	TIME		M	1	2	3	4	5	6	7	8	9	10	11	N	1	2	3	4	5	6	7	8	9	10	11
	SPONTANEOUS	4																								
EYE	TO SPEECH	3																								
	TO PAIN	2																								
OPENING	NONE	1																								
BEST	ORIENTED	5																								
	CONFUSED	4																								
VERBAL	INAPPROPRIATE	3																								
	INCOMPREHENSIBLE	2																								
RESPONSE	NONE	1																								
BEST	OBEYING	5																								
	LOCALIZING	4																								
MOTOR	FLEXING	3																								
	EXTENDING	2																								
RESPONSE	NONE	1																								

FIGURE 7-4
Glasgow coma scale.

Another scoring system employed in PACU settings is the Glasgow coma scale (GCS) (Figure 7-4). This scale was developed as a prognostic indicator of outcome in head injury but has been used as a simple assessment of level of consciousness as well. When used in PACUs, it is a part of a larger assessment procedure. The GCS consists of three areas of assessment: response by opening eyes, verbal response, and motor response. Scoring at five levels is provided for verbal and motor response, and at four levels for the opening of eyes. Measurements are recorded at predetermined intervals, usually every 15 minutes in PACU and more (or less) frequently as indicated by the patient's condition. In and of itself, the scale is not sufficient for use as the criterion for discharge, but may be a useful adjunct, particularly in assessing neurosurgical patients.

DISCHARGE BY ANESTHESIOLOGIST

Many PACUs operate under a policy that requires an anesthesiologist's assessment, discharge note, and signature before the release of any patient. This works well in a setting where an anesthesiologist is always readily available to the PACU; it is not a workable solution in many instititions.

When an anesthesiologist writes the discharge order, according to the ASA, the vital signs are stable and an evaluation of the patient's status has been made by a responsible physician or designee. The discharge order requires a signature. Any other requirements, such as assessments, notes, or destination, should be determined by the individual institution. ASA will be issuing updated standards for anesthesiologists soon.

DISCHARGE CRITERIA

Some hospitals have opted for an across-the-board minimum stay in PACU, generally based on length of surgical procedure: for example, 1 hour in PACU for every hour in the operating room (OR), or 2-hour minimum stay for adult patients and 1-hour minimum stay for children under 12 years of age. These arbitrary lengths of stay may vary among institutions and may refer exclusively to patients receiving general anesthetics. Other time restrictions may be assigned after general anesthesia or for alternate techniques of anesthesia administration.

Other factors that may be considered for imposing a waiting period before discharge include the following:

A minimum 30-minute observation period after

administration of intravenous narcotics, anti-biotics, or naloxone (Narcan)

A 1-hour observation period after administration of intramuscular antibiotics, antiemetics, or narcotics

Other medication-related observation periods as determined by the department of anesthesiology

A 30-minute observation period after discontinuance of oxygen therapy

A 1-hour observation period after extubation

Writing Discharge Criteria

In assessing a patient's eligibility for discharge from PACU, the nurse must consider the complete physiological response of the patient to the effects of anesthesia and surgery.

At University Hospitals in Cleveland, all of the following constitute criteria or considerations for discharge:

A minimum stay of 1 hour

Stability of vital signs (blood pressure, pulse rate, respiratory rate)

Body temperature

Level of consciousness

Complications related to:
  Pain
  Wound drainage
  Nausea and vomiting
  Urinary output
  Specific surgical procedure

Patency of tubes and catheters

Postoperative orders

Ongoing nursing care needs

Standards for each of these criteria have been developed. For example, stability of vital signs is measured by three consecutive 15-minute interval readings immediately before discharge that are in the same range, as well as in the patient's normal range (as determined by preoperative and intraoperative values). Standards include written postoperative orders that have been reviewed, stat orders carried out, and parenteral medications started unless contraindicated in the immediate postanesthetic period.

In New York State, representatives of the Society of Anesthesiologists, Post Anesthesia Nurses Association, and Association of Nurse Anesthetists have published *Guidelines for Post Anesthesia Care*. In their introduction, they state, "No two hospitals are alike . . . No guidelines can possibly fit all situations." Application of the guidelines is recommended to be adapted by individual institutions.

Regarding responsibilities of the PAN at the time of discharge, their guidelines say the following:

Appropriate criteria for discharge . . . should be detailed in the PACU Procedure Manual. When the patient meets these criteria, an anesthesiologist or surgeon should be notified to verify and approve his or her discharge. A discharge note including time and level of consciousness should be written and signed. The individual discharging the patient should determine the type and number of personnel required for transport to the floor or special unit. The PAN should report to the floor nurse the patient's general condition, operation, postanesthesia progress, fluid and blood replacement, urine output, drainage, and any other pertinent information.

Each PACU is responsible for establishing written criteria for discharge and standards for these criteria.

In assessing the patient's readiness for discharge to a hospital room after general anesthesia, certain parameters seem evident and universally accepted.

1. The patient is able to maintain his own airway, clear secretions, and deep breathe and cough on command. The patient can turn to his side in the event of vomiting and summon assistance when needed.

2. The hemodynamic status of the patient has stabilized. Blood pressure and pulse are stable and correlate with the preoperative measurements.

3. The fluid balance status of the patient is equilibrating. The patient is neither hypovolemic nor hypervolemic, urinary output is adequate according to the standards of that institution (usually 25 to 50 ml per hour), and electrolyte levels are within normal limits (or are being treated).

4. The postsurgical status of the patient is pointing toward recovery. There is no evidence of active bleeding. All tubes, drains, catheters, intravenous lines, etc., are patent, working properly, and connected according to physician instructions. Where indicated, the ordered fluids are infusing or irrigating.

5. The continuing care needs of the patient have been identified and implemented as indicated. Ice has been applied where ordered, stat and other medications have been administered, and the patient's responses to treatment have been observed and documented. Physician orders to be initiated in the PACU have been implemented.

6. Pain has been assessed and treated, and the patient's response to treatment documented.

7. The patient's temperature is stable within defined limits. If necessary, treatment has been started to control hypothermia or hyperthermia.

8. Potential problems have been forestalled, and no active problems (that is, any not undergoing treatment) are apparent.

Special Discharge Criteria

In the PACU, there are also patients who have special discharge criteria needs.

Ambulatory patients

The ambulatory surgery patient (phase Two in the ASPAN Standards of Nursing Practice) is assessed and evaluated for the following, as applicable, before discharge home:

Adequate respiratory function

Stability of vital signs, including temperature

Level of consciousness and muscular strength

Ability to ambulate consistent with developmental age level

Ability to swallow oral fluids, cough, or demonstrate gag reflex

Ability to retain oral fluid

Skin color and condition

Pain minimal

Adequate neurovascular status of operative extremity

Ability to demonstrate proper use of crutches

Ability to demonstrate proper care of drains and catheters

Ability to describe care of and changing of dressings

Ability to demonstrate proper method of administering eye and ear drops

Ability to describe the "proper" taking of prescribed medications

Ability of patient and home care provider to understand all home care instructions

Written discharge instruction given to patient/family

Concur with prearrangements for safe transportation home

Some PACUs keep ambulatory surgery patients for 4 to 6 hours postoperatively and serve a meal. Others may elect to discharge the patient home in 1 to 2 hours, provided other criteria have been met. PACUs have also reported that a first voiding is a requirement before discharge.

Discharge planning for the ambulatory surgery patient is integral to the care.

An example of detailed post anesthesia and postsurgical instructions that is provided to the ambulatory surgery patient in writing at AMI Doctors Hospital of Prince Georges County, Lanham, Maryland, is shown in Figures 7-5 and 7-6.

Critical care patients

The patient who will be transferred from the PACU to another critical care area may not achieve the levels of stability anticipated in a patient returning to a hospital room. The continued intense nursing care provided to these patients enables the transfer of patients still intubated, of hemodynamically and surgically unstable patients, and of patients with multisystem problems. Criteria for discharge to critical care areas need to be developed by each PACU. For example, if a unit uses a PAS system as a discharge criterion, the departmental policy may state, "Patients with a PAS of 5 or below must be transferred to a critical care area." Discharge policy will also indicate who must accompany the patient during transfer, and any other precautions deemed necessary.

OUTPATIENT POSTANESTHESIA AND POSTSURGERY INSTRUCTIONS AND INFORMATION

1. Although you will be awake and alert in the recovery room, small amounts of anesthetic will remain in your body for at least 24 hours and you may feel tired and sleepy for the remainder of the day. Once you are home, take it easy and rest as much as possible. It is advisable to have someone with you at home for the remainder of the day.
2. Eat lightly for the first 12 to 24 hours, then resume a well-balanced, normal diet. Drink plenty of fluids. Alcoholic beverages are to be avoided for 24 hours after your anesthesia or intravenous sedation.
3. Nausea or vomiting may occur in the first 24 hours. Lie down on your side and breathe deeply. Prolonged nausea, vomiting, or pain should be reported to your surgeon.
4. Medications, unless prescribed by your physician, should be avoided for 24 hours. Check with your surgeon and/or anesthesiologist for specific instructions if you have been taking a daily medication.
5. Your surgeon will discuss your postsurgery instructions with you and prescribe medication for you as indicated. You will also receive additional instructions specific to your surgical procedure prior to leaving the hospital.
6. Your family will be waiting for you in the hospital's waiting room area adjacent to the outpatient surgery department. Your surgeon will speak to them in this area prior to your discharge.
7. **Do not operate a motor vehicle or any mechanical or electrical equipment for *24 hours* after your anesthesia.**
8. Do not make any important decisions or sign legal documents for 24 hours following your anesthesia.

FIGURE 7-5

Outpatient post anesthesia teaching information
(AMI Doctors Hospital of Prince Georges County).

Pediatric patients

Pediatric patients constitute another group with special discharge criteria needs. Further subdivision may be made into ambulatory surgery, in-house, and critical care patients. Adjustments in the discharge criteria may need to reflect the indications for measurement of blood pressure and its effect on the PAS (if this system is used). Depending on the needs of a particular PACU, all discharge criteria employed for adult patients are established with reference to pediatric patients.

The pediatric ambulatory surgery patient should have no nausea or vomiting and, depending on age, should cry lustily, talk and be oriented, and walk. The patient should have no nystagmus. Clear fluids should be retained.

Regional anesthetic techniques

The patient who has received any of a variety of regional blocking techniques requires specific assessment of recovery from the effects of those agents.

Discharge instructions:

___Keep limb elevated, apply ice packs if ordered. Instructions given.

___If dressing on extremity is "too tight" and swelling occurs, or discoloration, loosen and contact private physician.

___If "redness, numbness, unusual swelling" occur either in suture line or on operative extremity, contact private physician.

___Prescription given by private physician.

___Other instructions given by private physician.

___Keep dressing dry and clean. Instructions given.

___Reinforce dressing if necessary. Instructions given.

___Contact private physician if bleeding occurs. Instructions given.

___Make appointment with private physician for postoperative visit in _____

_____ (Days or Weeks)

Additional Comments:_____

_____

Signature of Discharge R.N./L.P.N._____ Date _____

I have reviewed and understand the instructions listed above:

Signature of Patient and/or Guardian_____ Date_____

FIGURE 7-6

Outpatient postsurgical instruction information
(AMI Doctors Hospital of Prince Georges County).

DISCHARGE (TRANSFER) OF PATIENTS FROM PACU

The post anesthesia care record must contain a discharge summary and transfer note. The PAN documents how the patient has met established criteria. Areas that require documentation, when applicable, include the following:

The patient's level of consciousness and degree of orientation

The patient's response to regional anesthetics, if applicable

Vital signs at discharge, and indication of pattern of stability

Cardiac rhythm(s) observed in the postanesthetic period

Status of all peripheral lines, such as amount remaining and patency

Status of surgical dressing(s) or operative area, such as drainage and swelling

Patient's level of pain perception or response to pain medication, if administered

Voiding status of the patient

Continuing care to be provided during the transfer process, for example, oxygen, cardiac monitor, traction

Mode of transfer, for example, stretcher, wheelchair, ICU bed

Patient teaching accomplished and reinforced

Time of discharge

Signature and title of PACU nurse writing the discharge summary

Name and title of the nurse on the patient's care unit who has received a verbal report on the patient's status

The PACU nurse should provide a verbal report to a nurse on the patient's assigned care unit. In addition to the information on the written transfer note, the verbal report includes the following:

Medications administered in the PACU and the patient's response to medications

Medications administered in the OR that have continuing implications for the patient's care

Equipment that must be obtained by the nursing unit for the continuing care of the patient

Interactions of the OR and PACU staff with the patient's family and significant others

Physician's orders, particularly those that have been clarified by the PAN

Any other pertinent information

Each PACU should develop written standards for documentation on the post anesthesia care record. This provides completeness and consistency and a uniform standard of care. These charting criteria also serve as the basis for an audit tool, providing quality assurance. Written standards are also a valuable teaching tool during the orientation phase of new PACU staff members, and for nursing student experiences in the PACU.

SUMMARY

Discharge criteria should be developed by each PACU to meet its own needs and standards. Several published models are available for reference. The benefits of written standards and criteria include the following:

Consistent application of quality care for all patients

Improved relations between the department of anesthesiology staff and the PACU staff

Professional application of abilities and accountability for the PAN

Fulfillment of JCAHO guidelines for discharge criteria

Available standards and retrievable data for audit purposes

SUGGESTIONS FOR FURTHER READING

Aldrete JA: Assessment of recovery from anesthesia, Curr Rev Recov Room Nurses 1(21):161, 1980.

Aldrete JA: Recovery room scorecard, AORN J 17:79, 1973.

Aldrete JA and Kroulik D: A postanesthetic recovery score. Anesth Analg 49:924, 1970.

Andrews IC: Criteria for discharge from the recovery room, Curr Rev Recov Room Nurses 2(7,8):49, 1980.

Bakutis AR: Assessing the anesthesia patient, J Am Assoc Nurs Anesth June:255, 1975.

Bushong MW: Principles of postanesthetic recovery room management: criteria for patient discharge. Curr Rev Recov Room Nurses 1(10):75, 1980.

Carignan G, Keeri-Szanto M, and Lavelee J-P: Postanesthetic scoring system, Anesthesiology 1964; 25(3):396, 1964.

Danner CA et al: Recovery scoring revisited. S Med J 66:865, 1973.

Drain CB and Christoph SB: The recovery room: a critical care approach to post anesthesia nursing, ed 2, Philadelphia, 1987, WB Saunders Co.

Dripps RD, Eckenhoff JE, and Van Dam LO: The immediate postoperative period: recovery and intensive care. In Introduction to anesthesia: the principles of safe practice, ed 6, Philadelphia, 1982, WB Saunders Co.

Figueroa M: The postanesthesia recovery score: a second look, S Med J 65(7):791, 1972.

Guidelines for recovery room care. Task Force of the Anesthesia Care Team Committee of the New York State Society of Anesthesiologists, 1983.

Hartwell PW: Discharge criteria. In Frost E, Andrews IC, editors: International anesthesiology clinics: recovery room care, Boston, 1983, Little, Brown & Co. Inc.

Holzgrafe RE: A postanesthesia recovery score, Wis Med J, p. 239, 1972.

Joint Commission for Accrediation of Health Care Organizations: Accreditation Manual for Hospitals, 1988.

Jones C: Glasgow coma scale. Am J Nurs, 1551, 1979.

Practice advisory for recovery room, American Society of Anesthesiologists, no 2, May 1978.

Schneider M: Meeting the criteria for discharge, Curr Rev Recov Room Nurses 4(6):41, 1982.

Selvin BL: Recovery room policy manual: a model, Md St Med J, Oct, 1981.

Standards of Nursing Practice, American Society of Postanesthesia Nurses, 1986.

Suggestions for a record of anesthesia care to facilitate medical audit, American Society of Anesthesiologists, October 1977.

PART II

PATIENTS WHO REQUIRE SPECIAL CONSIDERATION

CHAPTER 8

Children in the PACU

Nirmala Balan
Ingrid Hollinger

Infants and children require special attention by the post anesthesia care team because of anatomical, physiological, and psychological differences when compared with adults. Familiarity with these problems, as well as the surgical problems specific for this age group, is essential for rational management by the PACU staff.

ANATOMY

Although the difference in size is the most striking feature when comparing pediatric and adult patients, it is the difference in the anatomy of the airway that is responsible for most of the problems encountered in recovering from general anesthesia. Although the actual size and weight are much smaller, the body surface to weight ratio increases as size diminishes. The result is a much greater propensity for heat loss. There is also a difference in the relative proportion of body structures. For instance, the newborn has a relatively large head, with a small thorax and a protuberant abdomen.

AIRWAY

The anatomical configuration of the pediatric airway predisposes to upper airway obstruction and hypoventilation. The main problems are as follows:

- The head is large with a short neck.
- The tongue is relatively large.
- The epiglottis is longer and stiffer, U-shaped, and located higher.
- The larynx is located approximately one vertebral body higher at approximately the interspace between the third and fourth cervical vertebrae when compared with the adult, and the glottis is tilted cephalad posteriorly.
- The airway is small in diameter, with the narrowest area at the cricoid ring; minimal mucosal swelling can critically decrease diameter and increase airway resistance.
- The thorax is narrow and compliant, leading to a reduction in functional residual capacity.
- The diaphragm is the major muscle of respiration; any increase in the size of the abdominal contents or in intraabdominal pressure may readily lead to ventilatory embarassment.
- Muscle tone is poorly developed, and accessory muscles may be unable to stabilize the airway.

PHYSIOLOGICAL DIFFERENCES
Cardiovascular System

The cardiovascular system is not fully matured in the infant. The heart contains less contractile elements, and cardiac output is rate dependent. The sympathetic innervation is also incomplete, predisposing to exaggerated vagal responses. Cardiac output under basal conditions is, however, twice that of an adult because of high energy demands. Because of the heart rate dependency of cardiac output, bradycardia is more worrisome than tachycardia. The neonate has an average heart rate of 120 to 140 beats per minute, which progressively decreases to 80 beats per minute by 12 years of age. At birth, the right ventricle is larger than the left ventricle, with greater wall thickness, but by 6 months of age, the adult ratio of ventricular size is reached. Blood pressure measurement is especially important in children because it has been shown to correlate well with the circulating blood volume. Because the heart rate response to hypovolemia is unpredictable, it is necessary to rely on blood pressure as a guide to the adequacy of intravascular volume. The blood volume in children is relatively larger when based on body weight (Table 8-1).

TABLE 8-1

Comparisons of blood volume based on weight in children and adults

Newborn	85 ml/kg
Infant (12 months)	80 ml/kg
Child (1-12 years)	75 ml/kg
Adult	65 ml/kg

Respiratory System

The thoracic cage of a newborn is small, with horizontally placed ribs, which limit expansion. The motion of the highly placed diaphragm is easily restricted by any increase in the volume of the abdominal contents or increases in intraabdominal pressure. Several other differences in respiratory parameters exist (Table 8-2).

The large body surface to weight ratio results in increased oxygen consumption to maintain normal body temperature and increased minute ventilation requirements. Both predispose the pediatric patient to the ready development of hypoxemia. Although the chest wall is compliant, the compliance of the lung itself is only one-tenth to one-twentieth that of an adult. The lung contains only about 8% of the adult alveolar number at birth, and alveolar growth continues until approximately 8 years of age. Large airways contribute 80% of the total airway resistance in adults, whereas small airways contribute a large fraction of total airway resistance in patients younger than 5 years. Thus the signs and symptoms of small airway disease (bronchiolitis) are marked in children. The tidal volume is the same in both children and adults (6 to 7 ml/kg), but the respiratory rate is higher in children. The alveolar ventilation of the newborn is twice that of the adult (V_a expressed as ml/kg per minute is 60 in adults and 100 to 150 in a newborn). The closing volume is increased and is above functional residual capacity

TABLE 8-2

Differences in respiratory parameters between adults and neonates

	Adult	Neonate
Respiratory rate (per minute)	20	40
Tidal volume (ml/kg)	6-7	6-7
Alveolar ventilation (ml/kg/min)	60	100-150
Dead space (ml/kg)	2.2	2.2
FRC (ml/kg)	34	34
PaO_2 mm Hg	80-100	60-80
$PaCO_2$ mm Hg	38-40	32-35
pH	7.38	7.38

FRC, Functional residual capacity.

until about 6 years of age, contributing to the development of hypoxemia.

Kidneys

The differences in renal function include the following:

1. Glomerular filtration rate is reduced at birth because of an increased resistance of afferent renal arteries resulting in inability to secrete large volume loads rapidly; the permeability of the glomerular capillaries is also decreased.
2. Glomerulotubular imbalance exists secondary to a more rapid development of the glomeruli as compared with the proximal tubule.
3. The concentrating power of urine is reduced in neonates to approximately half of adult values: urine specific gravity of 1.025 compares with 1.040 in adults; this impairs the neonatal compensatory mechanisms in the face of dehydration.
4. Neonates are obligatory sodium losers, which means that they are unable to conserve sodium.

These functional limitations are most marked during the first 4 to 6 weeks of life, after which time renal function is 80% to 90% of that in the adult.

The rate of fluid metabolism is 2 to 3 times faster in infants than in adults. Thus after 24 hours of starvation, an adult loses 4% of his body weight, whereas a newborn loses 10%. The metabolic rate for oxygen utilization is higher also in children. The basal oxygen requirement in infancy is 6 ml/kg per minute, whereas it is 3 to 4 ml/kg per minute in adults. In addition, the infant has only small glycogen stores, which, combined with the high metabolic demand, predisposes to the development of metabolic acidosis and hypoglycemia.

Temperature Regulation

Infants, particularly exprematures, are susceptible to developing hypothermia for the following reasons:

- They have a large body surface area relative to body weight: the body weight of a full-term newborn is 5% that of an adult's, but the body surface area is 15%.

TABLE 8-3	
Recommended environmental temperatures for various ages	
Premature or neonate	27° C
Infant 1-6 months	26° C
6 months-2 years	25° C

- The subcutaneous fat is thin, leading to a fourfold increase in core conductance in an infant.
- They have a higher metabolic rate.
- The hypothalmic temperature control center is immature.
- Infants depend on nonshivering thermogenesis as a source of heat production in response to cold; metabolism of this fat is stimulated by norepinephrine and occurs only with adequate levels of oxygen—that is, hypoxia will prevent this response to cold. Nonshivering thermogenesis is less efficient in producing heat than a shivering response and results in metabolic acidosis.

To avoid the metabolic stress of temperature maintenance, it is important that not only core but also skin temperature is maintained. A decrease in skin temperature will increase an infant's oxygen consumption and may result in metabolic acidosis even without a fall in core temperature. Recommended environmental temperatures for various ages are listed in Table 8-3. The use of overhead infrared lamps can mitigate the affects of a cool environment to a large extent.

Central Nervous System (CNS)

Inadequate neurological function causes instability of respiration and muscular activity. However, the minimum alveolar concentration (MAC) of inhalational anesthetics is higher in children, which means that more drug is required to achieve the same depth of anesthesia. Emergence is rapid because of the high fraction of minute ventilation to FRC. The increased permeability of the blood-brain barrier and the lack of myelination lead to accumulation of drugs, such as barbiturates, in higher concentration in the CNS in children than in adults. Despite this, higher doses of all anesthetic agents are required for pediatric patients except during the newborn period.

Autonomic Nervous System

Parasympathetic and α-sympathetic innervation occurs earlier in gestation than β-sympathetic innervation, which is incomplete at birth and continues to develop in early life. The infant responds to hypoxemia and shock by bradycardia caused by vagal preponderance rather than by the initial tachycardia seen in adults. The adrenals, although oversized at birth, have little functional activity. It has been shown that norepinephrine plays a more important role than epinephrine in neonatal life and that the norepinephrine is produced solely by the organs of Zuckerkandl along the sympathetic chain.

Fluid and Electrolyte Metabolism

The relative size of fluid compartments differs. In the newborn, total body water and extracellular fluid volume are larger (Table 8-4). There is a gradual decrease in the proportion of the extracellular fluid volume so that by the time the child is 2 years of age, adult values are reached.

TABLE 8-4		
The percentage of body weight of fluid compartments in the newborn and adult		
Compartment	Newborn	Adult
ECF $\begin{cases} \text{Plasma volume} \\ \text{ISF} \end{cases}$	5 35	5 15
ICF	40	40
TBW	80 (2L)	60 (40L)

ECF, Extracellular fluid; ISF, Interstitial fluid; ICF, Intracellular fluid; TBW, Total body water.
TBW = ECF (plasma volume + ISF) + ICF.

Psychological Differences

The child characteristically has lack of self-control, and it is usually difficult to persuade children in the preschool age to act against their will. Induction of anesthesia and the waking-up process in the PACU are critical times. Whereas the infant less than 1 year old recovering from surgery is often satisfied with a loving hug to make him comfortable, the toddler waking up in strange surroundings requires comforting and compassionate care by the PACU staff to avoid lasting psychological sequelae. Causes of hypoxia or hypoventilation should be excluded before sedating an agitated child. Protection from self-inflicted injury during a period of disorientation is important. Presence of a parent may be the best sedative for the child.

TRANSFER TO THE PACU

The recovery process begins in the operating room when surgery and anesthesia are terminated. Transport from the operating room to the PACU is a critical period for the development of hypoxia in particular. Heart and breath sounds should be monitored with a precordial stethoscope if possible. The patient should be transported on his side to prevent airway obstruction and aspiration of gastric contents and to allow secretions to escape. The use of pulse oximetry in transport will alert the anesthesiologist to the development of hypoxemia and hypotension. On arrival in the PACU, the airway and ventilation should be rechecked. The nurse should receive a full report of events during surgery, the patient's medical problems, and any special measures to be taken. The anesthesiologist should remain with the patient until the vital signs have been taken and the patient is in stable condition and well attended.

MONITORING

The process of awakening begun in the operating room continues in the PACU, where the patient regains full consciousness and cardiopulmonary stability. In the majority of cases, the patients are retained in the PACU for a minimum of 1 hour after any general anesthetic. During this period, close observation includes monitoring of the following:

1. Pulse: rate, rhythm, and pulse volume.
2. Respiration: rate and depth, freedom from obstruction, good bilateral breath sounds on auscultation.
3. Oxygenation: in unconscious or deeply sedated patients, pulse oximetry is indicated to assess adequacy of oxygenation.
4. Blood pressure: proper width of the cuff should equal two-thirds the length of the upper arm: a narrow cuff will give an erroneously high reading; in older children who have undergone relatively simple procedures, systolic blood pressure alone may be measured by the palpatory method or by watching the bounce of the needle on the pressure gauge as the cuff is deflated; in infants, blood pressure can be measured accurately by either the Doppler or electronic ausculatory or plethysmographic methods.
5. Color of the skin.
6. Temperature.
7. Level of consciousness: awake and alert, drowsy, disoriented, or unconscious.
8. Intake (fluid and blood replacement) and output (gastric, urinary, wound drainage, or active bleeding).

RESPIRATORY COMPLICATIONS

In all children the major respiratory complications encountered in the PACU include the following:
- Airway obstruction
- Postextubation croup
- Respiratory depression
- Pulmonary aspiration
- Acute respiratory failure

Airway Obstruction

In the early postoperative period, the most frequent and serious complication is airway obstruction. Etiological factors are as follow:
- Soft tissue obstruction of the upper airway; although infants are often obligatory nasal breathers, the relatively large tongue tends to fall back and produce pharyngeal obstruction
- Enlarged tonsils and adenoids
- Laryngeal spasm
- Laryngeal edema
- Surgery of the airway or surrounding tissues

Hallmarks of airway obstruction are retractions (suprasternal, subcostal, intercostal), nasal flaring, inspiratory stridor or crowing, and decreased or absent air entry.

Obstruction of the upper airway may follow surgery for cleft palate repair, tongue resection, resection of a cystic hygroma, or tonsillectomy. Bleeding from the surgical site may lead to the development of a clot, causing complete airway obstruction. Positioning of the patient so that drainage is away from the glottis or inserting nasopharyngeal airways may ameliorate the problem. After surgical procedures in which large oozing surfaces are left behind (cleft palate), careful sedation and positioning are important to minimize bleeding from the surgical site and allow for natural clotting over the raw surface.

Airway obstruction should be relieved promptly. Arterial carbon dioxide tension ($PaCO_2$) rises 6 mm Hg during the first minute of total obstruction and then rises at a rate of 3 to 4 mm Hg per minute, along with a progressive fall in arterial oxygen tension (PaO_2) as a result of a decrease in alveolar oxygen tension. Airway obstruction caused by pharyngeal obstruction by the tongue can be effectively overcome by hyperextension of the head with anterior displacement of the mandible. If obstruction is still not relieved, a nasal or oral airway can be inserted. The nasal airway is preferred because it is better tolerated by patients. The oral airway may stimulate gagging, vomiting, and laryngospasm. Oxygen (100%) should be administered by face mask until the obstruction is relieved.

Laryngeal spasm is defined as laryngeal obstruction caused by partial or complete spasm of the intrinsic or extrinsic muscles of the larynx. Two mechanisms are in effect as follows:
- Reflex closure of the glottis is caused by a shutterlike adduction of the vocal cord; that is, it involves the intrinsic laryngeal muscles. The

resulting airway obstruction is incomplete and intermittent and occurs during inspiration or expiration. It usually occurs in response to somatic sensory stimulation, such as suctioning or the presence of an airway during light planes of anesthesia and during recovery. Treatment includes discontinuation of the stimulus and application of positive pressure with bag and mask, and administration of 100% oxygen.

- Reflex closure of the larynx is caused by a ball valve mechanism involving the extrinsic muscles and occurs in response to visceral sensory stimulation. It results in complete laryngeal obstruction. To treat the laryngeal spasm, the stimulus should be stopped or any irritant removed from the larynx, such as secretions, blood, or a long airway. Oxygen (100%) should be administered. This spasm cannot be broken by positive pressure. Forcing the chin forward by strong pressure applied behind the angles of the jaw is often an effective maneuver. A small dose of succinylcholine (10 to 20 mg) may be necessary. Respiration must then be supported by positive-pressure ventilation (for example, Ambu bag) until full muscle function has been recovered.

Postextubation Croup

Laryngeal or, more accurately, subglottic edema leads to the clinical picture of postextubation croup. Infants are more prone to postintubation complications for the following reasons (in order of decreasing importance):

1. Small size of the larynx: in the adult, 1 mm of edema produces only slight hoarseness; in the infant, the same amount of edema reduces the lumen by 75% and produces serious airway obstruction
2. Loose areolar tissue in the submucosa of the subglottic area, where edema fluid easily accumulates
3. Complete ring formed by the cricoid cartilage

The incidence of postextubation croup varies between 1% to 4% of intubated patients. It is most common in children 1 to 3 years of age. Contributory factors include the following:

- Tight-fitting endotracheal tube
- Trauma during intubation
- Long duration of intubation (more than 48 hours)
- Movement of the head and therefore of the endotracheal tube during positive-pressure ventilation
- Surgery of the head or neck, or bronchoscopy
- Concomitant airway infection
- Hypotension
- Anticoagulant therapy

Symptoms of postextubation croup usually occur within 30 minutes after extubation, peak at 6 to 8 hours, and usually subside in the next 24 hours. The diagnosis is made on the basis of stridor, thoracic retraction, hoarseness, crouplike cough, and varying degrees of respiratory obstruction.

Treatment includes the following:

1. Upright position
2. Cool, humidified oxygen
3. Inhalation of racemic epinephrine (in a 1:8 proportion; the 2.25% solution is diluted with distilled water or saline to reach a volume of 4 ml; for older children, a 1:4 dilution is used). it is administered by nebulization for 15 minutes

If symptoms cannot be controlled with inhalation every 30 minutes, if hypoventilation with rising $PaCO_2$ occurs, or if the patient appears obtunded, reintubation is necessary to stabilize the airway. Reintubation should be performed with an endotracheal tube at least one size smaller than the original endotracheal tube, and an auscultatory air leak should be detectable over the larynx at 25 to 30 mm H_2O airway pressure after reintubation to avoid long-term sequelae. The use of steroids for the treatment of postextubation croup remains controversial. The drug and dosage most commonly recommended is dexamethasone 0.2 to 0.5 mg/kg.

Respiratory Depression

Respiratory depression in the PACU may occur for a variety of reasons. The most common are the following:

- Residual anesthetic effect. All inhalational agents are respiratory depressants. Barbiturates produce depression of both tidal volume and respiratory rate. Narcotic overdosage shows marked pupillary constriction and a slow rate of respiration with full tidal exchange. Narcotics, particularly morphine, are more potent in infants when given on a weight basis than in older children or adults.
- Residual neuromuscular blockade caused by inadequate reversal of muscle relaxants administered intraoperatively. Insufficient reversal of neuromuscular function may lead to fatigue and respiratory failure. The neuromuscular junction is immature in the infant, and adequacy of reversal should be assessed by the use of a nerve stimulator.
- Preexisting pulmonary disease.

Treatment of respiratory depression involves the following:

1. Stir-up regimen by the PACU personnel stimulates spontaneous respiration and is often sufficient. This involves verbal and tactile stimulation.
2. Naloxone (Narcan) may be used to reverse narcotic-induced respiratory depression. It is a pure narcotic antagonist and acts by competitive inhibition. Its duration of action is short-lived (30 to 60 minutes) and, hence, respiratory depression may recur. Thus patients must be observed closely, or an intravenous dose of naloxone must be followed by an intramuscular dose to provide a longer-lasting effect.
3. Residual muscle relaxant may be reversed with an anticholinesterase and anticholinergic combination.
4. Controlled ventilation may be indicated to maintain a normal $PaCO_2$ and to enhance the excretion of inhalational anesthetics by increasing alveolar ventilation.

Pulmonary Aspiration

Factors that make the infant more vulnerable to regurgitation and aspiration include the following:

- The resting intragastric pressure may be higher in infants than in adults because of (1) the rel-

atively small size of the stomach, (2) excessive air swallowing during crying, (3) encroachment of other abdominal organs, and (4) strenuous diaphragmatic breathing.
- Short esophagus.
- Relaxation of the gastroesophageal junction; regurgitation after feeding is considered normal during the first 6 months of life.
- Cough reflex may not be well developed.
- Incoordination of breathing and swallowing mechanisms may occur in premature and dyspneic infants.
- Atropine relaxes the tone of the esophageal-gastric junction.

Anesthetic deaths for the pediatric age group are 2 to 3.3 per 10,000 anesthetics. Of these deaths, 26% are the result of aspiration of vomitus and blood.

Acid aspiration produces a chemical burn of the lungs. The critical gastric pH and volume necessary for the development of this lesion are a pH of less than 2.5 and a volume of 0.4 ml/kg (25 ml for the average adult patient). Particulate food stuff aspiration or a high bacterial count of the aspirated material, such as from bowel obstruction, may produce lethal results, regardless of the pH.

The diagnosis is made on the basis of tachypnea, dyspnea, bronchospasm, cyanosis, shock, and pulmonary edema. Arterial blood gases reveal hypoxemia, initial hypocapnia secondary to tachypnea, and later hypercapnia caused by increased work of breathing. The arterial pH may be decreased because of respiratory or metabolic acidosis. Chest x-ray examination reveals irregular, mottled densities, but changes may not be apparent until at least 8 hours later, typically involving the apical segment of the right lower lobe when aspiration occurs in the supine position.

Treatment is as follows:

1. Position the patient with a head-down tilt, with the head turned to one side to aid drainage of gastric contents.
2. Suction the mouth and oropharynx to remove residual material.
3. Administer 100% oxygen by face mask.
4. Intubate the trachea if the patient is not alert and cooperative.

5. Perform arterial blood gas analysis and obtain a chest x-ray.
6. Apply continuous positive airway pressure (CPAP) to increase FRC and improve ventilation-perfusion ratios.
7. Support the cardiovascular system and the acid-base balance as necessary.
8. Steroids are no longer recommended because studies have not shown improved survival.
9. Prophylactic antibiotics are advocated only after aspiration of primary infected material.

Acute Respiratory Failure

Acute respiratory failure is defined as an impairment of alveolar ventilation and pulmonary gas exchange sufficient to pose an immediate threat to life. Etiological factors include the following:

- Lung disease (bronchiolitis, status asthmaticus, viral pneumonia)
- Central nervous system dysfunction (encephalitis, drug overdosage, Reye's syndrome)
- Circulatory failure (congestive heart failure)

Clinical criteria for diagnosis of acute respiratory failure in infants and children include the following:

- Severe inspiratory retractions and use of accessory muscles of respiration
- Irregular respiration or apneic spells
- Diminished or absent breath sounds on auscultation
- Decreased or absent blood pressure
- Poor skeletal muscle tone
- Decreased level of consciousness and response to painful stimuli

Physiological criteria include the following:

- Hypercapnia ($Paco_2 > 60$ mm Hg)
- Hypoxemia ($Pao_2 < 100$ mm Hg with fraction of inspired oxygen (Fio_2) = 1.0)
- Persistent and severe metabolic acidosis

The diagnosis of acute respiratory failure is made based on the finding of any three clinical and one physiological criteria.

Treatment aims are as follows:

1. Improve pulmonary gas exchange by administration of 100% oxygen by positive-pressure ventilation and suctioning of upper airway secretions.
2. Administration of sodium bicarbonate may be necessary to increase arterial pH to 7.2.
3. Insertion of an artificial airway is essential unless there is dramatic improvement with the above measures.

Special Circumstances
The former premature

The incidence of complications in the group of infants born prematurely and undergoing anesthesia and surgery within the first few months of life is significantly higher than in full-term infants. All the complications seen involve the respiratory system and include the following:

Apnea
Postoperative atelectasis
Aspiration pneumonia
Extubation stridor
Excessive secretions
Coughing and cyanosis

Apnea is the most common complication and occurs most frequently in infants with a history of apnea or periodic breathing. It occurs up to 12 hours postoperatively and can be treated by manual stimulation and/or by administration of 100% oxygen by mask. The cause of the apnea is uncertain and may be related to the depressant effect of inhalation anesthetics or the depressed chemoreceptor response to hypoxia. Apnea occurring several hours after the anesthetic may be secondary to ventilatory muscle fatigue. Thus preterm infants should be carefully and closely observed for 24 hours postoperatively with an apnea monitor. The period at risk does not appear to extend beyond the fiftieth week of postconceptual age.

Sleep apnea

Sleep apnea syndromes occur not infrequently in young, overweight males. Frequently these children have undergone tonsillectomy. Use of long-acting hypnotics and analgesics may result in prolonged apnea in the postoperative period even after relief of the obstructive component. Patients who exhibited preopative hypoxemia may develop postoperative apnea in the presence of uncontrolled inspired oxygen concentrations, since ventilatory control remains abnormal for weeks. Ventilation should be controlled. At the end of the operative procedure, the residual effects of neuromuscular blocking agents should be reversed and the patient completely awakened before the endotracheal tube is removed. Nasopharyngeal airways inserted by the surgeon should be maintained for 24 hours after nasopharyngeal surgery. All patients require intensive monitoring for apnea in the 48 hours after surgery. Only if apnea or obstruction does not occur during sleep postoperatively may patients be discharged to their hospital room. These patients are not good candidates for ambulatory surgery.

RESPIRATORY SUPPORT

Endotracheal Intubation in Children
Size

The optimal size of endotracheal tube is one that passes easily through the glottic and subglottic regions and produces a small leak of gas around the tube at 25 to 30 cm of water peak inspiratory pressure. The formula for calculation of the size of endotracheal tube is:

$$\text{Internal diameter (mm)} = \frac{\text{age (years)}}{4} + 4$$

This formula is for uncuffed endotracheal tubes and is applicable for children older than 2 years. A few patients will require an endotracheal tube that is smaller or larger.

Cuffed endotracheal tubes should not be used in children younger than 7 to 8 years, since they reduce the size of the lumen, thereby increasing airway resistance and putting pressure on the delicate tracheal mucosa, thus increasing the incidence of subglottic damage. The correct size of a cuffed endotracheal tube is 0.5 mm internal diameter less than that calculated by the above formula.

Composition

The composition of endotracheal tubes is important. Toxic substances form on gamma ray steril-

ized PVC (polyvinyl chloride) tubes after resterilization with ethylene oxide. The clear, polyvinyl disposable tubes that have been tissue implant-tested (ANSI Z 79) are the most satisfactory ones for general use.

Laryngoscope

Miller zero blade (straight) is used for newborns and Miller one blade for larger infants. For older chidren, a Wis Foregger blade is preferable because the flange is wide, improving visibility. Macintosh curved blades are suitable for children older than 3 years.

PAIN AND AGITATION
Pain

Postoperative pain is a very common problem, the consequences of which are the following:

   Agitation
   Hypertension
   Hypoventilation as a result of splinting of abdominal muscles
   Hypoxemia secondary to hypoventilation and atelectasis

Factors that influence the incidence and severity of pain are the following:

- Age—pain appreciation is less at extremes of age.
- Psychological factors, including the personality traits of the patient and the degree of anxiety and apprehension before the operation—adequate preoperative preparation of the patient about postoperative pain has been shown to decrease significantly the requirement for morphine in the postoperative period.
- Site of operation—in children, pain is more severe after perineal and orthopedic operations.
- Anesthetic techniques—inhalation anesthetics have no analgesic properties and may lead to a stormy recovery; if no narcotics have been administered preoperatively or intraoperatively, early use of narcotics in the postoperative period is necessary; the use of a narcotic as a premedicant delays the first postoperative re-

TABLE 8-5

Dosages of drugs commonly used for children in the PACU

Drug	Common dosage
Analgesics	
Morphine sulfate	0.05 to 0.1 mg/kg IM (maximum = 10 mg)
Meperidine hydrochloride (Demerol)	1.0 to 1.5 mg/kg IM (maximum = 100 mg)
Codeine phosphate	1.0 to 1.5 mg/kg IM (maximum = 60 mg)
Acetaminophen (Tylenol)	5 to 10 mg/kg orally or rectally
Acetysalicylic acid (aspirin)	60 mg/year of age orally or rectally
Sedatives	
Diazepam (Valium)	0.1 to 0.2 mg/kg IV or orally
Droperidol	0.05 to 0.1 mg/kg IM or IV
Pentobarbital (Nembutal)	2 to 5 mg/kg orally or IM
Secobarbital (Seconal)	2 to 4 mg/kg orally or IM
Others	
Atropine	0.02 mg/kg (maximum = 0.6 mg)
Lidocaine	1 mg/kg
Epinephrine	10 μg/kg or 0.1 ml/kg of 1:10,000 solution
Dopamine	1 to 10 μg/kg/min (maximum = 50 μg/kg/min)
Isoproterenol (Isuprel) infusion	1 μg/kg/min
Propranolol (Inderal)	0.05 to 0.1 mg/kg
Calcium chloride	10 to 20 mg/kg
Sodium bicarbonate	1 to 2 mEq/kg
Furosemide (Lasix)	0.5 to 1.0 mg/kg
Naloxone hydrochloride (Narcan)	5 μg/kg

quest for pain medication, whereas preoperative medication with barbiturates appears to worsen postoperative pain, especially after short procedures.

Both pain and anxiety are more easily prevented by medication than controlled after their onset. Thus it is recommended that narcotics be given preoperatively or intraoperatively to ease the early pain and anxiety on awakening.

1. Narcotics provide excellent analgesia and control excitement. It is preferable to use the intravenous route of administration because this provides more rapid and effective pain relief, enables titration of smaller doses of the drug, and is painless compared with intramuscular administration. The first postoperative dose should be reduced by one-half the regular dose, and the drug should be readministered only if needed, rather than on a regular dosage schedule. Patients should be carefully observed for the side effects of narcotics, including dose-dependent respiratory depression, excessive sedation, nausea, and vomiting. The presence of pain does not prevent narcotic-induced respiratory depression. It is prudent to avoid narcotics in patients who weigh less than 10 kg, for fear of profound depression.

2. Regional blocks of the surgical area (inguinal nerve block, dorsal penile block, intercostal block) given before emergence from anesthesia will result in significant pain relief and reduction of postoperative restlessness and crying. Caudal analgesia is one of the most frequently performed blocks to reduce the postoperative pain of circumcision, hypospadias repair, and orchiopexy. It is relatively simple to perform and provides good analgesia, without delaying discharge from the ambulatory surgery unit.

3. In children older than 8 years, patient-controlled analgesia (PCA) may be used, resulting in excellent pain relief without depression.

4. For major thoracic or abdominal procedures, epidural morphine (0.1 mg/kg) can be used even in small children to provide long-lasting

postoperative pain relief. These children, however, require monitoring for late respiratory depression.

Agitation

Postoperative excitement is a fairly common problem in pediatric patients, particularly in the 3 to 9 year age group. The patient may awaken from anesthesia in a violent and agitated state. The etiology is multifactorial and is as follows:

- Drug response is a frequent cause of excitement. Barbiturates may lead to postoperative restlessness and may make some children wild and uncontrollable, especially in response to pain. This reaction is seen more commonly in the PACU if the patient has not been given narcotics at the end of the operation. Anticholinergics also increase the incidence of postoperative excitement and may lead to emergence delirium, an effect seen more with scopolamine than with atropine. After ketamine anesthesia, hyperactivity may be prolonged. Halogenated agents have also been related to awakening delirium, with significantly greater excitement after enflurane than halothane anesthesia.
- Pain.
- Hypoxemia.
- Hypercarbia.
- Gastric distension.
- Urinary retention with bladder distension.
- Separation anxiety from parents and waking up in a strange room puts an appreciable emotional strain on a child.

Treatment involves the following:

1. Before giving narcotics, ascertain the adequacy of ventilation and exclude hypoxemia.
2. Relieve gastric or urinary distension.
3. Relieve pain with analgesics (Table 8-5). Prevent pain by judicious application of local anesthetics before emergence.
4. Control continued excitement by simple measures, such as the parent's presence at the patient's bedside.
5. Control anxiety with small doses of a benzodiazepine (diazapam, midazolam).

TEMPERATURE REGULATION
Hypothermia

Infants are more likely than adults to develop hypothermia for reasons mentioned earlier. The effects of hypothermia (35° C) include the following:

Increased oxygen consumption (to reverse a 1° C fall in temperature, metabolic rate increases by 10%).

Hypoxemia may develop because of the increased oxygen consumption if supplemental oxygen is not given.

Anaerobic glycolysis occurs secondary to hypoxia, which dissipates glycogen 20 times faster than aerobic glycolysis. Thus hypoglycemia may develop.

Increased lactic acid production and metabolic acidosis may develop because of the anaerobic glycolysis and poor tissue perfusion secondary to the vasoconstriction produced by cold.

Dysrhythmias.

Irregularity of respiration and apnea.

Pulmonary vasocontriction, leading to right-to-left shunting of blood through the foramen ovale and ductus arteriosus.

Increased viscosity of blood.

Hypocalcemia.

Delayed anesthetic arousal.

Increased morbidity and mortality in the postoperative period.

Hypothermia treatment is as follows:

1. Monitor body temperature.
2. Provide supplemental oxygen.
3. Cover the patient with warmed blankets, wrap the extremities with cotton, and cover the head with a Stockinette cap.
4. Use a warming mattress for children weighing less than 10 kg.
5. Use overhead infrared lamps.
6. Warm intravenous fluids before administration.

Hyperthermia

Etiological factors related to hyperthermia are as follows:

- Elevated ambient temperature
- Dehydration

- Carbon dioxide retention
- Preexisting infection and fever
- Bacteremia, especially after urinary tract operations
- Transfusion reaction
- Atropine—temperature elevation secondary to atropine has been difficult to document
- Malignant hyperthermia

Fever increases oxygen consumption and carbon dioxide production, stimulates the cardiorespiratory system, and causes metabolic and respiratory acidosis. If uncorrected, convulsions, hypoxic brain damage, arterial hypotension, and cardiac arrest may occur. To treat the patient the following measures should be taken:

1. Cool the room.
2. Uncover the patient as much as possible.
3. Apply ice bags to the neck, groin, and axillae.
4. Infuse cold intravenous fluids.
5. Administer antipyretic agents, such as aspirin, acetaminophen, or chlorpromazine.

Malignant hyperthermia

Malignant hyperthermia is a syndrome of hypermetabolism, both aerobic and anaerobic, resulting in an intense production of heat, carbon dioxide, and lactate, and generally accompanied by tachycardia and other signs of circulatory and metabolic stress.

The defect in malignant hyperthermia appears to be an abrupt loss of control of intracellular calcium levels, resulting in a rise of sarcoplasmic calcium. The consequences of the increased calcium levels are the following:

Glycolysis secondary to activation of phosphorylase kinase

Hydrolysis of adenosine triphosphate (ATP) to adenosine diphosphate (ADP) as a result of activation of myosin adenosine triphosphatase (ATPase)

Troponin inhibition, leading to muscle contraction

Membrane instability

Possible uncoupling of oxidative phosphorylation

The incidence of malignant hyperthermia is 1 per

15,000 anesthetics in children and 1 per 50,000 anesthetics in adults.

Diagnosis is based on unexplained tachycardia; dysrhythmias; generalized rigidity and masseter spasm; hyperventilation; flushing, sweating, and skin mottling; cyanosis; unstable blood pressure; hyperthermia; and cardiac arrest.

To treat malignant hyperthermia the following measures should be taken:

1. Call for help.
2. Change the breathing tubing from the oxygen supply.
3. Hyperventilate with 100% oxygen at 3 times the normal minute ventilation.
4. Apply external and internal cooling measures.
5. Give sodium bicarbonate, 2 to 4 mEq/kg, titrated by monitoring of arterial blood gases and pH.
6. Maintain intravascular volume; administer iced saline at 2 to 8 ml/kg per hour.
7. Maintain urinary output at 2 ml/kg per hour with fluid infusion, furosemide (1mg/kg), and mannitol (1g/kg).
8. To treat dysrythmias occurring during the acute episode, give procainamide.
9. Give dantrolene sodium 1 to 10 mg/kg, up to a maximum total dose of 300 mg; the average recommended dose is 3 mg/kg, which may be repeated every 5 to 10 minutes.
10. Monitor vital signs, electrocardiogram, temperature, arterial blood gases, urinary output, and central venous pressure.
11. Send blood and urine specimens for serum electrolytes, enzymes (CPK, LDH, SGOT, aldolase), blood sugar, urea, creatinine, lactate, pyruvate, clotting studies, and urinary hemoglobin and myoglobins.
12. Avoid calcium salts, cardiac glycosides, vasopressors, and lidocaine.

FLUID MANAGEMENT

The physiological differences in body fluid compartments, limited renal function, a higher metabolic rate, and an increased incidence of vomiting influence fluid therapy in infants and children. Fluid management falls into three categories as follows:

1. Maintenance fluid requirement: estimated fluid requirement (EFR) and estimated fluid deficit (EFD)
2. Replacement fluid therapy (third-space loss and vomitus)
3. Blood replacement

Maintenance Fluid Requirement

The aim is to provide replacement of insensible fluid losses, which includes evaporative losses through the respiratory tract to humidify the inspired gas, insensible cutaneous loss, and the minimal urine volume necessary to excrete the normal solute load of the kidney.

Type of fluids

Because these losses are essentially sodium-free, maintenance fluids should be hypotonic with respect to their sodium concentration. A suitable maintenance fluid is a solution of 5% dextrose in 0.25% saline. The solution should contain glucose to provide energy, prevent depletion of glycogen in the liver, prevent ketosis, and spare endogenous proteins. Five grams of glucose per 100 calories expended is the standard amount of glucose given for intravenous support.

Amount

EFR may be calculated on the basis of the following:

Body weight
Body surface area
Estimated metabolic rate or caloric expenditure (the most accurate method)

The following is a formula for pediatric fluid therapy based on caloric expenditure, arrived at indirectly by relating weight to caloric expenditure.

$$EFD = EFR \times \text{number of hours fasted}$$

Information in the chart should indicate the number of fasting hours; one half of this deficit is replaced in the first hour with a maintenance fluid but should not exceed 10 ml/kg per hour to avoid an excessive glucose load. With large fluid deficits, non–glucose-containing solutions are necessary to avoid hyperglycemia with glucosuria. The other half is replaced as a quarter each in the second and third hours after the intravenous infusion is started. Much of this replacement should be completed intraoperatively.

Replacement Fluid Therapy

The purpose of replacement fluids as opposed to maintenance fluids is to correct body fluid deficits caused by external losses (vomiting, nasogastric suction) or internal sequestration (burns, loss into the bowel wall and lumen in intestinal obstruction). These losses usually cease 3 to 5 days after injury.

Type of fluids

Third-space fluid is derived initially from the plasma volume, which in turn is replenished from the interstitial fluid. Thus this fluid loss is nearly isotonic, and suitable replacement fluids include lactated Ringer's solution, normal saline, and Normosol.

The amount of third-space loss and therefore the amount of replacement required depend on the severity of trauma, but large amounts may be required to maintain blood pressure and urine output (Table 8-6). A minimal urine output of 0.5 to 1 ml/kg per hour should be maintained under any circumstances.

TABLE 8-6	
Estimate of amount of third-space loss based on type of surgery performed	
Surgery	**Third-space loss**
Minimal surgical trauma (hernia repair)	1 to 2 ml/kg/hour
Moderate surgical trauma (pyloromyotomy)	2 to 4 ml/kg/hour
Major surgical trauma (bowel resection)	4 to 6 ml/kg/hour

Blood Replacement

The allowable whole blood loss in pediatric surgical patients is calculated to attain a final postoperative hematocrit of not less than 30% for infants and children and 40% for prematures and newborns (see box below).

$$EBV = wt \text{ in } kg \times y \text{ ml/kg}$$
$$\text{where } y = 85 \text{ for newborn, 80 if 6 months,}$$
$$75 \text{ if 12 years.}$$

$$ERCM = EBV \times \frac{Hct\ (A)}{100}$$

$$ERCM_{30} = EBV \times \frac{30(B)}{100}$$

$$ARCL = (A) - (B)$$

$$AWBL = (A) - (B) \times 3$$

EBV, Estimated blood volume
ERCM, Estimated red cell mass (depends on patient's preoperative hematocrit)
$ERCM_{30}$, Estimated red cell mass at a hematocrit of 30%
ARCL, Allowable red cell loss
AWBL, Allowable whole blood loss

The assumption is that blood loss is occurring at a hematocrit of 30%. For practical purposes:

Amount of blood loss	Therapy
Blood loss is less than one third of AWBL	Lactated Ringer's solution
Blood loss is more than one third but less than total AWBL	Colloid, preferably 5% albumin
Blood loss is equal to or more than AWBL	Blood

When replacing blood loss with isotonic electrolytes solution, each milliliter of blood must be replaced with 3 ml of crystalloid, since the latter is redistributed to the interstitial fluid volume as well.

VOMITING

Vomiting is a common and unpleasant sequel of general anesthetics in children. It is more common after certain procedures, particularly strabismus repair. Vomiting is more common in the presence of surgical pain. Severe vomiting may preclude patients' discharge after a planned outpatient surgery and in the early stages of recovery may lead to aspiration and development of aspiration pneumonitis. Unconscious patients should be positioned on their sides to prevent aspiration if vomiting should occur. Administration of droperidol intravenously (0.075 mg/kg) during surgery significantly lowers the incidence of postoperative vomiting. Droperidol may be given in the PACU in case of vomiting but is less effective under these circumstances. Children undergoing surgical procedures as outpatients cannot be discharged home unless able to tolerate oral feeding.

DRUG DOSAGES

Response to drugs is different in children than in adults. Some of the reasons for these observed differences are the following:

There are differences in body fluid compartments (larger total body water and larger extracellular fluid volume) that affect the apparent volume of distribution of drugs, resulting in lower plasma concentrations.

The gastric pH is higher, reaching adult levels by 2 years of age; this relatively higher pH results in a better absorption of orally administered drugs (for example, ampicillin).

Gastric emptying time is longer in infancy and reaches normal adult values by 6 to 8 months of age, which may slow the absorption of drugs such as acetaminophen.

Infants have a decreased plasma protein concentration, resulting in a higher serum concentration, resulting in a higher serum concentration of unbound drugs and a narrower therapeutic range; the protein binding of drugs reaches adult levels by 1 year of age.

The increased permeability of the blood-brain barrier and the lack of myelination in neonates allow drugs such as phenobarbital to accumulate in the central nervous system in concentrations 20% to 100% higher than in adults.

Pathways for drug biotransformation are immature in infants younger than 3 months, prolonging the half-life of drugs and increasing their sensitivity to drugs such as morphine.

Reduction in renal clearance may also lead to an altered response to drugs in infants (for example, increased susceptibility to ampicillin toxicity).

Larger doses of sedatives are required during childhood because of the higher metabolic rate.

Barbiturates and narcotics are more potent in neonates than in adults because not only does more drug enter the central nervous system, but there is an increased sensitivity to the drugs themselves and decreased metabolism and excretion.

Two formulas for pediatric drug dosages have been described:

Formula 1 is derived on the basis of age, weight, and body surface area (Clark formula):

$$\text{Child dose} = \frac{\text{child's weight (pounds)} \times \text{adult dose}}{150}$$

Formula 2 is calculated from the body surface area rule:

$$\text{Child dose} = \frac{\text{body surface area (m}^2) \times \text{adult dose}}{1.7}$$

Dosages of commonly prescribed drugs are listed in Table 8-5.

It is important to note that, although not a drug, the defibrillation dose in a child should be calculated at 2 watt-sec/kg.

SPECIAL SITUATIONS
Plastic Surgery

Children undergo plastic surgery to correct congenital anomalies and acquired lesions, such as burn scars and contractures. The points to be remembered are the following:

Other defects should be suspected in the presence of one congenital anomaly.

If the child has congenital heart disease, antibiotics should be given perioperatively for prophylaxis against infective endocarditis.

The potential for preexisting airway problems in these patients is high; in addition, the head and neck are common sites for reconstructive surgery, which impose further problems of airway management.

It is essential that emergence from anesthesia be quiet and smooth to lessen the risk of damage to grafted areas and delicately sutured repairs.

Cleft lip and palate

The incidence is 1 per 1000 live births. Associated anomalies include the following:

Congenital heart disease

Subglottic stenosis

Pierre Robin's syndrome (micrognathia, glossoptosis, high arched palate, congenital heart disease)

Treacher Collins' syndrome (malar and mandibular hypoplasia, microstomia, choanal atresia, congenital heart disease)

Cleft lip repair is usually performed at 10 to 12 weeks of age. The recovery phase is the most critical period and involves several potential problems.

Airway obstruction is the primary problem postoperatively. The patient should be extubated awake. At the end of the operation, a long silk stitch is placed deep in the tissue of the tongue. Pulling on this traction suture is a very effective means of maintaining an adequare airway after extubation; additionally, it provides a stimulus for the patient to breathe.

Restlessness is common. To prevent damage to the repaired area, the infant should be restrained. The use of jackets with sleeves splinted to prevent elbow flexion is helpful in keeping the patient's hands away from his face. The Logan bow is used by some plastic surgeons for protection and relief of tension.

Cleft palate repair is usually performed at 18 to 24 months of age. This repair is more tedious than repair of a cleft lip and involves more blood loss during and after surgery. Blood pools in dependent areas, such as the hypopharynx and trachea. Postoperatively, the patient should be cared for in a croup tent and in the prone position to prevent aspiration of blood. The child should be restrained and observed closely for blood loss. Because large areas of raw surface are left behind in these repairs, it is important that these children remain quiet in the first few hours postoperatively to prevent excessive oozing caused by straining and coughing. With large, obstructing pharyngeal flaps, severe airway obstruction may occur after extubation. Nasopharyngeal airways inserted by the surgeon and intensive nursing care are required for the first 24 to 48 hours until the patient has adjusted to the altered airway anatomy.

Burns

This topic is more completely covered in Chapter 14. However some special points pertain to children. We depend on the skin for thermal regulation, fluid and electrolyte homeostasis, protection against bacterial infection, as well as our own recognition as individuals. A peculiar aspect of burns is that no matter how small the area involved, there are systemic ramifications.

Estimating the percent of surface burns is done by the rule of nines: head, 9%; neck, 1%; upper extremity, 9% each; lower extremity, 18% each; anterior trunk, 18%; and posterior trunk, 18%. However, this rule is modified for children because a small child has a proportionately larger head (head, 18% in infants) and less surface area on the extremities, particularly the lower extremities, than an adult. This larger head and neck area, when burned, is more susceptible to edema formation, leading to airway obstruction. Prognosis and fluid therapy are based on knowledge of the area burned.

Anesthesia may be required for initial débridement and escharotomy, followed by skin grafts and plastic repair of burn scars and contractures. Discussion of special problems related to burned patients follows.

Fluid therapy

Fluid requirement is increased in burned patients as a result of: (1) fluid shifts secondary to changes in vascular integrity remote from the injured area; (2) evaporative fluid losses; (3) higher metabolic rate. Depending on the magnitude of the injury, the metabolic rate doubles or triples at the time of injury and remains elevated for weeks or months until the burn is healed.

A burned child may lose as much as 20% to 30% of his lean body mass; calories are lost because of evaporative and radiation losses. Thus the potential for hypovolemia and hypotension exists.

The Parkland formula for fluid resuscitation in burns is 4 ml/kg per 1% body surface area burn, up to a maximum of 50% burns. One half to two thirds of this requirement of crystalloids is given in the first 8 hours and the remainder over the rest of the first day. The aim is to give lactated Ringer's solution in sufficient quantity to maintain urinary output with a specific gravity of 1.010 to 1.020. By the second day after the burn, fluid requirement decreases as capillary integrity improves. Albumin (1 g/kg per day) should be administered to attain a serum albumin level of at least 2 g per 100 ml. Vital signs, urinary output, and central venous pressure should be monitored along with serial weights and laboratory tests (hematocrit, serum electrolytes, and albumin levels).

Airway problems

Head and neck burns may be associated with edema of lips, tongue, and the airway. Airway burns produce laryngeal and tracheal edema, the major portion of which forms within 8 hours of injury but may continue to accumulate slowly for 12 to 24 hours. Such an airway should be protected immediately, if only for prophylactic reasons. Increasing edema in the first few hours may make intubation hazardous, if not impossible.

Pulmonary problems

Hypoxemia may occur as a result of: (1) increased metabolic rate and oxygen consumption; (2) bronchospasm caused by inhalation of smoke, copious secretions, desquamation of the epithelium of the airways; (3) pulmonary edema caused by increased pulmonary capillary permeability; (4) atelectasis and pneumonia; (5) carboxyhemoglobin formation, which shifts the oxyhemoglobin dissociation curve to the left and therefore decreases oxygen availability.

Psychological problems

These problems stem from both the disfiguring nature of the injury and the need for repeated anesthetics and surgery during the prolonged phase of therapy.

Pain

The pain resulting from a second-degree burn is more severe and longer lasting than pain from a full-thickness third-degree burn.

Technical problems

Intravenous sites may be difficult to secure, and a surgical cutdown may be necessary. Monitoring may also be difficult because of lack of intact sites. Blood pressure reading will usually be 20 to 30 mm Hg higher in the lower extremity than in the upper extremity.

Temperature regulation

It is impaired and, hence, measures should be undertaken to maintain body temperature and prevent hypothermia (such as the use of radiant lamps, warm fluids).

Infection

Aseptic techniques should be employed even for insertion of an intravenous cannula because of the increased susceptibility to infection.

OUTPATIENT SURGERY

Outpatient surgery has become popular in the pediatric population because it minimizes emotional disturbances, reduces the cost of treatment, and decreases the risk of nosocomial infection. Hospital-acquired upper respiratory and gastrointestinal infection may be reduced by 50% to 70% in children when operations are performed on a 1-day-stay ambulatory basis.

Factors influencing selection of patients for outpatient surgery are the following:

Physical status of the patient. Healthy patients or patients with well-controlled systemic disease (for example, bronchial asthma, epilepsy) are considered suitable candidates.

Age of the patient. All age groups may be considered suitable for outpatient surgery except the expremature infant (less than 37 weeks at birth) if less than 50 weeks postconceptual age at surgery.

Parents. The parents should be willing and capable of caring for the child after the operation. They should live within a reasonable distance from the hospital, generally no more than a 1-hour drive. They should be informed about the possibility of overnight hospitalization of the patient.

Type of operation. A variety of surgical procedures are performed on an outpatient basis and include those associated with minimal bleeding and minimal physiological derangements.

Duration of operation. Four hours is generally considered the upper limit for outpatient surgery.

Premedication should be avoided or minimal, using short-acting drugs.

Postoperative Care

Before discharge from the outpatient unit, the patient should be awake, alert, with stable vital signs, and without anesthetic or surgical complications. Various scoring systems and discharge criteria have been set up for evaluating postanesthetic recovery in ambulatory surgical units. Those for children place greater emphasis on the adequacy of motor strength and physiological functions, whereas evaluation of adults emphasizes mental acuity and driving fitness. The patient should be examined by a physician, preferably the anesthesiologist, before he is sent home in the care of an adult. The parents must be provided with written instructions for home care. Patients are usually detained for 4 hours when endotracheal anesthetic has been administered.

Complications after outpatient surgery are as follows:

- Nausea and vomiting is commoner in children than in adults and in association with certain procedures (strabismus). Whereas barbiturates are associated with minimal postoperative vomiting, narcotic premedication increases the incidence, which also appears to be directly related to the duration of anesthesia. Low-dose droperidol (0.05-0.075 mg/kg) may be useful in reducing postoperative vomiting. If oral intake of fluids becomes a problem, an antiemetic should be prescribed, such as dimenhydrinate (Dramamine) (2mg/kg intramuscularly or rectally).
- Postoperative headache occurs in 10% to 20% of patients. It occurs more commonly after use of inhalational than intravenous anesthetic agents.
- Croup.
- Sore throat is common even without endotracheal intubation.
- Loss of appetite.
- Muscle pain.
- Dizziness.
- Behavioral changes and bad dreams occur in 15% to 20% of young children hospitalized for surgery.
- Postoperative surgical bleeding.

Although this list may seem formidable, these complications have all been identified and may be minimized by careful attention to fluid replacement and careful surgical and anesthetic technique. The overall hospitalization rate secondary to these complications is less than 2%.

SUGGESTIONS FOR FURTHER READING

Berde CB, Todres ID, and Cote CJ: Recovery from anesthesia and the postoperative recovery room. In Goudsouzian N, editor: A practice of anesthesia for infants and children, Orlando, 1986, Grune & Stratton, Inc, 263-272.

Bennett EJ and Bowyer DE: Fluid balance in pediatric anesthesia. In Sumner E and Hatch D, editors: Clinics in anaesthesiology 3, Philadelphia, 1985, WB Saunders, Co, pp. 569-596.

Beyer JE and Levin CR: Issues and advances in pain control in children In Donovan M, editor: Nursing clinics of North America 22, New York, 1987, Harcourt Brace Jovanovich, Inc, pp. 661-676.

Charney JR: Postanesthesia care after pediatric surgery. In Luczum ME, editor: Handbook of postanesthesia nursing. Rockland, Md, 1987, Aspen Publishers, Inc, pp. 191-215.

Duncan A: The postoperative period in pediatric anesthesia, In Summer E and Hatch D, editors: Clinics in anesthesiology 3, Philadelphia, 1985, WB Saunders, Co, pp. 619-632.

Freeley TW: The recovery room, In Miller RD, editor: Anesthesia 3, New York, 1986, Churchill Livingstone, Inc. pp. 1921-1948.

Smith RM: Anesthesia for infants and children, ed 4, St. Louis, 1980, The CV Mosby, Co, pp. 216-228 and 587-615.

CHAPTER 9

Postoperative Care of Neurosurgical Patients

Somasundaram Thiagarajah

Commonly performed neurosurgical procedures include (1) craniotomy for removal of an intracranial tumor, clipping of cerebral aneurysm or arteriovenous fistula, and evacuation of a blood clot or an abscess; (2) cranioplasty for correction of a deformed or defective skull; (3) surgery on the vertebral column, including cervical or lumbar laminectomy, cervical osteophytes or fractures, and thoracic arteriovenous malformation and scoliosis; and (4) ventriculoperitoneal shunt, lumbar-peritoneal shunt, and placement of Omaya reservoir.

After any surgery, swelling of tissues in and around the surgical site as a result of edema formation and minimal bleeding is usual and normally has no serious sequalae. If bleeding is exessive, it is usually easily detected by observing the wound dressings or drainage tubes. But after neurosurgery, because the operative field is covered beneath a rigid cranium, not only is detection of bleeding difficult, but the increasing volume because of tissue swelling or bleeding will raise the intracranial pressure and thus decrease the blood flow to the brain, compress vital centers, or even cause herniation of the brain tissue. All of these effects adversely affect the neurological function of the patient. Furthermore, after general anesthesia, if cardiovascular and respiratory function are unstable, any hypotension, hypoxemia, or hypercapnia may decrease intracranial compliance and neurological function.

These complications in the postoperative period are amenable to therapy if detected and treated early. Therefore vigilance by trained staff in a well-equipped area is important. The quality of the outcome from the surgery depends largely on the care of these patients in the immediate postoperative period.

During transportation of the patient from the operating room to the PACU, he should be positioned 30 degrees head up (unless contraindicated, for example, after shunt procedures, lumbar laminectomy) (Figure 9-1). Breathing should be supplemented with oxygen and vital signs constantly monitored.

On the patient's arrival in the PACU, the nurse should continue oxygen administration and assess respiration; measure and record the baseline vital signs; determine serum electrolytes, hemoglobin, and arterial blood gases (ABG); and assess neurological function. The important factors to monitor in these patients are the following:

1. Neurological status
2. Intracranial pressure (ICP)

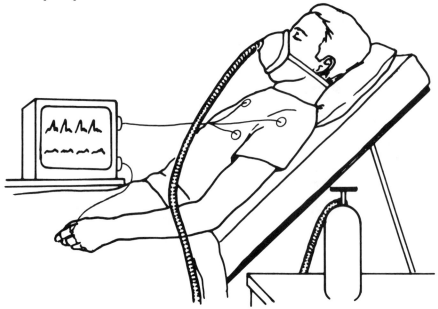

FIGURE 9-1

Transportaion of patients after craniotomy. Note the head-up position, monitoring of vital signs, and oxygen supplementation.

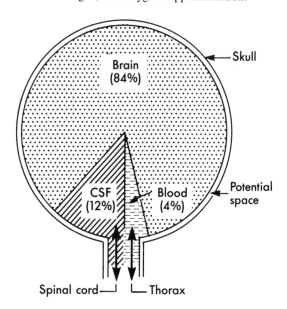

ICP 10 mm Hg

FIGURE 9-2

Intracranial contents: brain (84%); CSF (12%); and blood (4%). Communication is with CSF and blood in the thorax.

3. Respiratory system: rate, tidal volume, ABG's, and pulse oximetry
4. Cardiovascular system: blood pressure (BP), electrocardiogram (ECG), and pulse

PATHOPHYSIOLOGY

Within the rigid cranium are the following: (Figure 9-2)

- Brain tissue, 84%
- Cerebrospinal fluid (CSF), 12%
- Arterial and venous blood, 4%
- A small potential space
- Communication with the spinal column via spinal canal and with the thorax via the venous system

The normal ICP is less than 15 mm Hg. Uncompensated increase in the volumes of any of the above components will raise the ICP. Maintenance of the flow of oxygenated blood to the brain tissue is the most important factor in the care of these patients. It depends on:

Cerebral perfusion pressure (CPP) = mean BP − ICP

CAUSES OF ↑ICP

SURGICAL:

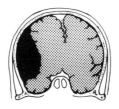 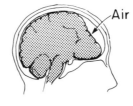 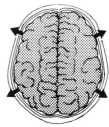

Air

Blood clot   Pneumocephalus   Edema

↑CEREBRAL BLOOD FLOW

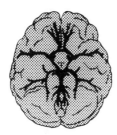

↑ BP
↑ $PaCO_2$
↓ PaO_2
Vasodilators
• Nitroprusside
• Nitroglycerine

| ↑ INTRATHORACIC PRESSURE | IMPAIRMENT OF CEREBRAL VENOUS DRAINAGE |

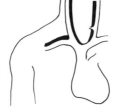

Coughing
Straining
Suctioning
PEEP

Supine
Head low
Twist neck

FIGURE 9-3
Schematic representation of the different causes of increased intracranial pressure.

where the normal range of CPP is 70 to 100 mm Hg. CPP decreases with hypotension, increased ICP, cerebral vessel spasm, and congestive heart failure.

Several pathophysiological changes may occur in the PACU and cause increased ICP (Figure 9-3).

These include the following:
1. Surgical dissection in brain substance → edema
2. Bleeding at the operative site → intracranial hematoma

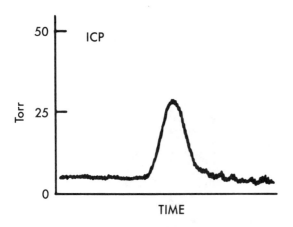

FIGURE 9-4
The ICP tracing shows the rise in the ICP when the head is lowered. On raising the head, the ICP returns to the baseline.

3. Obstruction to CSF drainage (tumor, surgical dissection, bleeding, edema)
4. Infection (intracranial or systemic)
5. Increase in cerebral blood caused by hypotension, hypercapnia, hypoxia, or cerebral vasodilation (drugs)
6. Obstruction to cerebral-venous drainage caused by increased intrathoracic pressure, coughing, suctioning, positive-pressure ventilation (PEEP), head down position (Figure 9-4)

TABLE 9-1

Glasgow coma scale

Eyes	open	spontaneously	4
		to verbal command	3
		to pain	2
		no response	1
Best motor response	to verbal command	obeys	6
	to painful stimulus	localizes pain	5
		flexion-withdrawal	4
		flexion-abnormal (decorticate rigidity)	3
		extension (decerebrate rigidity)	2
		no response	1
Best verbal response		oriented and converses	5
		disoriented and converses	4
		inappropriate words	3
		incomprehensible sounds	2
		no response	1
TOTAL			3-15

From Jennet B and Teasdale G: Aspects of coma after severe head injury, Lancet, April 23, 1977, pp. 878-881.

MONITORING

On admission to the PACU, baseline neurological function should be assessed, recorded, and retested at 15-minute intervals. In assessing neurological function, level of consciousness, motor activity, response to commands, and pupillary size, equality, and reaction to light are the usual parameters to observe. Immediately after anesthesia, pupillary size and its reaction to light may be the only parameters available. The Glasgow coma scale is used both as a prognostic indicator and as a monitor of neurological status (Table 9-1) after head trauma and in the postoperative period after craniotomy.

Deterioration in neurological function usually indicates that perfusion and oxygenation are decreasing to the brain and are either the result of decrease in BP, increase in ICP, or spasm of cerebral vessels. A common cause of postoperative deterioration is hematoma, a formation that compresses the brain tissues and increases ICP. Less common causes are cerebral edema or pneumocephalus (see Figure 9-3).

INTRACRANIAL PRESSURE

Direct monitoring of ICP in the postoperative period enables early detection of any changes in ICP before clinical manifestations on pupils, sensorium, or vital signs become evident. The immediate response, if any, to therapeutic intervention is also apparent if ICP is directly monitored.

Three systems have been described to monitor ICP: intraventricular cannulation, subarachnoid bolt, and an epidural device (Figure 9-5). These systems are connected by a transducer to a graphic recorder or an oscilloscope. Advantages of the ventricular catheter include (1) withdrawal of CSF in an emergency, (2) simple calibration, and (3) easy calculation of compliance. Disadvantages include (1) liability to infection (5%), (2) blockage of the catheter by the choroid plexus, (3) hemorrhage, and (4) difficulty in placement within ventricles compressed by edema. The subarachnoid bolt has less chance of causing bleeding, but swollen brain or blood clots can occlude the end. Focal seizures can also occur, and CSF cannot be drained. Compliance measurements are less reliable.

All systems must be closed and aseptic conditions maintained. No heparin or external pressure is required. No more than 0.1 ml of lactated Ringer's solution should be used to clear any obstruction.

For the reference point (zero point), the base of the skull or the external auditory meatus should be used. Because of the narrow range of normal values, careful calibration is important (Figure 9-5).

CT scan affords a one-time assessment of cerebral edema and is frequently used if a direct monitor has not been placed.

Patients who have increased ICP preoperatively or cerebral vasospasm or those in whom extensive surgical resection was required may develop cerebral edema, making ICP monitoring desirable.

The normal ICP tracing shows a pulsation with each heart beat and with respiration. Lundberg classified ICP values into four groups:

Normal	0-10 mm Hg
Slight increase	11-20 mm Hg
Moderate increase	21-40 mm Hg
Severe increase	>40 mm Hg

As the volume in the closed intracranial system increases, ICP remains constant as long as CSF is moved from the cranium to the spinal subarachnoid space and venous blood is displaced into the chest (Figure 9-6). However, a rapidly growing lesion

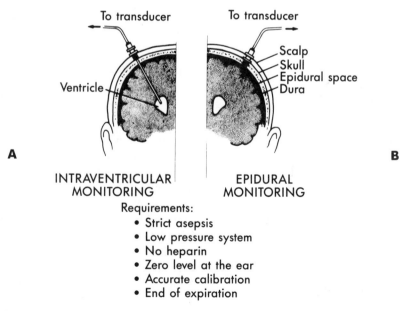

A INTRAVENTRICULAR MONITORING

B EPIDURAL MONITORING

Requirements:
- Strict asepsis
- Low pressure system
- No heparin
- Zero level at the ear
- Accurate calibration
- End of expiration

FIGURE 9-5

Commonly used clinical modes to measure intracranial pressure: **A,** Intraventricular cannulation of the anterior horn of the right ventricle. **B,** Epidural space monitor.

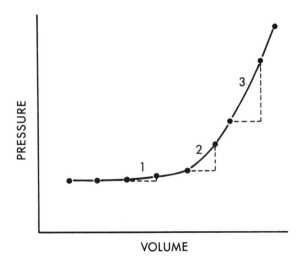

FIGURE 9-6

The classical intracranial pressure volume curve: *1,* On the flat portion of the curve any increase in the intracranial volume hardly affects the ICP. *2,* Later, a small increase in the intracranial volume produces a rise in the ICP. *3,* On reaching the steeper part of the curve, any increase in volume causes a steep increase in the ICP.

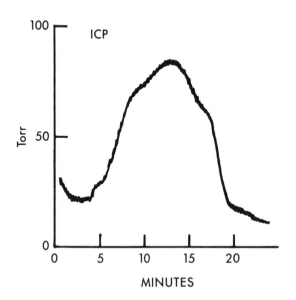

FIGURE 9-7

Type A (plateau wave).

will quickly exhaust the compensatory buffer mechanisms. As compliance decreases, a modest increase in intracranial volume produces a rise in ICP, and when the steepest part of the curve is reached, a further small increase in volume results in a massive increase in ICP. In Figure 9-6, the flat portion of the intracranial compliance curve reflects the elastic properties of the CSF space. The steep portion represents progressive loss of CSF buffering as the elastic properties of the cerebral tissue become the main buffer. Because of this exponential curve of the pressure-volume relationship, a knowledge of ICP alone cannot define the actual tightness or decrease in reserve of the intracranial space. Reserve can be assessed by eliciting the response to removing or adding 1 ml saline through the catheter. The immediate change in ICP provides an index of intracranial compliance. The amplitude of the arterial pulsation of an ICP tracing can be used also as a guide to intracranial compliance (higher peaks are associated with reduced compliance).

Sometimes neurological deterioration cannot be correlated with increasing ICP. Lesions in the medial temporal lobe and in the posterior fossa are life threatening because of their proximity to the brain stem. In the presence of such lesions, ICP may remain normal until death.

Types of Waves

Lundberg described three types of waves, designated A, B, and C waves. A waves (plateau waves) (Figure 9-7) are associated with increased ICP up to 80 mm Hg and may persist for 15 to 20 minutes. These waves indicate that the patient is nearing the limits of compensatory mechanism on the compliance curve. They may be associated with clinical signs of an acute increase in ICP and may be precipitated by several factors, such as pain, surgical stimulation, tracheal intubation, positive-pressure ventilation, or laryngoscopic examination. B waves are smaller, 20 to 25 mm Hg, occur once per minute, and are thought to be precursors of A waves. The less-sustained C waves occur at a rate of six per minute. Their significance presently is not known, although they seem to be benign.

EFFECTS OF ↑ ICP

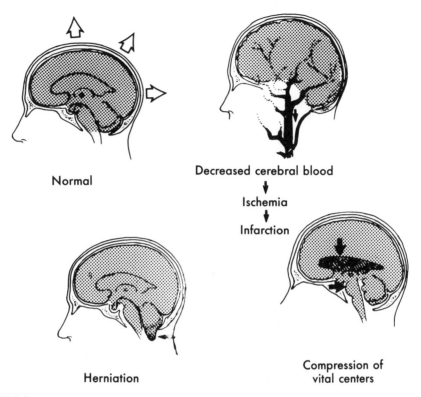

Normal

Decreased cerebral blood
↓
Ischemia
↓
Infarction

Herniation

Compression of
vital centers

FIGURE 9-8
Effects of increasing ICP. Decrease in cerebral blood flow will cause ischemia or infarction
of the brain tissue. Acute compression of the vital centers or herniation of the medulla is
catastrophic.

Effect of Rising ICP

Increasing ICP decreases blood flow to the brain,
compresses vital centers, and may cause herniation
of brain tissue (Figure 9-8). Herniation of brain tissue around the tentorium compresses the oculomotor nerve and causes dilation of the pupil on the
ipsilateral side.

Management of Increased ICP (Table 9-2)

Once an increase in ICP is suspected, the cause
should be determined after skull roentgenograms,
arterial blood gas estimations, and computed tomography scans. Hematomas require immediate
surgical evacuation. Coagulation profiles should be
recorded. Pneumocephalus can be released through
a twist drill hole. Cerebral edema is treated with
intubation, hyperventilation, and diuretics. Routine
use of steroids and/or barbiturates is highly controversial. If a ventricular drainage system has been
placed, removal of 5 to 10 ml of CSF may be life
saving. Mannitol is administered in doses of 0.5 to
2 g/kg infused over 30 minutes. The onset of action
is within 20 minutes, and the maximum effect is
seen in 1 to 2 hours.

TABLE 9-2		
Increase in ICP		
Cause	**Diagnosis**	**Treatment**
Hematoma	CT scan, coagulation profile	Surgery
Pneumocephalus	Skull x-ray, CT scan	Twist drill
Edema	CT scan, ICP monitoring	Hyperventilation, steroids, diuretics
Hypoxia and hypercapnia	Arterial blood gas	Respiratory support
Spasm of cerebral vessels	Clinical deterioration, angiogram	Hydration, maintain BP, ? vasodilators

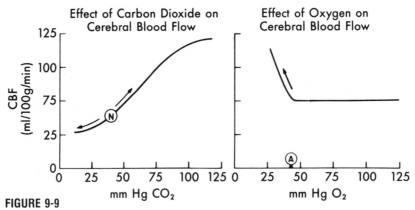

FIGURE 9-9

A, Arterial CO_2 ($Paco_2$) is a potent cerebral vasodilator. Any increase in $Paco_2$ will increase cerebral blood flow and thus the ICP. **B,** When the arterial oxygen (Pao_2) declines below 45 mm Hg (A), there is an increase in the cerebral blood flow leading to increasing ICP.

RESPIRATORY SYSTEM

Respiratory inadequacy of any degree is undesirable in this group of patients because both hypoxia and hypercapnia increase cerebral blood flow and ICP and may lead to edema formation. A rise of 1 mm Hg in arterial CO_2 increases cerebral blood flow by 4% (Figure 9-9).

Anesthetic-related causes of respiratory insufficiency in the postoperative period include the following:

1. Residual effects of relaxants, anesthetics, narcotics.
2. Diffusion hypoxemia, usually a brief period related to the use of nitrous oxide.
3. Hyperventilation hypoxemia. Intraoperative hyperventilation depletes CO_2 stores, which are replenished by spontaneous hypoventilation with concurrent development of hypoxemia.
4. Reduced functional residual capacity associated with general anesthetics.
5. Mechanical factors: shivering, secretion, atelectasis.

Neurological causes are as follows:
• Damage to vital centers
• Damage to both carotid bodies, after bilateral carotid endarterectomy

Cardiovascular and pulmonary causes are as follows:

- Heart failure; may be associated with infusion of hyperosmolar solutions like mannitol
- As postoperative sequelae of intraoperative air embolism during operations performed in the sitting position
- Neurogenic pulmonary edema after a variety of neurological conditions
- Microaggregates in pulmonary vessels after massive transfusion

Most of these causes of hypoxemia will respond to oxygen therapy (supplemental oxygen 30% to 50% by face mask), tracheobronchial toilet, and chest physiotherapy.

Management of respiratory insufficiency involves the monitoring of respiratory rate, tidal volume, inspiratory force, chest x-ray, and arterial blood gases. Pulse oximetry is invaluable.

Patients with airway edema, gross obesity, or preoperative pulmonary problems may require positive-pressure ventilation to achieve normocapnia and adequate oxygenation.

CARDIOVASCULAR SYSTEM

Cardiovascular instability leading to hypotension, hypertension, or dysrhythmias is a common com-

plication in the postoperative period, and therefore monitoring of BP and ECG is imperative.

Autoregulation

Over a wide range of systemic blood pressures, blood flow to the brain is maintained constant because of the ability of the cerebral blood vessels to change their caliber (Figure 9-10). Autoregulation in normotensive patients is limited to a range from 50 to 150 mm Hg of mean blood pressure. Above and below this range, cerebral blood flow passively follows changes in systemic blood pressure. Autoregulation is impaired by the following:

1. Surgical intervention
2. Head trauma
3. General anesthesia
4. Drug therapy
5. Diabetes mellitus
6. Hypertension

Hypotension

Hypotension decreases CPP. Causes must be identified by assessing the fluid intake, urine output, urine osmolarity, central venous pressure, pulmonary capillary wedge pressure, or cardiac output

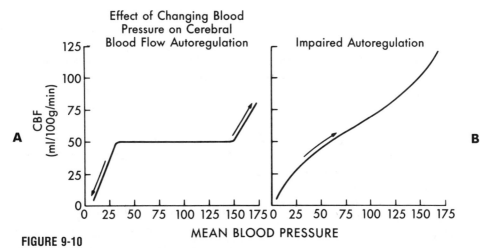

FIGURE 9-10

Blood flow to the brain is maintained constant during changes in the mean blood pressure from 50 to 150 mm Hg, **A.** After surgery, general anesthetics, or medications, the autoregulation is impaired, **B.**

and the appropriate therapy instituted. Causes of hypotension include the following:

1. Inadequate blood replacement
2. Fluid restriction compounded by diuresis
3. Hypovolemia associated with intracranial aneurysm and prolonged diuretic administration
4. Myocardial failure, dysrhythmias
5. Hypoxemia
6. Brain stem damage

Hypertension

Hypertension is claimed to be the most common nonneurological complication in neurosurgical patients in the postoperative period. Several causes have been identified and are as follows:

1. Vasoconstriction caused by hypothermia
2. Fluid overload
3. Emergence from anesthesia, pain, and shivering
4. Hypercapnia and early stages of hypoxia
5. Cushing's reflex caused by intracranial hypoxia
6. Medications, for example, dextran, naloxone, or rebound effect after nitroprusside infusion or withdrawal of antihypertensive medication
7. Revascularization techniques; alteration of cerebral blood flow patterns
8. Preexisting disease

An increase in blood pressure of more than 20%, if not treated, may lead to cerebral hemorrhage, myocardial failure, or myocardial infarction and can increase ICP by increasing the tendency to bleed at the operative site, increased cerebral blood volume, and edema formation (vasogenic edema).

Because of the serious consequences of hypertension, it should be treated aggressively. However, one cause of hypertension, Cushing's reflex, is a protective mechanism to improve cerebral perfusion. Therefore identification of the cause is important before treatment (see Table 9-2). Therapy includes the following:

1. Propranolol 1 mg or labetolol, 5 to 10 mg intravenously

2. Reinstitution of previous medications as soon as possible
3. Correction of fluid imbalance
4. Optimization of arterial blood gases

Hydralazine, nitroprusside and nitroglycerine all cause cerebral vasodilation, increase ICP, and markedly reduce CPP. They should be avoided except in extreme cases.

Cardiac Dysrhythmias and Electrocardiogram Change

Cardiac dysrhythmias and acute ECG changes (T wave inversion, ST segment elevation) are not uncommon. Hyperventilation and diuresis are common modes of therapy in neurosurgical patients, and both can lead to hypokalemia and associated supraventricular dysrhythmias.

In these patients, particularly after head trauma and ruptured cerebral aneurysm, acute ECG changes similar to myocardial ischemia have been observed. The need for ECG monitoring and electrolyte measurements are underscored.

TEMPERATURE

During anesthesia, heat loss as a result of convection, conduction, and radiation (cold room, infusion of refrigerated blood or cool fluids) decreases body temperature. In the immediate postoperative period when the hypothalamus regains its function, patients begin to rebuild the lost heat by shivering. This shivering is associated with an increase in oxygen consumption (400% to 700% of the basal metabolic rate), and if respiratory and cardiac reserves are borderline, hypoxia and heart failure may follow. In anticipation of this impingement on the reserves of the vital functions, temperature should be monitored and external sources of heat made available.

FLUID AND ELECTROLYTES

Disturbances in fluid and electrolyte balance are common after neurosurgical procedures and are associated with surgery in and around the hypothalamus and pituitary areas, or hypokalemia resulting from hyperventilation, diuretics, and steroid therapy. The injured brain is especially subject to deleterious effects of hyperglycemia, increased by steroids or inappropriate intraoperative replacement. Blood sugar levels should be maintained below 150 mg/dl, by administration of insulin if necessary. Fluid replacement is best managed by colloid administration or slow infusion of a saline solution.

Monitoring the intake of fluids, urine output, and electrolytes is important. Diabetes insipidus is diagnosed by the presence of hypernatremia, extreme polyuria, and low urinary specific gravity. Therapy involves replacement of urinary losses with 0.25% saline solution and administration of pitressin (either as DDAVP nasal insufflation or injection of pitressin tannate).

SEIZURES

Approximately 20% of untreated patients develop seizures within the 24-hour period after intracranial surgery. Seizures cause hypoxia and may result in aspiration. Intravenous phenytoin, with careful ECG monitoring, is the drug of choice. To obtain therapeutic levels, 18 mg per kilogram diluted in normal saline is infused at 50 mg per minute. This dose maintains a therapeutic level for 24 hours. Phenytoin must not be given faster than a rate of 50 mg per minute to minimize cardiovascular depression.

RESTLESSNESS AND PAIN

Restlessness of neurosurgical patients in the postoperative period needs careful evaluation to exclude cerebral hypoxia. Other causes include cardiac or respiratory dysfunction. Postoperative pain in this group of patients is not a major problem, and pharmacological pain relief is generally not required. However, if necessary, mild analgesics ranging from acetaminophen to codeine phosphate are adequate. Narcotics should be used cautiously and only if facilities are available for immediate CT scan in view of the depressing effect on the central nervous system and pupillary constriction. Both effects

mask the changes of rising intracranial pressure. In addition, rising CO_2 as a result of respiratory depression caused by narcotics increases ICP.

SPINAL COLUMN SURGERY

Spinal column surgery is performed in the cervical, thoracic, and lumbar regions. The problems related to this type of surgery are shown in the box below.

Pain

These operations cause muscle spasm and pain in the immediate postoperative period, requiring analgesics. Unlike patients after craniotomy with compromised intracranial compliance, narcotics can be given for pain relief.

Position

In the immediate recovery period, the head-elevated position increases the functional residual capacity and thereby improves oxygenation and cerebral venous drainage. In patients who had surgery in the lower thoracic or lumbar spine area, keeping the head elevated leaves the operated site at the most dependent level. This impairs drainage of venous blood from the wound, leading to edema formation, bleeding, and poor healing. Therefore the supine position is more appropriate.

Problems related to spinal column surgery

Pain
Venous stasis
Respiratory function
   Phrenic nerve palsy
   Auxiliary muscle spasm
   Infection
   Bronchospasm
Central nervous system
   Hallucinations
Cardiovascular system
   Bradycardia
   Pulmonary edema
   Autonomic hyperreflexia

Respiratory Function

Respiratory distress can occur because of a number of reasons.

Phrenic nerve damage. The diaphragm is the primary respiratory muscle and derives its nerve supply from cervical segments C3 to C5. Patients are liable to experience respiratory distress either because of structural damage or if ascending edema after surgery encroaches on these segments. Therefore careful assessment and monitoring of respiration is necessary before extubation. If worsening of respiratory function is anticipated, as in surgery on the cervical vertebrae particularly after an anterior approach, extubation of the trachea should be delayed.

Auxiliary muscle spasm. Preoperatively, if the patients had compromised respiratory function and depended on auxiliary muscles to maintain adequate ventilation, in the immediate postoperative period, spasm, edema, and pain in these areas may further decrease this marginal reserve. Respiratory distress should be anticipated and supportive measures made available for several hours or days postoperatively.

Respiratory infections. Accumulation of secretions and regurgitation of gastric contents into the tracheobronchial tree will lead to pulmonary infection. Effective coughing can prevent both complications. However, neurological deficits decrease abdominal and chest wall muscle action, and active physiotherapy is necessary.

Bronchoconstriction. After sympathetic denervation caused by high spinal cord injury, patients tend to develop bronchoconstriction. Bronchodilators and respiratory support may be necessary.

Central Nervous System

Patients with spinal cord damage develop hallucinations and psychiatric problems because of decreased sensory input. Music, a clock, and a window in their surrounding environment increase sensory input and probably decrease psychological complications.

Cardiovascular System

Patients sympathectomized because of high spinal cord injury are liable to develop severe bradycardia, and even minimal vagal stimulation (for example, suctioning the trachea or distended stomach) may lead to cardiac arrest, especially if some degree of hypoxia exists. Prior administration of atropine and limiting the period of suctioning to 10 seconds will eliminate this catastrophic event.

Autonomic hyperreflexia

In patients with complete transection of spinal cord at or above T5 segment

Causes

Viscous distension
Anogenital stimuli

Manifestations

Hypertension, bradycardia
Flushing above the level of lesion
Pallor below the level of lesion

Complications

Cerebral hemorrhage
Retinal hemorrhage
Myocardial failure and infarction

Patients are liable to develop pulmonary edema easily, and therefore fluid management should be carefully guided, if necessary, with monitoring of central pressures.

Patients with complete transection of the spinal cord at or above T5 are liable to develop autonomic hyperreflexia some weeks after the injury. Discomfort caused by visceral distension (for example, bladder) may cause severe hypertension and reflex bradycardia requiring immediate hypotensive therapy and sedation to prevent cerebral hemorrhage or myocardial infarction (see box). Sedation, α-adrenergic blockade, and even general anesthesia are indicated before performing painful maneuvers below the level of injury.

SUGGESTIONS FOR FURTHER READING

Cottrell JE and Newfield P: Neurosurgical and anesthetic aspects of recovery room care. In Israel JS and Bekornfeld TJ, editors: Recovery room care, Chicago, 1989, Year Book Medical Publishers, Inc.

Frost EAM: Control of intracranial pressure, Curr Rev Clin Anesth 1:16, 1981.

Lappas DG, Powell WM Jr, and Daget WM: Cardiac dysfunction in the perioperative period: pathophysiology, diagnosis and treatment, Anesthesiology 47:117, 1979.

Lundberg N: Continuous recording and control of ventricular fluid pressure in neurosurgical practice, Acta Psychiatr Neurol Scand 36:149, 1960.

Lundberg N: Monitoring of the intracranial pressure. In Critchley M and O'Leary JL editors: Scientific foundation of neurology. Philadelphia 1972, FA Davis Co.

Marshall BE and Wyche MQ Jr: Hypoxemia during and after anesthesia, Anesthesiology 37:178, 1972.

Miller JD: Intracranial pressure monitoring. Br J Hosp Med 19(50):497, 1978.

Miller JD and Garibi J: Intracranial volume pressure relationship during continuous monitoring of ventricular fluid pressure. In Brock IM and Dietz H editors: Intracranial pressure, Berlin 1972, Springer Publishing Co. Inc.

Shoemaker WC eta al, editors: Textbook of critical care, Philadelphia, 1987, WB Saunders Co.

Smith DS: Perioperative management of the patient with acute spinal cord injury, Amer Soc Anes Refresher Courses, San Francisco, 1988.

Thiagarajah S: Postoperative care of neurosurgical patients. In Frost EAM and Andrews IC editors: International anesthesiology clincs. Recovery Room Care. 21(1):139, 1983.

CHAPTER 10

Recovery from Regional Anesthesia

Richard B. Patt
Laurent Kaleka

GENERAL CONSIDERATIONS

Regional or conduction anesthesia refers generically to the application of local anesthetic agent to block nerve impulses and render a surgical site insensible to pain without obligate loss of consciousness. Regional anesthetic techniques include spinal, epidural, and caudal blocks, as well as peripheral nerve blocks, field block, and local infiltration anesthesia. Traditionally, a local anesthetic is used, either injected locally at the surgical site (minor conduction block) or proximally, near the nerves that supply the surgical site (major conduction block). The administration of narcotics directly to spinal and epidural sites is a related modality that has been recently introduced. Spinal and epidural opiate therapy produces selective analgesia that is insufficient to block surgical stimulus but is useful to alleviate postoperative and chronic cancer pain.

NURSING CONSIDERATIONS

Current medical practice dictates that levels of monitoring and vigilance be applied equally for patients, without regard to their status as ambulatory or inpatients, or whether they have undergone general anesthesia, regional anesthesia, or local anesthesia with sedation. Relaxation of vigilance by nurses and physicians involved in the care of patients recovering from regional anesthesia represents a great danger. There is a tendency for reduced watchfulness because patients usually are alert and breathing spontaneously and invasive physiological monitoring is less commonly applied than after general anesthesia. Although in the past some authors have advocated discharging selected patients directly to their hospital rooms, the current trend is for all patients who have undergone major conduction anesthesia to be admitted to the post anesthesia care unit (PACU).

Although it is difficult to show statistical differences in morbidity and mortality in patients who have had general versus regional anesthesia, most anesthesiologists and surgeons share strong impressions that regional anesthesia is associated with less physiological stress and is safer than general anesthesia. For this reason, regional anesthesia is frequently the technique of choice for high-risk surgical patients with advanced systemic disease, thus intensifying the need for aggressive post anesthesia nursing care. The intraoperative administration of narcotics and major sedatives as supplements to regional anesthesia is common practice and may result in additive cardiorespiratory depression and the need for airway support and fluid resuscitation, in even young, healthy subjects.

Regional anesthesia is associated with physiological changes that, if unrecognized, have the potential to result in serious morbidity. Moderate to high levels of spinal and epidural anesthesia can compromise respiratory function through paralysis of the intercostal muscles and even the diaphragm. Sympathetic nerves and sensory nerves are blocked, and hypotension may result from sympathetically mediated vasodilation and bradycardia. These alterations in physiology may be compounded by changes induced by surgery, including unrecognized or persistent loss of blood, atelectasis and pneumothorax. In particular, these physiological changes may be poorly tolerated by elderly patients with limited cardiorespiratory reserves. Occasionally a local anesthetic is applied to the nerves supplying the larynx (superior laryngeal and recurrent laryngeal nerves) as a supplement to general anesthesia. In this setting, protective airway reflexes may be inadequate, and suctioning is required to prevent aspiration of blood and secretions. To prevent self-injury, reinforcement of limb protection is important in patients who have received major conduction anesthesia for extremity surgery. Finally, early recognition of rare but potentially serious complications, such as epidural hematoma, central nervous system toxicity, and phrenic nerve paralysis, is essential.

Thus the recovery of patients who have received regional anesthesia requires additional nursing skills and knowledge of applied anatomy and physiology. Patients are usually less obtunded than their counterparts recovering from general anesthesia. With increased use of long-acting local anesthetics (bupivacaine, etidocaine), patients can often be spared pain in the immediate post anesthesia period. Combined, these factors create an excellent opportunity for enhanced personal contact between the post anesthesia care nurse and the recovering surgical patient.

SPINAL, EPIDURAL, AND CAUDAL ANESTHESIA

Spinal and epidural blocks are the most common forms of conduction anesthesia administered to surgical patients, particularly for lower extremity and pelvic surgery. Because multiple nerves are anesthetized including sympathetic fibers, clinically significant derangements of cardiac and respiratory function may occur and a high degree of vigilance is required in the PACU.

Anatomical and Technical Considerations

Subarachnoid (spinal) and epidural anesthetic techniques involve the injection of local anesthetic solutions close to the spinal cord, interrupting the transmission of nervous impulses to and from neighboring spinal segments. Developmentally, the rate of growth of the bony vertebral column exceeds that of the spinal cord, which in the adult finally terminates at about the L1 vertebral level. Although epidural and spinal blocks are sometimes performed at higher levels for special purposes (pain management, thoracic surgery), injections are usually performed in the lower lumbar region to reduce the risk of spinal cord trauma (Figure 10-1).

Spinal anesthesia involves the introduction of a small-caliber needle through intervening midline structures in the back so that the tip of the spinal needle is finally located just beyond the dura (Figure 10-1). A small volume of anesthetic solution is injected into the cerebrospinal fluid surrounding the targeted nerves and produces anesthesia. For epidural anesthesia, the needle tip is localized just superficial to the dura, within the epidural space. Because direct contact between the drug and nervous tissue is less than with spinal anesthesia, large volumes of local anesthetic are required. Anesthesia is usually less complete or dense than that observed after spinal injection. Small-caliber needles (25- to 26-gauge) are preferred for spinal anesthesia to reduce the risk of post-dural-puncture headache. Larger-bore needles (17- to 18-gauge) are used for epidural anesthesia to facilitate location of the epidural space and to permit passage of a catheter that may be used to increase the height of aesthesia or extend its duration, intraoperatively and postopera-

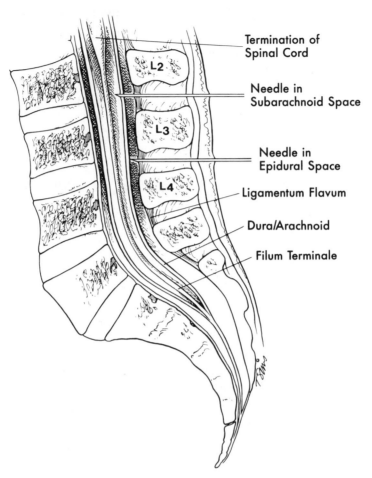

FIGURE 10-1

Diagrammatic representation of the sagittal section showing needle placements in both the subarachnoid and the epidural space. (From Raj P: Handbook of regional anesthesia, New York, 1985, Churchill Livingstone, Inc.)

tively. Caudal block, now waning in popularity, refers to epidural anesthesia administered distally through the sacral hiatus. Saddle block, that is, low spinal anesthesia limited to the perineal area, is rarely associated with alterations in cardiorespiratory function.

Physiological Considerations

Local anesthetics block sensory, motor, and sympathetic fibers indiscriminately, although unequally.

Differential block refers to the disparity frequently observed between levels of sympathetic, sensory, and motor blockade and is related to the variable sensitivities of nerves of different caliber to local anesthetics. Anesthetic action is more profound on thin, nonmyelinated (sympathetic) nerves, whereas thick, heavily myelinated (motor) nerves are more resistant to blockade. Clinically, loss of sympathetic tone is the first sign of effective spinal or epidural anesthesia, and sensory and motor anesthesia follow sequentially (Figure 10-2). Recovery usually

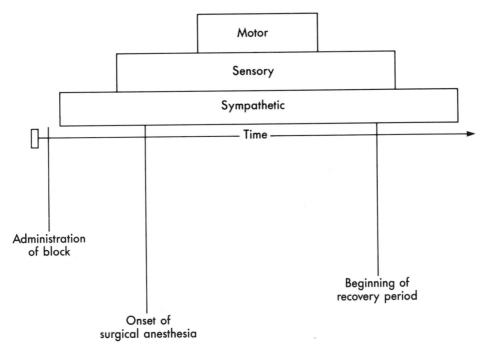

FIGURE 10-2

Relative onset and duration of sympathetic, sensory, and motor block with spinal and epidural anesthesia *(schematic)*.

occurs in the reverse order, with the return of motor function followed by regression of sensory and then sympathetic block (Figure 10-2).

POSTANESTHETIC MANAGEMENT

On the patient's admission to the PACU, a full history and an account of intraoperative events are obtained, vital signs are determined, and a physical survey, including assessment of dermatomal levels and inspection of the surgical wound, is performed.

The extent of sensory, motor, and sympathetic block should be evaluated separately because each component has a different clinical significance. Nursing personnel should become familiar with the spinal dermatomes (Figure 10-3), and a simple chart should be readily available for reference. It is useful to form a mental association between the key dermatomes and major anatomical landmarks of the trunk (that is: T12, pubis; T10, umbilicus; T8, cos-

tal margin; T6, xiphoid; T4, nipples; T2, sternal angle).

Sensory level can be assessed by determining the level at which dullness to pinprick (hypalgesia) is present on each side of the midline. Care must be observed not to injure the skin in anesthetized regions. Once the level of sensory anesthesia has been determined, sympathetic and motor levels can be estimated. The height of sympathetic block usually exceeds that of sensory block by two to four segments, and the height of motor block usually lies a few spinal segments below the sensory level (Figure 10-4). Sympathetic level usually corresponds to the level at which the application of an alcohol swab no longer feels cold to the patient.

Expected duration of analgesia can be roughly estimated by considering the drug used, time it was administered, route of administration, and the addition or omission of epinephrine (Table 10-1). Discharge criteria vary among institutions, but the

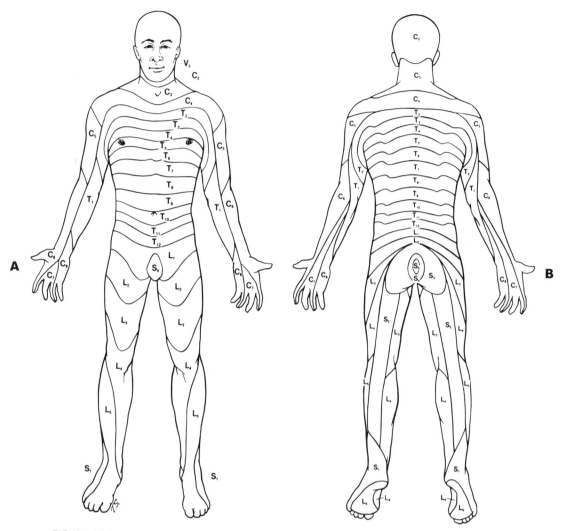

FIGURE 10-3

A, Dermatomal distribution of the body wall, anterior view. **B,** Dermatomal distribution of the body wall, posterior view. (From Raj P: Handbook of regional anesthesia, New York, 1985, Churchill Livingstone, Inc.)

most important factors are the presence of hemodynamic stability and regression of sympathetic block. In an otherwise stable inpatient, a descending sensory level to T12 and the absence of orthostatic changes are reasonable criteria for postanesthetic discharge.

INDWELLING CATHETERS

A catheter may be inserted while performing a nerve block to facilitate repeat dosing of local anesthetic or narcotic for postoperative analgesia. Catheter techniques are used most commonly after epidural anesthesia but are readily adaptable to other blocks, including brachial plexus and intercostal blocks.

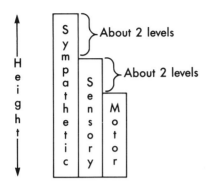

FIGURE 10-4

Relative dermatomal distribution of sympathetic, sensory, and motor block after spinal and epidural block *(schematic)*.

To reduce the risks of infection, catheters should incorporate a bacterial filter. Unlike an intravenous cannula, a catheter for a nerve block can be capped for an indefinite period between doses, and flushing is unnecessary. A local anesthetic agent or preservative-free preparation of a narcotic can be infused continuously with a calibrated pump or can be injected intermittently as needed by a physician.

Injection is preceded by careful aspiration and observation for the return of blood or cerebrospinal fluid to detect catheter migration. Another important precaution is the use of a small "test dose" before administration of the complete dose of drug. When the catheter is removed, its tip should be inspected to ensure that it is intact. If shearing has occurred, x-ray examination of the area and documentation are required. Rarely are neurological or infectious sequalae caused by small pieces of plastic in the epidural space, and the patient should be so informed.

SEQUELAE SPECIFIC TO SPINAL AND EPIDURAL ANESTHESIA
Circulatory Insufficiency

The differential diagnosis of hypotension in the postsurgical patient after a moderate-to-high spinal or epidural block must include consideration of relative hypovolemia from extensive sympathetic blockade (Figure 10-5). As much as one liter of the circulating blood volume can pool in relaxed venous capacitance vessels, which alone may produce hypotension or may exacerbate coexisting hypovo-

TABLE 10-1

Average duration of local anesthetic agents used for spinal and epidural anesthesia		
	Spinal average duration	Epidural average duration
Short-acting agents		
Procaine (Novocain)	no longer used	not used
2-chloroprocaine (Nesacaine)	not used	30-90 min
Intermediate-acting agents		
Lidocaine	60-90 min	60-120 min*
Mepivacaine (Carbocaine)	not used	60-150 min*
Long-acting agents		
Bupivacaine (Marcaine, Sensorcaine)	90-110 min	120-140 min
Etidocaine (Duranest)	not used	120-240 min
Tetracaine	90-180 min*	not used

*Duration of anesthesia prolonged from 25% to 50% by the addition of epinephrine.

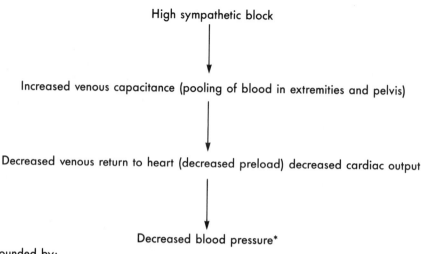

High sympathetic block

↓

Increased venous capacitance (pooling of blood in extremities and pelvis)

↓

Decreased venous return to heart (decreased preload) decreased cardiac output

↓

Decreased blood pressure*

* May be compounded by:
   impaired compensatory tachycardia
   bradycardia from blockade of cardioaccelerator fibers (T1-T4)

FIGURE 10-5
Physiology of circulatory insufficiency after high spinal or epidural block.

lemia or surgical blood loss. High sympathetic block can impair compensatory tachycardia, masking an important early sign of hypovolemia. If surgery predisposes to occult blood loss, the post anesthesia nurse must be alert to subtle signs of hypoperfusion, including pallor, reduced pulse pressure, and disorientation.

A further mechanism by which sympathetic block may decrease blood pressure is through bradycardia, related to blockade of sympathetic cardioaccelerator fibers (T1-T4).

Once other correctable causes of hypotension have been excluded, treatment is symptomatic. The responsible physician is notified, and treatment started with elevation of the legs and rapid infusion of a balanced salt solution. If patient response is inadequate, treatment is with a vasopressor, such as phenylephrine or ephedrine. Bradycardia is generally regarded as significant when the pulse rate falls below 50 beats per minute or is associated with reduction in blood pressure. Intravenous administration of atropine (0.2 to 0.8 mg) is indicated.

Respiratory Insufficiency

True respiratory insufficiency is uncommon after spinal or epidural block unless a severe, preexisting pathological condition of the lung is present. It is not uncommon for patients to experience dyspnea that is primarily subjective with a high (T2) anesthetic. This syndrome results from a combination of reduced ventilatory strength from intercostal paralysis (usually subclinical) and reduced awareness of chest wall movement because of sensory loss (Figure 10-6). In extreme cases, muscle weakness may impair the patient's ability to cough and can reduce phonation to a hoarse whisper, contributing to patient unease. It should be ascertained that levels of blockade do not extend to include the cervical segments, since in the absence of pulmonary disease, the diaphragm (C3 to C5) compensate readily for accessory muscle weakness. If there are no overt signs of hypoxia or hypercarbia, treatment is primarily supportive: the patient is reassured and encouraged not to hyperventilate. Supplemental oxygen may be administered, and if blood pressure is stable, the head of the bed is elevated as tolerated to

Intercostal muscle paralysis

$+/-$

Decreased sensation of chest wall movement (subjective dyspnea)

$+/-$

Diaphragmatic paralysis

FIGURE 10-6
Physiology of respiratory insufficiency after high spinal or epidural block.

reduce abdominal resistance to diaphragmatic excursion. Light sedation may be beneficial, providing hypoxia and hypercarbia have been excluded, and oxygen saturation is continuously measured.

Post-dural-puncture Headache

Headache occurring after spinal anesthesia is often the result of persistent leakage of cerebrospinal fluid (CSF) through a dural tear. It is postulated that CSF hypotension reduces support for cerebral structures so that in the erect posture, traction on pain-sensitive structures (dura and blood vessels) causes symptoms. A small-bore needle or epidural anesthesia (that does not violate the dura) is often elected to reduce the incidence of post-dural-puncture headache. When headache occurs, it is severe, postural, and may be accompanied by nausea, vomiting, and visual symptoms. Characteristically, symptoms do not appear until the first or second postoperative day and are not present during the immediate postanesthetic period.

Vigorous intravenous and oral hydration is effective treatment and may help prevent symptoms. This measure may be elected in the early perioperative period in patients who are prone to headache, including young individuals or those who have experienced an accidental dural puncture with a large epidural needle. In the past, it was believed that maintenance of a horizontal position in the immediate postoperative period would reduce the incidence of headache. Although this practice is effective

treatment for a headache already in progress, several large studies have shown that maintenance of the supine position is of no prophylactic value and postural restrictions are no longer considered useful to prevent headache. If post-dural-puncture headache occurs and has not responded to conservative therapy (hydration, bed rest, abdominal binder, analgesics), the sterile injection of autologous blood (epidural blood patch) usually relieves symptoms promptly. When the risk of spinal headache is high, such as after dural puncture with a 17- or 18-gauge needle, prophylactic blood patch is occasionally performed in the immediate postanesthetic period. Alternative treatments include intravenous infusion of caffeine sodium benzoate and epidural infusion of preservative-free saline.

Epidural Hematoma

Epidural hematoma is a rare but potentially devastating complication of epidural or spinal block. Diagnosis early in the recovery period is essential to prevent permanent neurological injury (Figure 10-7). All reported cases have been associated with the rapid onset of neurological deficit and/or severe back pain. Patients who have received anticoagulants or who have coagulation defects are at greatest risk. In the presence of suspected epidural hematoma, anticoagulants are discontinued and an emergency myelogram or CT scan is obtained. If radiological studies are corroborative, early laminectomy and decompression is imperative. The majority

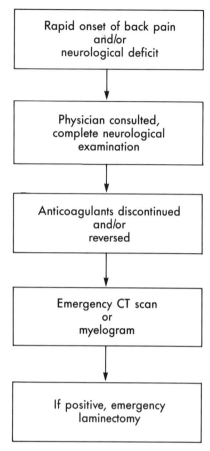

FIGURE 10-7
Recognition and management of suspected postoperative epidural hematoma.

of patients who have recovered after epidural hematoma have done so when surgery has been performed within 12 hours of the onset of symptoms.

PERIPHERAL NERVE BLOCKS

Local anesthetic blockade of peripheral nerves may be performed to produce complete surgical anesthesia or as an adjunct to general anesthesia to reduce postoperative pain. Nerves may be blocked individually or, alternatively, more proximally where they lie together in a plexus. Infiltration of the surgical wound with local anesthesia or field block is another, usually less effective, means of blocking postoperative pain.

Brachial plexus block is by far the most frequently used peripheral block. The brachial plexus innervates the upper limb and can be accessed by the anesthesiologist from several routes. Above the clavicle, the intrascalene or supraclavicular approaches are used, primarily for surgery of the shoulder and upper arm. Axillary block is used for surgery of the lower arm and hand. Occasionally an infraclavicular approach is used.

The supraclavicular approaches are more frequently associated with pneumothorax, which, if small, may not be apparent until late in the recovery period. A careful clinical examination is essential to exclude pneumothorax. A postoperative chest x-ray film should be obtained. Supraclavicular approaches are also associated with higher incidences of spread of local anesthetic to neighboring structures. Unintentional involvement of the cervical plexus may produce a higher level of anesthesia but is usually not associated with ill effects. Anesthesia of the third, fourth, and fifth cervical nerve roots or, alternatively, spread of anesthetic to the nearby phrenic nerve results in hemidiaphragmatic paralysis. Phrenic nerve involvement probably occurs more often than is clinically realized. Although fit patients usually compensate adequately through the use of accessory respiratory muscles, patients with preexisting pulmonary disease or patients who have been heavily sedated may experience respiratory insufficiency. Phrenic nerve paralysis can be confirmed by clinical examination, chest x-ray examination, or fluoroscopy and usually responds to supplemental oxygen and nursing in the head-up position. Spread of anesthesia to the recurrent laryngeal nerve is associated with hoarseness, dysphagia, and subjective dyspnea. Spread to the stellate ganglion (cervicothoracic sympathetic ganglion) is followed by ipsilateral Horner's syndrome (miosis, enophthalmos, ptosis, anhidrosis).

Nerve blocks to the lower extremity usually involve combination of blocks of the femoral, sciatic, obturator, and lateral femoral cutaneous nerves. Because superior and more reliable anesthesia is usually obtained with spinal or epidural techniques, which are also less stressful to the patient, blockade of the individual nerves is performed infrequently. As with brachial plexus block, nursing considerations include protection of the extremity, inspection for hematoma, and concern for local anesthetic toxicity because large volumes of local anesthesia are used (30 to 50 ml).

Multiple intercostal nerve blocks are frequently performed, either to provide anesthesia for superficial procedures on the chest or abdominal wall or to reduce the pain associated with cholecystectomy and other upper abdominal surgery. Because the intercostal artery and vein lie proximate within the neurovascular bundle, systemic absorption of anesthetic is higher after this block than after others. Other possible complications include hematoma formation and pneumothorax.

Epidural and Spinal Opiate Therapy

Research into endogenous opiate-like substances and the discovery of central nervous system opiate receptors has led rapidly to the clinical administration of exogenous opioids directly to central nervous system sites for the relief of chronic and postoperative pain. The hallmark of spinal opiate therapy is selective analgesia, that is: pain relief without motor, sensory, or sympathetic blockade.

The use of spinal opiates is new and is expanding so rapidly that protocols for drug administration are still emerging. One important criterion for drug administration is that medication be free of

preservatives. If morphine is used, a special formulation is required (Duramorph, Astramorph), whereas standard commercial preparations of meperidine, fentanyl, and sufentanil are all preservative-free. Although only morphine has been approved by the FDA for intraspinal use, there has been widespread clinical experience with a variety of other opiates and their use is not considered experimental.

The physiochemical properties of the opiates, in part, determine their clinical effects. As with opiates administered by other routes, morphine has emerged as the standard with which other drugs are compared (Table 10-2). Morphine is poorly lipid soluble, and intraspinal injection absorption is slow compared with that of more lipid-soluble drugs (meperidine, fentanyl, sufentanil). Delayed absorption produces a ''reservoir effect,'' accounting for morphine's extended duration of action (about 24 hours) and a propensity for late respiratory depression (at 8 to 12 hours) as a result of rostral migration of morphine to brainstem respiratory centers. In contrast, the analgesic effects of fentanyl and sufentanil range between 2 and 4 hours and late respiratory depression probably does not occur. Early respiratory depression occasionally occurs as a result of venous absorption or accidental intravascular injection.

Side effects of intraspinal narcotics are similar to those of opiates administered by other routes and include pruritus, nausea and vomiting, urinary retention, dysphoria, and biphasic respiratory depres-

---

TABLE 10-2

Profiles of narcotics commonly used for epidural and spinal analgesia

Drug	Lipid solubility	Duration	Potential side effects	Reversible with naloxone
Morphine	+	20-24 hr	Urinary retention, pruritis, early and late respiratory depression	+
Fentanyl	+++	2-4 hr	Same as with morphine, except late respiratory depression has not been reported	+
Sufentanil	++++	2-4 hr		
Meperidine	++	3-5 hr		

sion. Side effects can be reversed by the intravenous injection of a narcotic antagonist (naloxone, nalbuphine), administered in small doses to preserve analgesia. A dilute infusion of naloxone (0.4 mg/1000 ml at 50 to 100 ml/hr) may be administered prophylactically. Late respiratory depression has not been reported in narcotic-tolerant patients and is uncommon in parturients. Guidelines for ventilatory monitoring are still emerging. If epidural or spinal morphine is administered, a protocol for monitoring ventilatory status on the postsurgical ward is mandatory. Options include frequent nursing checks and the use of apnea monitors and pulse oximeters.

COMPLICATIONS OF REGIONAL ANESTHESIA
Systemic Toxicity

Largely preventable, toxic reactions may occur either (1) during the performance of a nerve block, because of accidental intravascular injection or (2) within the first 5 to 30 minutes after a block is placed, because of vascular absorption of large quantities of local anesthetic. Except after reinjection through an indwelling catheter, systemic local anesthetic toxicity is unlikely to occur *de novo* in the recovery period. There is, however, occasionally a need for continued nursing care of a patient with a reaction that occurred intraoperatively.

Direct intravascular injection can produce immediate neurological signs including twitching, loss of consciousness, and seizure, as well as cardiovascular instability. Prophylactic measures include careful aspiration and the use of a local anesthetic test dose. All but urgent surgery is postponed in the event of significant intravascular injection. Treatment priorities are airway control, oxygenation, treatment of seizures, and restitution of normotension and a regular cardiac rhythm. Ordinarily, major symptoms will have been controlled by anesthesia personnel before the patient's admission to the PACU. Nursing considerations may include the management of an intubated, postictal patient who, in the most extreme cases, has undergone cardiopulmonary resuscitation. Although toxic reactions to local anesthetics are primarily neurological, bupivacaine has recently received attention for its cardiotoxic potential, particularly in obstetric patients.

More common, toxicity is related to the slow vascular absorption of a relative overdose of anesthetic, and symptoms are mild, gradual in onset, and often self-limited. Early signs and symptoms include circumoral numbness, tinnitus, mild intoxication, and other signs of CNS irritability or depression. The likelihood of delayed toxicity increases with techniques that require large volumes of injectate (brachial plexus block, high epidural block, sciatic femoral block) and also is more likely with injections into highly vascular regions (intercostal block). The addition of epinephrine produces local vasoconstriction and, by decreasing the venous absorption of the local anesthetic, results in lower plasma levels and a reduced risk of toxicity. The low volume and dose of drugs used for spinal anesthesia mitigate toxicity by this mechanism.

Treatment of gradual-onset toxicity is reassurance, supplemental oxygen, and the administration of a benzodiazepine to elevate the seizure threshold. After surgery of short duration, nursing personnel may be involved in the care of these patients and close observation is required to monitor for progression of symptoms.

Total or High Spinal Block

A high or total spinal anesthesia results from relative overdosage, usually by the spinal route and most often when an epidural dose of drug has been accidentally injected intrathecally. This complication can almost always be avoided by careful observation of the patient's reaction to a test dose of local anesthetic. Anesthesia of the nervous outflow to the diaphragm and accessory muscles results in rapid onset of respiratory insufficiency that progresses to apnea if anesthesia ascends to involve medullary respiratory centers. Similarly, hypotension resulting from sympathetic paralysis and venous pooling may be exacerbated by involvement of medullary structures. Hemodynamics may be further affected by bradycardia associated with paralysis of cardioaccelerator fibers (T1 to T4) and medullary centers. Ability to phonate diminishes with loss of strength

oliguria, may be an appropriate response of a normally functioning kidney to volume depletion. A seemingly normal urine volume may be seen in patients with "nonoliguric" acute tubular necrosis.

Urine specific gravity

Urine specific gravity is often measured to evaluate adequacy of hydration. This may be misleading in the patient with renal failure who is unable to concentrate or dilute urine and in the patient who is excreting large amounts of solute (for example, glucose, mannitol).

Other laboratory tests

Complete blood count (CBC)

Hemoglobin	normal = 14-16 g/dl ± 2
Hematocrit	normal = 42-47% ± 5

Serum electrolytes

Potassium	normal = 3.5-5.0 mEq/L
Sodium	normal = 135-145 mEq/L
Bicarbonate	normal = 24-30 mEq/L

Serum osmolality

normal = 280-300 mOsm

Clinical Symptomatology (see box)
Cardiovascular

Many problems in the patient with chronic renal failure arise from decreased ability to excrete water and sodium, or from complications of chronic hypertension. These patients respond slowly to changes in sodium intake, and urinary sodium excretion reflects chronic intake rather than acute needs. To maintain sodium balance, a nonedematous patient with renal insufficiency should receive approximately as much sodium as his chronic intake. The 24-hour urinary sodium content can be used to establish this level, although a daily intake of 2 to 3 g sodium chloride (approximately 1 to 1.5 g Na$^+$, or 35 to 50 mEq) is adequate in most patients. As a reference, 500 ml of 0.9% NaCl contains 4.5 g Na$^+$. If salt intake exceeds excretory ability, circulatory overload may develop (peripheral edema, pulmonary congestion, hypertension). Treatment includes salt restriction and administration of diuretics. Caution should be used in diures-

---

Clinical symptomatology found in the patient with chronic renal disease

Cardiovascular	**Neurological**
Hypertension	Confusion
Peripheral edema	Disorientation
Pulmonary congestion	Coma
	Convulsions
	Peripheral neuropathy
Hematological	**Musculoskeletal**
Anemia	Associated with hyperparathyroidism
Platelet function	
Metabolic	**Gastrointestinal**
Acidosis	Bleeding
Hyperkalemia	Nausea and vomiting

Only those symptoms relevant to the PACU setting are discussed in the text.

---

ing edematous patients with hypoalbuminemia who may also have intravascular volume depletion. Measurement of central venous pressure is a useful guide in treating these patients.

A person with normal renal function rapidly decreases urinary sodium excretion almost to zero when faced with dietary sodium restriction or extrarenal sodium losses. In chronic severe renal disease, urinary sodium excretion cannot be decreased rapidly, and the kidneys continue to excrete sodium, leading to extracellular fluid (ECF) volume depletion, hypotension, and a further decrease in glomerular filtration rate (GFR). Patients with severe renal disease who sustain significant unreplaced volume loss (such as trauma, diarrhea, surgery, or inadequate intake) may suffer further deterioration of renal function on a temporary or even permanent basis.

Patients with severe renal disease excrete urine that is more or less the same osmolality as plasma. They dilute and concentrate urine poorly in response to alterations in water intake. Urine volume will be 1.5 to 2 L per day as long as the GFR exceeds 3 to 5 ml per minute. Hypothalamic osmoreceptors control water intake by alterations in thirst to maintain serum osmolality and sodium concentration.

Surgical patients with renal insufficiency may develop hyponatremia from water overload or sodium depletion. Water overload results when sodium-containing losses (urine, "third-space") are replaced only with water or as the result of inappropriate antidiuretic hormone (ADH) secretion (positive-pressure ventilation, neurological lesion). This is best treated by restricting the amount of free water the patient receives. If the patient is symptomatic (confused, lethargic, convulsing), hypertonic saline is administered at 50 ml per hour up to ~200 ml. In addition, the actual seizure activity is treated with anticonvulsants. Diuretics are also administered to the volume-overloaded patient to speed the removal of water from the body. Sodium depletion is infrequently seen as an acute postoperative event. It is best treated with isotonic sodium chloride or, in acidotic patients, sodium bicarbonate.

Hypernatremia is most commonly the result of water depletion and thus should be treated by increasing the amount of free water administered to the patient.

Hematological

The anemia of chronic renal insufficiency is caused by decreased erythrocyte synthesis (in part the result of decreased renal erythropoietin) and shortened erythrocyte life. Patients in an unstressed situation may tolerate hemoglobin levels as low as 5 g/dl, but blood oxygen-carrying capacity is markedly reduced and increased heart rate, intravascular volume, and cardiac output maximize oxygen delivery to tissues. Perioperative decreases in cardiac output as seen with myocardial depressant drugs (for example, anesthetic agents) or increases in tissue oxygen requirements (shivering, hyperthermia) may decrease tissue oxygenation to dangerously low levels in such anemic patients. Administration of humidified oxygen to the postoperative anemic patient is essential.

Although transfusion is not without risks (including volume overload, disease transmission, and transfusion reaction), hemaglobin levels of 10 g/dl are often necessary to provide an adequate oxygen-carrying capacity. The possibility of stimulating antibody formation, which was thought to increase the risk of rejection of future transplants, is no longer a contraindication.

Metabolic acidosis

Metabolic acidosis is relatively benign at a bicarbonate level of 15 mEq/L or above, although it prolongs the effect of nondepolarizing neuromuscular blocking agents (curare and pancuronium) and decreases buffer reserve. Acidosis may be treated with sodium bicarbonate (1 ampule of $NaHCO_3$ will increase the plasma HCO_3^- of a 70 kg person by about 1 mEq/L). This treatment carries with it the risk of sodium overload.

Potassium

The ability to excrete a normal daily potassium intake is usually preserved in severe renal disease as long as urine output is maintained; however, rapid changes in potassium excretion cannot be made. Hyperkalemia is seen in the perioperative period when large potassium loads (cellular breakdown, blood transfusion) occur. A serum potassium > 5.5 mEq/L is associated with an increased risk of life-threatening dysrhythmias in the surgical patient with renal insufficiency. Electrocardiographic evidence of hyperkalemia includes T-wave peaking with modest elevations and loss of P waves with widening of QRS complexes as the hyperkalemia becomes more severe. As cardiac muscle function is impaired, cardiac output is severely compromised.

The most rapid treatment of hyperkalemic cardiac toxicity is the slow infusion of 10 to 20 ml of 10% calcium gluconate, which should be reserved for the patient with severe hyperkalemia (>7.5 mEq/L). Calcium infusions do not alter serum potassium concentrations, but decrease the neuromuscular irritability seen with hyperkalemia. Electrocardiogram (ECG) monitoring should be continuous, particularly in the patient who is receiving digitalis and who may respond to calcium infusion with an increase in the frequency of digitalis-related dysrhythmias (for example, premature ventricular contractions [PVCs]). The effects of calcium infusions are rapid (< 5 minutes) but short-lived, and more definitive treatment should begin immediately.

Administration of 50 ml of 50% glucose with 10 units of regular insulin to move potassium into cells from the ECF is indicated for K^+ levels < 7.5 mEq/L. If acidosis is present in addition to hyperkalemia (in the normovolemic patient), infusions of sodium bicarbonate at a rate of 1 ampule (44 mEq) per hour for 2 to 3 hours are beneficial. However, the potassium will return to ECF after several hours.

Removal of potassium from the body is accomplished by using cation exchange resins administered orally or rectally (for example, Kayexalate) to slowly exchange sodium for potassium in the gastrointestinal tract. A discussion of the use of dialysis in the hyperkalemic patient follows.

Medications
Antibiotics

Many antibiotics are excreted by the kidney and may accumulate to toxic levels in patients with impaired renal function. This is particularly important for the nephrotoxic aminoglycosides (for example, kanamycin, gentamycin) and tetracyclines where excessive plasma levels can further impair renal function. Tetracyclines are best avoided in patients with decreased GFR because of their antianabolic effect (increased BUN, hyperkalemia, and acidosis) with the exception of doxycycline, which is excreted by the liver. Aminoglycosides should be carefully monitored with plasma levels. As a rule of thumb, the physician increases dosage intervals in proportion to the fall of GFR (that is, a patient with a GFR one-third normal should be given aminoglycosides one-third as often as normal). A detailed description of drug dosage may be found in the review by Anderson et al.

Antihypertensive agents

These agents alter the responsiveness of the autonomic nervous system both to normal homeostatic stimuli and to exogenously administered drugs.

Morbidity is increased in the patient whose hypertension is poorly controlled (diastolic blood pressure greater than 110 mm Hg). Antihypertensive therapy should not be discontinued in the perioperative period.

Reserpine and guanethidine deplete peripheral catecholamine stores and reduce the response to indirect-acting vasopressors (for example, ephedrine) but increase sensitivity to exogenously administered norepinephrine. Clonidine and α-methyldopa are centrally acting α-agonists, and their abrupt discontinuation may cause rebound hypertension, especially in the PACU.

β-adrenergic blocking agents (for example, propranolol, metoprolol) decrease blood pressure by decreasing myocardial contractility, decreasing plasma renin levels, and also acting in the central nervous system. Patients chronically maintained on these drugs may be unable to increase heart rate in response to volume depletion, hypoglycemia, or other sympathetic stimuli. Therefore a slow, stable heart rate cannot always be regarded as a reassuring sign.

Postoperative hypertension is frequently seen in patients with chronic renal disease. The differential diagnosis includes hypoxia, hypercapnia, pain, volume overload, and "inadequately" treated preexisting hypertension. Therapy should be directed at the etiological factors: improvements in oxygenation and ventilation, administration of analgesics or diuretics, institution of dialysis. In the acute setting, vasodilators, such as hydralazine or nitroglycerine, may be used. Sodium nitroprusside should be avoided in these patients because thiocyanate, a metabolite of nitroprusside, is excreted by the kidney and can accumulate to toxic levels.

Corticosteroids

Corticosteroids are frequently prescribed either as a treatment for glomerulonephritis or as immunosuppression after renal transplantation. Because of chronic suppression of adrenal steroid synthesis, these patients may not be able to respond to the stresses of the perioperative period with a release of endogenous glucocorticoids. Supplementation using a total parenteral steroid dose of 300 mg hydro-cortisone per day (which is equivalent to the amount of endogenous steroid normally released in response to stress) in divided doses is recommended in the immediate perioperative period.

Digitalis preparations

Digoxin is excreted largely by the kidney, and its dosage should be decreased to prevent toxicity in the form of cardiac dysrhythmias. Serum digoxin levels can be monitored to ensure a proper therapeutic effect. Digitoxin is metabolized by the liver, and its dose need not be altered in renal insufficiency.

Diuretics

Diuretics, such as furosemide and hydrochlorothiazide, are used to treat both volume overload and hypertension. Excessive volume depletion may occur, further decreasing renal function and causing hypokalemia, which can precipitate digitalis toxicity.

Fluids

Fluid therapy is directed at replacement of losses. Insensible loss (sweat, respiratory) is replaced by free water as 5% dextrose in water (D_5W); ~500 ml/day is required for the 70 kg adult with no renal function. If the patient has a urine output, enough fluid should be given on a daily basis (as one-third or one-half normal saline) to provide for the anticipated urine output.

Blood loss must be replaced with blood. The use of triple-washed red blood cells allows the replacement of oxygen-carrying capacity without addition of excess volume or potassium. The amount of blood that may be lost before replacement is begun depends on the type of surgery and the individual patient.

Third-space losses should be replaced with a sodium-containing solution, preferably normal saline. If D_5W is given alone for replacement of third-space losses, hyponatremia may result. Colloid (5% albumin) may be given as part of the third-space replacement when the surgery involves viscera or

moderate blood loss. Third-space losses in the anephric patient are replaced at the rate of 1 to 5 ml/kg per hour depending on the extent of tissue trauma. Corresponding replacement rates in the patient with normal renal function and these losses are: as much as 5 ml/kg per hour for surgery involving minimal trauma (hernia repair, D&C); 5 to 10 ml/kg per hour for moderate trauma (cholycystectomy); and 10 to 15 ml/kg per hour for major trauma (bowel resection, burns). These numbers are only guidelines; volumes actually administered will be altered based on measurement of vital signs and central venous pressure (CVP). As mentioned, urine output may not readily reflect rapid changes in volume status in the patient with chronic renal disease.

Exogenous potassium should not be given to the patient with chronic renal disease unless the renal disease is mild or the patient has a specific potassium-losing renal defect. Preoperative or intraoperative tissue trauma and blood transfusions increase serum K^+ levels.

Monitoring

Monitoring of the patient with renal disease should include routine parameters, such as blood pressure, pulse, ECG, fluid intake and output, level of consciousness, and temperature. The pulse oximeter is a sensitive, noninvasive monitor of arterial oxygen saturation that is especially valuable in these patients who are often anemic. Where major blood loss or fluid shifts have occurred, a CVP or pulmonary artery catheter is useful. The need for an indwelling urinary catheter is controversial because urine output may not reflect acute changes in volume status or renal function and the risk of urinary tract infection is high.

A postoperative hemoglobin determination should be made and blood obtained for serum K^+, Na^+, and HCO_3^-. (An ECG may be useful here when looking for signs of hyperkalemia.)

The nondepolarizing muscle relaxants d-tubocurarine and pancuronium are excreted primarily via the kidney. Although biliary pathways are available for excretion of these drugs, half-lives will be pro-

overload whereas a large dose of furosemide (1 g) may cause deafness. It must be remembered that any diuresis in a volume-depleted patient must be accompanied by vigorous fluid replacement to prevent even more severe volume depletion with further diminution of renal function.

Treatment

Established postsurgical acute tubular necrosis carries a poor prognosis. About 60% of patients die, usually from infection of from the illness that precipitated the renal failure. Optimal patient survival requires careful management of fluids and medications, with timely use of dialysis. Fluid intake is limited to replacement of urinary and extrarenal losses. In the afebrile patient without diarrhea, a fluid intake limited to urine volume plus 500 ml per day is a reasonable regimen. Sodium should be provided in sufficient quantity to replace losses.

Potassium should not be given to the oliguric patient (volume < 400 ml per day). Kayexalate may be used to prevent or treat hyperkalemia. In the nonoliguric patient, urinary losses of potassium are replaced with careful monitoring of serum and urinary potassium.

Particular attention to detail should be paid to the postoperative monitoring and management of the patient with impaired renal function to preserve all remaining kidney function. It is important to be aware of the situations that place a patient at risk for developing acute renal failure. The early diagnosis and treatment of prerenal states may prevent acute tubular necrosis. Should acute renal failure occur, its prompt recognition and the institution of appropriate therapy will decrease morbidity and possibly mortality.

RENAL TRANSPLANTS
The Recipient

Patients who receive renal transplants usually have little if any remaining renal function. Postoperatively they present particular problems in terms of volume status and infection control.

Unlike the patient whose intravascular volume must be restricted to prevent volume overload, the transplant recipient needs an adequate circulating volume so that oliguria on the basis of volume depletion will not complicate the clinical picture. Moreover, almost all transplant recipients receive immunosuppressive drugs, and their ability to combat infection is impaired. Even greater attention than usual must be paid to aseptic technique.

The Donor

The PACU is often the site where patients whose kidneys are to be used as donor organs are cared for until criteria for brain death are met. These patients must be carefully monitored (urine output, blood pressure, temperature, arterial blood gases, and if available CVP or PCWP). Strict aseptic techniques should be adhered to because sepsis in the donor or the need to use potentially nephrotoxic antibiotics might render the kidneys unsuitable for transplantation. Particulars of drug therapy for organ preservation vary from center to center. A good review of the topic is presented by Slapak. The protocol followed at the Montefiore Hospital and Medical Center is a typical example (Figure 11-1).

SUGGESTIONS FOR FURTHER READING

Alfred HJ and Cohen AJ: Use of dialytic procedures in the intensive care unit. In Lippe JM et al: Intensive care medicine, Boston, 1985, Little, Brown & Co. Inc.

Anderson RJ et al: Fate of drugs in renal failure. In Brenner BM and Rector FC Jr, editors: The Kidney, ed 2, Philadelphia, 1981, WB Saunders Co.

Brenner BM and Lazarus JM: Chronic renal failure: pathophysiologic considerations. In Braunwald E et al, editors: Harrison's principles of internal medicine, ed 11, New York, 1987, McGraw-Hill, Inc.

Carpenter CB and Lazarus JM: Dialysis and transplantation in the treatment of renal failure. Ln Braunwald E et al, editors: Harrison's principles of internal medicine, ed 11, New York, 1987, McGraw-Hill, Inc.

Mazze RI: Anesthesia for the patient with abnormal renal function and genitourinary operations. In Miller RR, editor: Anesthesia, ed 2, Vol 3, New York, 1986, Churchill Livingstone, Inc.

Müller MC: Anesthesia for the patient with renal dysfunction. In Priebe H-J, editor: The kidney in anesthesia. Int Anesthesiol Clin 22:169, 1984.

Slapak M: The immediate care of potential donors for cadaveric organ transplantation, Anaesthesia 33(8):700, 1978.

CHAPTER 12

Post Anesthesia Care after Thoracic Surgery

Jonathan S. Daitch

Most patients who undergo pulmonary surgery have some degree of preoperative respiratory dysfunction. Sometimes surgery eliminates the problem, such as resection of a lung abscess. More often, though, patients have a long history of chronic pulmonary injury with a superimposed ailment, for example, emphysematous patient with lung cancer. Recovery after thoracic surgery depends not only on the type of surgery performed, but on the preoperative pulmonary status of the patient.

PREANESTHETIC ASSESSMENT

Preoperative pulmonary tests provide insight into a patient's anticipated postoperative course. Patients may have restrictive or obstructive lung disease, though obstructive pulmonary disease is more common. Patients with expiratory flow rates of at least 80% of predicted values have adequate pulmonary reserve and should recover uneventfully. However, reductions of 50% or more signify severe lung disease with little pulmonary reserve and predict the need for postoperative respiratory support. Preoperative arterial blood gas determinations may reveal hypoxemia or carbon dioxide retention, which indicates severe respiratory dysfunction.

A smoking history implies that a patient has early closure of small airways, which may lead to hypoxemia. Additionally, he has irritable large airways, which lead to excessive postoperative coughing. If lung damage from smoking has progressed to chronic obstructive lung disease, other problems may be anticipated. Emphysematous and bronchitic patients may retain CO_2. These patients have ineffective respiratory mechanics, and the work of breathing is increased, which promotes hypoventilation. Patients who retain CO_2 are at risk for severe hypoventilation from narcotics, and postoperative respiratory failure. In addition, hypercapnic patients may not respond to the normal stimulus that initiates ventilation, namely elevated $PaCO_2$. They respond, instead, to hypoxemia. If such patients receive high concentrations of oxygen, they may lose their last remaining stimulus to breathe, become apneic, and suffer cardiac arrest. Finally, those with a history of chronic bronchitis, by definition, have large amounts of secretions that must be cleared after surgery. These patients require intensive respiratory assistance from skilled nurses and respiratory therapists.

OPERATIVE TECHNIQUES

Many pulmonary procedures are performed routinely, ranging from diagnostic tests to major surgical undertakings. Requirements for PACU care vary considerably. After most diagnostic procedures, insertion of drainage systems are rarely indicated. However, after most lung and pleural surgery, chest tubes are inserted just before closure of the pleural cavity. Chest tubes reexpand the resected lung and allow drainage of blood and other fluid in the pleural space. One tube is usually placed at the anterior apex of the lung to remove air when the patient is sitting upright, while another is placed at the posterior base to drain fluid that accumulates.

Chest tube drainage systems employ three compartments (Figure 12-1). The first compartment is a graduated collection chamber that allows accurate measurement of drained fluid. The next chamber is an underwater seal that acts as a one-way valve. This design allows air to escape from the pleural space but prevents return of air to the drainage sys-

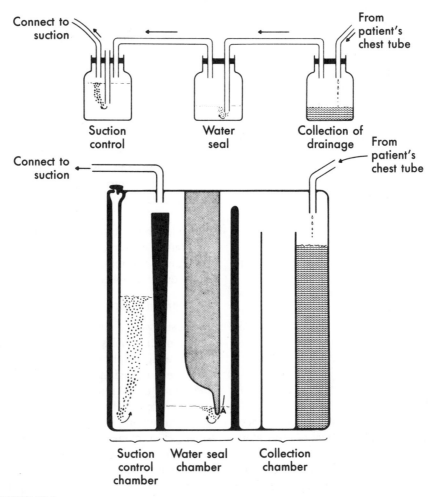

FIGURE 12-1

Schematic of a three-bottle chest tube drainage system *(top)*. Below are the corresponding chambers of the Pleur-evac unit.

tem on inspiration. The fluid in the second chamber should fluctuate with respirations. If the chest tubes become obstructed, fluctuations will cease. The third chamber contains a water column applied to suction. The height of the water column determines the amount of negative pressure that can be generated. A small port open to the atmosphere prevents additional pressure buildup.

After most pulmonary surgery, there is usually a small air leak in the lung that closes spontaneously. When the drainage system is attached to suction, air is evacuated from the pleural space. Air should bubble through the second chamber during expiration with spontaneous ventilation or during inspiration with positive-pressure ventilation. During transfer or if continued negative pressure is not required, suction should be discontinued, with the suction tubing left open to room air. This allows egress of air from the pleural space as is passes through the water-seal chamber.

Chest tubes are not usually inserted after pneumonectomy, since negative pressure applied to the empty hemithorax can pull the mediastinum toward the resected side, alter venous return to the heart, or overdistend the remaining lung.

Diagnostic Procedures

Diagnostic procedures are performed to evaluate the extent of disease, such as preoperative staging for lung cancer, and to obtain biopsy results for tissue diagnoses. They are used to visualize many areas of the thorax, such as the trachea, bronchi, mediastinum, and pleura. Several maneuvers have been described and are discussed in the following material.

Bronchoscopy

Bronchoscopy is the most common invasive procedure used for diagnosis and treatment of respiratory diseases. This procedure allows visualization of the oropharynx, larynx, trachea, carina, and large bronchi. Postoperative considerations depend on the indication for bronchoscopy. These indications include the following:

1. Preoperative surgical evaluation for patients with lung carcinoma or tracheoesophageal fistula
2. Evaluation of hemoptysis or inhalation injury
3. Removal of foreign bodies
4. Laser resection of bronchogenic carcinoma
5. Treatment of acute respiratory failure by removal of secretions and reversal of atelectasis

Patients in group 5 are usually critically ill and require intense monitoring of their cardiopulmonary systems.

Hypoxemia and dysrhythmias are very common during bronchoscopy. Most dysrhythmias are associated with a PaO_2 <60 mm Hg and resolve with improved oxygenation. Hypoxemia may persist for several hours after bronchoscopy, necessitating (1) oxygen supplementation and (2) close monitoring of the electrocardiogram for dysrhythmias, and pulse oximetry for decreased oxygen saturations.

Complications of rigid bronchoscopy include: airway bleeding; damage to the teeth, oropharynx, or vocal cords; and perforation of the tracheal mucosa with development of pneumomediastinum and subcutaneous emphysema. If high airway pressures were required intraoperatively or if transbronchial biopsies were performed, a chest radiograph should be obtained in the PACU to rule out pneumothorax. Flexible bronchoscopy is usually performed through an endotracheal tube to examine more distal bronchi and remove secretions and is associated with fewer complications.

Mediastinoscopy

Mediastinoscopy allows direct visualization of superior mediastinal structures, as well as biopsy of mediastinal lymph nodes or masses. The mediastinoscope is passed into the mediastinum through an incision at the sternal notch. Complications of mediastinoscopy include hemorrhage, pneumothorax, and recurrent laryngeal and phrenic nerve injury. A small, asymptomatic pneumothorax often occurs postoperatively. The vocal cords should be inspected at the time of extubation; if either recurrent laryngeal nerve has been damaged, the possibility of postoperative laryngeal obstruction must be considered. This may require reintubation or tracheostomy.

Thoracoscopy and esophagoscopy

Thoracoscopy allows inspection of the pleural cavity and its contents. An endoscope is passed through a small incision in the lateral chest wall. Samples of pleural fluid and biopsy specimens of the lung may be obtained. If biopsy specimens were not obtained, an insignificant amount of residual air may be left in the pleural space. Thoracoscopy usually presents no postoperative problems. Pleural or lung biopsies may lead to a pneumothorax. Esophagoscopy can result in esophageal perforation, aspiration, or hemorrhage from lacerations and biopsies.

Pulmonary resections (pneumonectomy and lobectomy)

Pneumonectomy and lobectomy are usually performed for removal of tumors and abscesses. The ability to take deep breaths after a thoracotomy is reduced by about 40%. This decrease is greatest for 3 days postoperatively and persists for over a week. In addition, total lung volume, functional residual capacity (FRC), and residual volume are significantly reduced.

Even resting tidal respirations can cause painful stretching of the incision. To avoid pain, patients reflexly contract their expiratory muscles near the incision (also known as "splinting"). Patients actively exhale to rapidly diminish the incisional stretching. Breathing is shallow, and coughing and sighing are avoided. Hypoventilation, retention of secretions, and atelectasis result. Adequate analgesia eliminates these problems. The relationship of the FRC to the closing capacity is extremely important. Closing capacity is the lung volume below which the small airways are not available for ventilation. Normally, closing capacity is well below FRC (Figure 12-2) and never reached during tidal respiration. However, because of the reduction in FRC after surgery, as well as the fact that closing

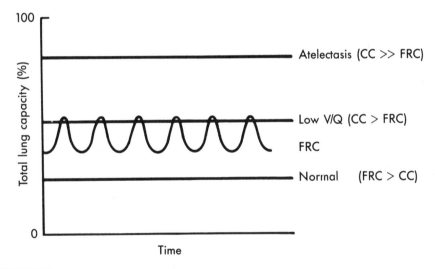

FIGURE 12-2

Relationship of FRC to CC. The sine wave represents changes in lung volume during tidal ventilation. Normally, CC is well below FRC. However, FRC declines after thoracotomy; CC may also be elevated (as occurs in heavy smokers, the supine position, and the elderly). Thus FRC may be less than CC. This can lead to low ventilation/perfusion (V/Q) ratios as blood is shunted past poorly ventilated alveoli. If the CC is extremely elevated, unventilated alveoli become atelectatic. *FRC,* Functional residual capacity; *CC,* Closing capacity.

(Reprinted with permission from Benumof JL: Anesthesia for thoracic surgery, p. 67, Philadelphia, 1987, WB Saunders Co.)

volumes are higher in smokers, the elderly, and patients in the supine position, the closing capacity may encroach on or surpass tidal ventilation after surgery.

Because these closed lung units are not ventilated, they can easily become atelectatic. Furthermore, closed alveoli are perfused. Thus hypoxemia secondary to atelectasis and intrapulmonary shunting can occur. Additionally, a reduction in FRC decreases pulmonary compliance and increases the work of breathing. All these combined changes result in problems not only in carbon dioxide elimination, but also in oxygenation. Sustained high alveolar inflating pressures should be used to reverse alveolar collapse and maintain a normal relationship of the FRC to the closing capacity. High inflating pressures can be achieved with mechanical ventilation or with maximum inspirations from incentive spirometry. Incentive spirometry inflates alveoli for about one hour and should be repeated 10 times each hour to maintain the highest possible FRC.

The diseased lung should always be placed in the nondependent (uppermost) position for several reasons. Placing the good lung in the dependent (downward) position promotes better ventilation/perfusion matching because the pulmonary blood flow is greater in the lower lung. Conversely, if the diseased lung is placed dependently, it will receive more blood flow and promote ventilation/perfusion mismatch. The dependent lung experiences higher pulmonary vascular pressures and has a tendency to transudate fluid, whereas the upper lung has a propensity to resorb fluid. If the diseased lung is placed in a dependent position, it may heal more slowly because additional fluid accumulates. Alternatively, if placed uppermost, it may heal faster because third-space fluid is resorbed more quickly. Although turning the patient hourly is advocated, the diseased lung should remain nondependent as much as possible.

COMPLICATIONS AFTER PULMONARY SURGERY

Several complications of pulmonary surgery may become apparent in the early postoperative period.

Complications after pulmonary surgery
Hypoxemia
Respiratory failure
Hemorrhage
Bronchopleural fistula
Herniation of the heart (pericardial approach)
Congestive heart failure
Intracardiac shunting
Dysrhythmias
Neural damage

Appropriate therapy in the early stages may prevent the development of more serious problems (see box above).

Hypoxemia and Respiratory Failure

The two major problems after pulmonary resection are hypoxemia and respiratory failure. Many methods are employed to improve alveolar ventilation and oxygenation (Figure 12-3). Frequent patient suctioning is required. Chest percussion and vibration serve to loosen and mobilize airway secretions. All patients must receive oxygen to compensate for shunting of blood through collapsed alveoli as a result of the diminished FRC. Inspired oxygen concentrations (FiO_2) of 0.40 in the PACU are indicated, and monitoring by pulse oximetry is essential. The patient must be encouraged to cough and eliminate secretions, which might otherwise obstruct bronchi and lead to atelectasis. However, incentive spirometry increases lung volumes and eliminates intrapulmonary shunting caused by atelectasis. Humidification of the oxygen helps to avoid drying of secretions. Administration of narcotics allows painless resting breathing and minimizes pain associated with coughing and incentive spirometry. If diseased lung remains, it should be kept nondependent. Then blood flow will be greater to the dependent good lung, maximizing ventilation/perfusion ratios. If all the diseased lung has been removed, the patient should be kept in an upright, reclining position to eliminate the pressure of abdominal contents on the lungs. Administration of bronchodilators, antibiotics, pulmonary vasodi-

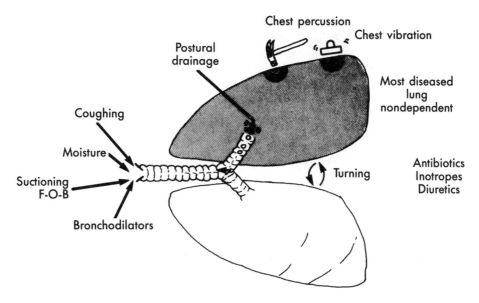

FIGURE 12-3

Regimen of aggressive respiratory therapy to diminish the risk of hypoxemia and respiratory failure. *FOB,* Fiberoptic bronchoscopy.

(Reprinted with permission from Benumof JL: Anesthesia for thoracic surgery, p. 458, Philadelphia, 1987, WB Saunder Co.)

lators, and inotropic agents as indicated will improve ventilation and perfusion. If a chest x-ray film indicates atelectasis of the right upper lobe, this may be caused by incorrect placement of a right-sided, double-lumen tube. Positive end-expiratory pressure (PEEP) or bronchoscopic reinflation should resolve the problem.

Hemorrhage

Significant hemorrhage is usually caused by dislodgment of a suture or clip around a pulmonary vessel or from bronchial or intercostal artery bleeding. Although the pulmonary vessels are not highly pressurized, bleeding into the thorax occurs into a low-pressure, high-volume cavity and may be massive. Intrathoracic bleeding may be detected in several ways. Patients may show signs of hypovolemia (hypotension, tachycardia, diminished urine output). The volume of blood in the chest drainage system may be excessive; bleeding greater than 150 to 200 ml per hour for more than 3 hours necessi-

tates further exploration. The hematocrit of normal chest tube drainage should be less than 20%. Higher hematocrits signify active bleeding. In patients without chest tubes, blood accumulates in the operated hemithorax, eventually resulting in a tension hemithorax with mediastinal shift. Exsanguination may occur very rapidly and necessitate immediate thoracotomy in the PACU to obtain vascular control. Later, the patient may be returned to the operating room for aseptic closure.

Bronchopleural Fistula

Disruption of a newly oversown bronchus leads to formation of a bronchopleural fistula. This complication may arise from a defective bronchial closure, from perforation of the bronchial stump by a suction catheter, or from high airway pressures. To reduce the possibility of a bronchopleural fistula developing, early extubation after pulmonary surgery is recommended. If a chest tube is not present, a bronchopleural fistula causes a tension pneumothorax, which presents suddenly with high inspiratory pressures, mediastinal shift, ipsilateral hyperresonance, circulatory collapse, and perhaps subcutaneous emphysema. Immediate decompression of the chest can be achieved by insertion of a large-bore needle or chest tube. If a chest tube is already in position, the occurrence of a bronchopleural fistula is heralded by massive bubbling of air through the drainage system. Patients quickly become hypoxemic and hypercarbic, since inspired air preferentially courses through the low-resistance fistula. When the leak is discovered, the chest tube should be removed from suction to minimize air loss through the fistula, and left to underwater seal only. Consideration should be given to insertion of a double-lumen endotracheal tube to prevent the escape of air through the fistula and improve ventilation to the intact opposite lung. Immediate reexploration and revision of the broncial stump are needed.

Herniation of the Heart

Rarely, an intrapericardial approach is used for a pneumonectomy to allow better surgical access to the hilum and great vessels. A large pericardial defect may be present that the surgeon is unable to close. Herniation of the heart through this pericardial defect may occur, causing acute cardiovascular collapse from twisting of the superior and inferior vena cavae. Alternatively, distortion of the trachea or mainstem bronchi may cause wheezing, whereas obstruction of the pulmonary veins may cause pulmonary congestion. The electrocardiogram may show ischemic changes or a shift in the electrical axis.

Herniation of the heart usually occurs when the patient is turned or during the first few hours of positive-pressure ventilation. If the empty hemithorax becomes dependent, gravity can pull the heart downward through the defect. Large tidal volumes and high airway pressures can push the heart into the empty hemithorax, as can chest tube suction. Upon diagnosis, help must be sought immediately. The operated side of the thorax should be placed uppermost so gravity returns the herniated heart to

its normal position. Tidal volumes and ventilatory pressures should be reduced, and PEEP and chest tube suction should be eliminated. Injection of 1 to 2 liters of air into the empty hemithorax may temporize the situation. However, preparation must be made for return to the operating room and reexploration.

Right Heart Failure

Right heart failure may occur after pulmonary resection. The decrease in the cross sectional area of the pulmonary vasculature after lung resection increases right ventricular afterload. Although patients who are prone to right heart failure are usually identified preoperatively, additional stresses (for example, pulmonary vasoconstriction caused by hypoxemia and acidosis) may precipitate this complication. The diagnosis is established when right atrial pressure exceeds left atrial pressure in the presence of an abnormally low cardiac output. Treatment follows that of left heart failure, with optimization of preload, afterload, heart rate, and contractility. Preload can be diminished by administration of nitroglycerin, whereas dobutamine is an ideal inotropic agent, since it also diminishes right ventricular afterload through pulmonary vasodilation. Other causative factors, such as hypercarbia, hypoxemia, shivering, fluid overload, bronchoconstriction, and infection, should be identified and treated appropriately.

Intracardiac Shunting

As many as 34% of adults have a probe-patent foramen ovale. Normally, no shunting occurs across this one-way flap-valve because left atrial pressure exceeds right atrial pressure. However, any increase in right atrial pressure can open the foramen, causing hypoxemia as poorly oxygenated blood from the right atrium enters the left atrium. Right atrial pressure may be increased by PEEP, pulmonary or air emboli, pulmonary hypertension, or congestive heart failure. After pneumonectomy and lobectomy, dyspnea and hypoxemia may be the first signs of right-to-left shunting. A progressive PEEP-induced decrease in arterial oxygenation suggests the diagnosis. Although not generally available in the PACU, contrast two-dimensional echocardiography noninvasively confirms the diagnosis as injected air bubbles are seen traversing the atrial septum as they bypass the pulmonary circulation. Initial therapy consists of decreasing pulmonary vascular resistance (by eliminating hypoxemia, hypercarbia, acidosis, and PEEP) and administration of pulmonary vasodilators and preload reducing agents. These manipulations usually permit functional closure of the foramen ovale and correction of the shunting.

Dysrhythmias

Supraventricular dysrhythmias, especially sinus tachycardia, are common after pulmonary resection. Possible causes include preexisting cardiovascular disease, trauma to the right heart from retraction, right atrial distention from increased pulmonary vascular resistance, infection, and sympathetic nervous stimulation (from hypoxemia, hypercarbia, and pain). Treatment of the underlying cause should resolve the problem.

Nerve Injuries

During hilar or mediastinal dissection, the phrenic or recurrent laryngeal nerves may be injured. Phrenic nerve injury causes immobility of the ipsilateral hemidiaphragm. It should be suspected in patients who have normal chest x-ray examinations and who cannot be removed from ventilatory support. Partial, bilateral injury to the recurrent laryngeal nerves may cause unopposed adduction of the vocal cords, resulting in complete upper airway obstruction after extubation. This is treated by immediate reintubation and possibly tracheostomy. The damaged nerves usually heal spontaneously within several weeks. Severance of the recurrent laryngeal nerves leaves a somewhat larger glottic opening, but turbulent air flow may cause stridor and necessitate reintubation.

OTHER TYPES OF THORACIC SURGERY

Although not directly involving the lungs, several other surgical procedures are commonly performed by thoracic surgeons. Discussion of some follows.

Tracheal Resection

Areas of the trachea may have been resected because of injury, chemical burns, or neoplasm. End-to-end anastomosis or insertion of a prosthesis is performed. Postoperatively, unique problems are encountered. The neck must remain in a flexed position to reduce tension on the tracheal suture line. Early extubation is desirable to minimize pressure on the sutures by the endotracheal tube cuff and to avoid high airway pressures. Usually only small amounts of narcotics are needed, since postoperative pain is not severe. Bucking and coughing must be meticulously avoided to protect the newly sutured trachea. Chest physiotherapy may be supplemented with fiberoptic bronchoscopy to remove secretions and minimize coughing. If massive airway bleeding occurs, it is most likely the result of erosion of a tracheal prosthesis into the pulmonary artery and is usually not treatable.

Thymectomy

Thymectomy is performed to achieve remission in patients with myasthenia gravis, a neuromuscular disease characterized by weakness of voluntary muscles. Antibodies are formed to the acetylcholine receptors in the postsynaptic cleft. In advanced myasthenia gravis, respiratory and bulbar muscle weakness occurs, resulting in dysarthria, dysphagia, and recurrent aspiration. Therapy includes the administration of anticholinesterase drugs, such as pyridostigmine (Mestinon) and neostigmine (Prostigmin), to improve muscle strength. Thymectomy results in remission or clinical improvements in more than 80% of patients.

Postoperative ventilatory support is usually required for patient with the following:

1. Myasthenia of more than 6 years duration
2. Concomitant pulmonary disease

3. Daily pyridostigmine dose greater than 750 mg

4. Preoperative vital capacity less than 40 ml/kg

Myasthenic patients are extremely sensitive to muscle relaxants and respiratory depressant drugs. Hence, ventilation should be supported postoperatively until the effects of inhalation agents and muscle relaxants have dissipated. A peripheral nerve stimulator must be used intraoperatively to monitor the effects of muscle relaxants. Muscle relaxation should be reversed with anticholinesterase agents at the conclusion of the operation.

The postoperative dose of anticholinesterase drugs requires individual titration. Usually, about one half of the regular dose is needed for the first 3 postoperative days, followed by the full dose thereafter. If the patient is unable to take medication orally, neostigmine 0.5 to 1.0 mg may be given intravenously or intramuscularly every 2 to 3 hours until oral pyridostigmine can be restarted. The anticholinesterase dose may be adjusted postoperatively by using the "Tensilon test." If muscle strength improves after administration of a small dose (5 to 10 mg) of edrophonium (Tensilon), the pyridostigmine or neostigmine dose should be augmented. However, if muscular weakness occurs, the patient has received an excess of anticholinesterase agents. Signs of cholinergic crisis (weakness), bradycardia, and salivation may then appear.

The thymus may be excised through a sternotomy, lateral thoracotomy, or cervical approach. The former incisions are quite painful. Adequate analgesia from narcotics is achieved at the expense of hypoventilation, and patients often require ventilatory assistance for 1 or 2 days postoperatively. The decision to extubate should be based on objective data, including the following:

1. Ability to follow commands

2. Need for a peak inspiratory force of less than -20 cm H_2O

3. Demonstration of a vital capacity of greater than 15 ml/kg

Ability to swallow must also be assessed; pharyngeal weakness can result in respiratory obstruction and aspiration after extubation. Myasthenic patients must be closely observed for respiratory muscle fatigue in a monitored setting after extubation.

VENTILATORY ASSISTANCE

Many patients need ventilatory assistance after thoracic surgery for reasons including the following:

Preexisting lung disease

Ventilatory depression from residual anesthetics or muscle relaxants

High-risk patients after pneumonectomy

Airway bleeding

Bronchopleural fistulas

Flail chest

Extensive surgical trauma

Poor arterial blood gas results

Poor medical or nutritional status

Acute respiratory insufficiency is the most common serious complication after pulmonary resection. The incidence is 4.4% with a mortality of 50%. The major cause of carbon dioxide retention is fatigue of the respiratory muscles. Respiratory work is greater because the lungs are stiff from operative trauma and fluid overload. In addition, airway resistance is greater, while the surface for gas exchange is diminished.

Advantages to postoperative ventilatory support include provision of adequate postoperative analgesia without the risk of respiratory depression, restoration of lung volumes by positive-pressure ventilation, and a more aggressive approach to hemodynamic support without excessive concern for an adverse effect on pulmonary function. Additionally, the presence of an endotracheal tube often facilitates pulmonary toilet.

If postoperative mechanical ventilation is planned, the patient should continue to receive narcotics, sedatives, and muscle relaxants. The double-lumen tube should be changed to a standard endotracheal tube to decrease the airway resistance and work of breathing. Peak inspiratory pressures should be minimized to reduce tension on bronchial sutures. Double-lumen tubes may be left in place if there is a large bronchopleural fistula or if unilateral PEEP or differential PEEP (for example, 5 cm H_2O to the resected side and 10 cm H_2O to the opposite side) is planned.

Intermittent mandatory ventilation (IMV) is desirable after the effects of muscle relaxant drugs have been reversed, because it allows the patient to breathe spontaneously between mechanical breaths. Patients breathing spontaneously generate more negative intrapleural pressure, which helps maintain venous return and cardiac output. Patients benefit psychologically from breathing spontaneously, and their respiratory muscles continue to be exercised. IMV weaning allows a gradual transition from mechanical ventilation to respiratory independence. Synchronized IMV (SIMV) is ideal, since it avoids superimposing a mechanical breath on a spontaneous respiration already in progress. Thus it avoids the attendant hazards of overinflation, and excessive airway pressures do not occur.

Large tidal volumes of 12 ml/kg of lean body weight are desirable after lung resection. Such volumes avoid the microatelectasis associated with smaller tidal volumes. Microatelectasis progressively decreases lung compliance and increases the alveolar/arterial oxygen gradient. Smaller tidal volumes (8 to 10 ml/kg) may be used in patients with bullous or cystic disease to minimize peak inspiratory pressures and the risk of tension pneumothorax. An adequate FiO_2 (at least 0.4) and pulse oximetry must be used initially to minimize the risk of hypoxemia.

Respiratory rates of 8 to 12 breaths per minute should be used to maintain a $PaCO_2$ of 40 mm Hg. Slow respiratory rates permit low inspiration/expiration (I/E) ratios of 1:2 or 1:3. A longer expiratory time facilitates complete exhalation, avoids air trapping, and allows more time for venous return. A slower inspiratory time promotes laminar flow, lowers airway resistance, and allows a better distribution of ventilation. Hypercarbia and concomitant acidosis should be avoided unless patients are chronic retainers of carbon dioxide. Hypocarbia and alkalosis are also undesirable, since they:

- Decrease cardiac contractility by diminishing sympathetic tone and the level of ionized serum calcium
- Shift the oxygen-hemoglobin dissociation curve to the left, causing increased affinity of hemoglobin for oxygen and less tissue oxygen delivery (Figure 12-4)
- Increase oxygen consumption by a pH-mediated uncoupling of oxidative phosphorylation

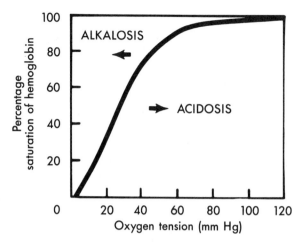

FIGURE 12-4

The oxyhemoglobin dissociation curve. Hemoglobin, the major carrier of oxygen in the bloodstream, achieves an oxygen saturation of 90% at a PaO_2 of 60 mm Hg. Because the curve begins to plateau at this level, higher oxygen tensions result in only small increases in oxygen saturation and therefore oxygen-carrying capacity. Alkalosis will shift the oxyhemoglobin dissociation curve leftward; this increases the affinity of hemoglobin for oxygen, resulting in less delivery of oxygen to vital tissues.

- Cause ventilation/perfusion mismatch by inhibiting hypoxic vasoconstriction
- Cause ventricular irritability perhaps caused by an associated hypokalemia

An FiO_2 of 0.5 or less with PaO_2 of greater than 60 mm Hg is desired for two reasons. First, an FiO_2 greater than 0.5 for an extended period is toxic to the lungs. Second, a PaO_2 of 60 mm Hg will achieve an oxygen-hemoglobin saturation of about 90%. Normally, about 98% of arterial oxygen is carried to the tissues and vital organs bound to hemoglobin. The remainder is dissolved in the plasma and creates an oxygen tension (PaO_2). For each PaO_2 there is a corresponding hemoglobin saturation as determined by the oxyhemoglobin dissociation curve (see Figure 12-4). A PaO_2 lower than 60 mm Hg will cause a marked decrease in oxygen-hemoglobin saturation and tissue oxygen delivery. Above a PaO_2 of 60 mm Hg however, large increases in PaO_2 produce only small increases in oxygen-hemoglobin saturation and tissue oxygen delivery. A PaO$_2$ of 70 mm Hg is adequate, since it provides a small margin of safety.

PEEP is the treatment of choice for arterial hypoxemia caused by ventilation/perfusion mismatching secondary to atelectasis or a low FRC. PEEP recruits alveoli and prevents early airway closure. It may be added sequentially in increments of 2.5 to 5 cm H$_2$O up to 20 cm H$_2$O. The end point for administration of PEEP is the lowest level that permits an adequate PaO$_2$ at an FiO$_2$ of less than 0.5.

Once a level of PEEP less than 10 cm H$_2$O has been achieved, the lung is functioning as an efficient gas exchange organ and weaning may proceed if the pathological condition of the lung is resolving. The IMV rate can be decreased at intervals of 2 breaths per minute, and the patient's progress can be followed by monitoring respiratory rate, arterial blood gas analysis, vital capacity inspiratory force, and pulse oximetry. If withdrawal is too rapid, the first sign is usually an increase in the respiratory rate and decrease in oxygen saturation. Vital capacity, inspiratory force, and arterial blood gas values deteriorate as the patient tires. Patients may also become hypertensive, tachycardic, diaphoretic, agitated, or develop dysrhythmias.

Once ventilatory assistance has been withdrawn and the patient is breathing independently on a T-piece for one hour, extubation is indicated (see box below). Throughout the weaning process it is important to administer adequate amounts of narcotics and sedatives so that the patient is comfortable and not resisting ventilatory assistance.

Before extubation, the oropharynx should be suctioned. If secretions are present, the endotracheal tube should be cleared. Tracheal suctioning should always be preceded and followed by several positive-pressure breaths with 100% oxygen. The lungs should be inflated to a pressure of 30 cm H$_2$O, the cuff rapidly deflated, and the endotracheal tube removed.

Thus the first event after extubation is a forceful exhalation from total lung capacity, which dislodges any material surrounding the vocal cords. The patient then receives oxygen via a face mask at an FiO$_2$ of 0.1 greater than previously. Continuous positive airway pressure (CPAP) may be required to maintain adequate oxygenation. After extubation, respiratory status must be closely followed by observation, pulse oximetry, and arterial blood gas measurements.

MANAGEMENT OF POSTOPERATIVE PAIN

There are many alternatives for alleviating incisional pain after thoracotomy (see box, next page). The two most commonly used methods are administrations of systemic and epidural narcotics.

Systemic Narcotics

Systemic narcotics have been used successfully for many years to control thoracotomy incisional pain. Nevertheless, patient comfort must be achieved without producing excessive respiratory depression or sedation. A 20% increase in arterial CO$_2$ tension may be expected to achieve adequate analgesia. The patient must be able to breathe easily without splinting and cough adequately without excessive pain to prevent retention of secretions, airway closure, and subsequent atelectasis. Small doses of narcotics (for example, morphine 2 to 4 mg) can be titrated intravenously to relieve pain.

Once analgesia has been established, it may be maintained by intermittent bolus administration or continuous infusion. Similarly, patient-controlled analgesia (PCA) can effectively treat postoperative pain once the patient has been discharged from the

---

Criteria for safe extubation

1. Adequate oxygenation
   PaO$_2$ > 70 when FiO$_2$ is less than 0.4
   PEEP < 10 cm H$_2$O
2. Adequate ventilation
   Vital capacity > 15 ml/kg
   Tidal volume > 5 ml/kg
   Respiratory rate < 25 per minute
   Negative inspiratory force > 25 cm H$_2$O
3. Acceptable mental status
   Conscious
   Following commands
   Reflexes (gag, swallow) intact
4. Active pathological condition of the lung resolving

Methods of postoperative analgesia

1. Systemic narcotics
   Intravenous
   Intramuscular
   Continuous intravenous infusion
   Patient-controlled analgesia (PCA)
2. Epidural narcotics
3. Intercostal nerve blockade
   Intermittent blocks
   Continuous catheter
4. Intrapleural catheter
5. Cryoanalgesia
6. Transcutaneous electrical nerve stimulation (TENS)

PACU. It is far better to administer narcotics to patients according to comfort rather than according to the clock.

Epidural Narcotics

Administration of epidural narcotics is the treatment of choice for postoperative pain when the patient is in a monitored setting. Epidural narcotics provide better pain relief with maintenance of adequate pulmonary function than occurs after administration of systemic narcotics. They enable long-lasting analgesia without sympathetic, motor, or sensory blockade. Epidural opiates diffuse across the dura and cerebrospinal fluid (CSF) to occupy opiate receptors in the substantia gelatinosa of the spinal cord dorsal horn. Opiate receptor stimulation in this area modulates transmission of pain signals from the incision traveling to the brain.

Many opiates have been administered epidurally. These can be classified into lipophilic (sufentanil, fentanyl, methadone, and Demerol) and low lipid-soluble (morphine) narcotics. Lipid solubility determines the onset, duration, and extent of analgesia. Epidural fentanyl results in a rapid onset, short duration (4 to 5 hours), and segmental location of analgesia. Epidural morphine, alternatively, has a slow onset (40 to 60 minutes) and results in a relatively nonsegmental block. However, its low lipid-solubility accounts for its extended duration of action (12 to 24 hours). It can be administered via the lumbar epidural route with 5 to 7.5 mg of morphine in 20 ml of sterile, preservative-free water or saline. Catheters have been left in place for 5 days without the development of opiate tolerance. Epidural fentanyl has been effectively used by continuous infusion (1 to 2 μg/kg per hour after a 2 μg/kg bolus) after thoracotomy.

There are important side effects of epidural opiate infusion. Intravascular absorption from epidural veins may result in early respiratory depression within 1 hour after administration. Late respiratory depression may result from spread of narcotics in the CSF to the medullary respiratory center. Rostral spread also accounts for the nausea and vomiting that is occasionally noted when narcotics reach the chemoreceptor trigger zone. Because of urinary retention, 15% of patients require bladder catheterization. Pruritus can also be present and may be generalized or localized. To treat such side effects, antihistamines and naloxone have been employed. Large amounts of naloxone also reverse the analgesic effect.

Other Modalities

Intercostal nerve blocks can be performed intraoperatively or postoperatively to improve lung function and arterial blood gases, and allow earlier hospital discharge. However, paravertebral spread may result in hypotension from sympathetic blockade. Performance of the block at least 8 cm from the posterior midline should prevent this complication. Nevertheless, the possibility of pneumothorax and rapid intravascular absorption of local anesthetic remains. Similarly, an intercostal catheter may be percutaneously placed to provide continuous postoperative analgesia.

Another recent technique involves the percutaneous insertion of an intrapleural catheter through which local anesthetics are instilled directly into the pleural space. As occurs after intercostal blockade, lung function and oxygenation are improved over that seen with systemic narcotics. Instillation of 20 ml of 0.5% bupivacaine allows 6 to 8 hours of unilateral pain relief. There is no respiratory depression or sympathetic or motor blockade.

Pleural pain from chest tubes can be alleviated—an effect not achieved with simple intercostal nerve block.

Cryoanalgesia provides extremely long-lasting intercostal neural blockade—lasting 6 weeks or more. Direct application of a cryoprobe to intercostal nerves during surgery results in freezing and degeneration of the nerve axons. However, because the supporting structures of the nerve are unaffected, a pathway for neuronal regeneration remains. Two to three weeks after freezing, neuronal function begins to recover. After 1 to 3 months there is complete restoration of nerve function and structure. Cryoanalgesia provides excellent pain relief, though pleural irritation from chest tubes may cause shoulder and arm pain.

Transcutaneous electrical nerve stimulation (TENS) can be used as adjunctive therapy to systemic narcotics although it is not usually available as initial therapy in the PACU. Low-voltage, high-frequency (80 Hz) transcutaneous electrical impulses stimulate large, myelinated A-fiber; these fibers inhibit small, unmyelinated C-fibers, which carry postoperative pain signals. When employed alone, however, TENS results in inadequate analgesia. It may be used as adjunctive therapy to any of the previously discussed methods. Close communication is essential to ensure that the nurse is aware of operative attempts to decrease postoperative pain so that she may appropriately modulate systemic narcotic administration and advise the patient.

SUGGESTIONS FOR FURTHER READING

Benumof JL: Anesthesia for thoracic surgery, Philadelphia, 1987, WB Saunders Co.

Benumof JL and Alfery DD: Anesthesia for thoracic surgery. In Miller RD, editor: Anesthesia, ed 2, New York, 1986, Churchill Livingstone, Inc.

Hurford WE: Anesthesia for thoracic surgery. In Firestone LL, Lebrowitz, PW, and Cook CE, editors: Clinical anesthesia procedures of the Massachusetts General Hospital, ed 3, Boston, 1988, Little, Brown & Co, Inc.

Kaplan JA: Complications of thoracic surgery. In Kaplan JA, editor, Thoracic anesthesia, New York, 1983, Churchill Livingstone, Inc.

Nakahara K, Ohno K, and Hashimoto J: Prediction of postoperative respiratory failure in patients undergoing lung resection for lung cancer, Ann Thorac Surg 46:549, 1988.

Nunn JF: Effects of anesthesia on the respiratory system. In 38th Annual Refresher Course Lectures, American Society of Anesthesiologists, Atlanta, 1987, no 254.

Reiestad F and Stromskag KE: Intrapleural catheter in the management of postoperative pain; a preliminary report, Reg Anaesth 11:89, 1986.

Shapiro BA: Evaluation of respiratory function in the perioperative period. In 31st Annual Refresher Course Lectures, American Society of Anesthesiolologists, St. Louis, 1980, no 107.

CHAPTER 13

The PACU as an Ambulatory and Special Procedures Unit

Elizabeth A.M. Frost

Medicosocioeconomic trends continue toward shorter hospital stays. An increasing number of surgical procedures are performed on a one-day stay, or ambulatory, basis. Frequently, because of space restrictions, other areas in the hospital are not available for care of these patients. The PACU therefore has assumed a critical role because it is here that many patients are monitored until they regain "street fitness" and may be discharged home.

Yet another role for the PACU has developed as that of a special procedures unit. It is difficult to predict operating times and thus PACU time on a daily basis. Periods occur in the PACU when, although staffing is available, there are few, if any, patients. This situation is most likely to occur early in the morning before the first operative procedures are completed. In many PACUs it has become routine to schedule certain procedures to fill these anticipated gaps. Other advantages of using the PACU as a special procedures unit are as follows:

1. Operating room proximity
2. Improved PACU utilization
3. Availability of intensive care nursing staff
4. Sterile area
5. Intensive care facility

6. Accessibility to anesthesiology and surgical departments

AMBULATORY SURGERY

Although 60% of all surgical procedures may be performed on an outpatient basis, the actual number is determined by several factors, including available supporting services, patient population and acceptability, and financial resources. Most frequently pediatric operations are suitable for ambulatory care because of short surgical duration and ready availability of family support. However, with increasing public awareness and involvement of close relatives, many other procedures may be treated safely on a one-day stay basis.

Operations most frequently performed on an ambulatory basis include the following:

Pediatrics	Adults
Hernia repair	D&C
Myringotomy and tube insertion	Breast biopsy
Circumcision	Varicose vein ligation
Cystometrics	Hernia repair
Endoscopy	Cystoscopy
Dental extraction	Cataract extraction

141

An area should be designated in the PACU or an adjacent room where these patients may be watched until they can be safely discharged home. Equipment requirements for such an area include the following:

- Stretchers
- Basic monitoring equipment: electrocardiogram (ECG); blood pressure
- O_2 supply, suctioning apparatus
- Lounge chairs
- Closets for storage of clothes
- Kitchen facilities to prepare light foods and beverages (for example, warm milk, tea, soda and ice)
- Drug cabinets
- Bathroom facilities
- Nearby waiting room for parents and relatives

Patients treated on an ambulatory basis should be given instructions, such as those outlined in the box below, before admission to the hospital. It is especially important to emphasize that patients must be accompanied home by a responsible adult. They should not drive within 24 hours of a general anesthetic procedure, nor should they be alone for the first day after surgery, especially if they received general anesthesia. One example of a consent form for day care surgery is illustrated in Figure 13-1.

Memory is considered to be an important function to retain in outpatients discharged shortly after general anesthesia. Test cards showing simple household items, such as shoes, fork, spoon, book, may be shown before and at varying periods after. Sufficient return of function is demonstrated by the patient's ability to recall new facts, that is, when a different memory card is identified as such. The factors affecting memory after general anesthesia are shown in Figure 13-2.

However, no single test can demonstrate accurately when the effects of anesthetic drugs have been sufficiently reversed to allow safe discharge of the patient to his home. There is no substitute for careful clinical evaluation.

The criteria that must be met before discharge

Instruction to be given to patients before admission for ambulatory surgery

Do

- Bring with you an early morning urine specimen.
- Bring someone with you to drive you home; if a child is having surgery, two adults are required: one to drive the car and one to care for the child.
- Wear loose-fitting, easy-to-put-on garments or a robe.
- Bring your insurance papers or their identifying numbers.

Do not

- Eat or drink anything after midnight before the day of surgery; take nothing by mouth; bring no food to the hospital.
- Bring jewelry or other valuables; we cannot be responsible for them.
- Bring pajamas, gowns, or slippers; the hospital supplies these.
- Bring children with you, since they may become apprehensive while waiting.

On discharge

- You will not be permitted to leave the hospital alone after administration of anesthetic; please have someone drive you home.
- You will be discharged on your physician's orders; do not drive or drink alcoholic beverages for at least 24 hours after discharge.
- You may be dizzy or drowsy; follow your doctor's orders regarding diet, rest, and medication.
- Please have a responsible adult stay with you for 24 hours after your operation.
- If you have medical problems, call your doctor (Tel. no._____) or Emergency Room (Tel. no._____), or Ambulatory Surgery Center (Tel. no._____).

I _____ agree to the operation
of _____ being performed on me under general/local
anesthesia

As instructed:

1. I have had no food or fluids for 6 hours before the general
   anesthetic.

2. I undertake not to drive my car, ride a bicycle, or operate
   machinery for 24 hours after the anesthetic.

3. I shall not drink alcohol for 24 hours after the anesthetic.

4. I shall be accompanied home by a responsible person.

5. I shall not be on my own when I return home.

6. I agree to contact the day surgical unit in the event of any
   postoperative complications arising.

Date_____

Patient's signature_____

Medical witness_____

Parent/Guardian's signature_____

FIGURE 13-1
A consent form for day care surgery.

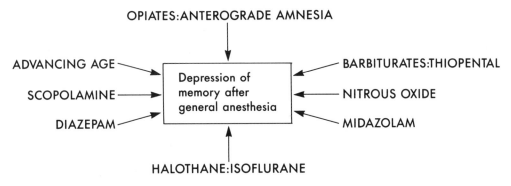

FACTORS THAT AFFECT MEMORY AFTER GENERAL ANESTHESIA

FIGURE 13-2
Several different factors may combine to contribute to decreased sensorium after general
anesthesia.

are outlined in Chapter 7. Patients should be able to tolerate fluids, dress themselves, and walk with minimal assistance. A sample discharge form is shown in Figure 13-3.

SPECIAL PROCEDURES

Procedures commonly scheduled for the PACU are as follows:

1. Electroconvulsive therapy
2. Cardioversion
3. Diagnostic nerve blocks
4. Blood patches
5. Blood transfusions
6. Monitoring placement

Staffing should be planned on a one-to-one basis. Most of these therapies, which usually do not require longer than 15 to 30 minutes, are performed by an anesthesiologist, assisted by a PACU nurse. During electroconvulsive therapy, a psychiatrist is present; during cardioversion, a cardiologist is usually in attendance.

Although epidural saline and blood patches can be completed in about 15 minutes, frequently a catheter is left in place should further administration be necessary. Patients should be observed for 1 to 2 hours.

Blood transfusions are administered slowly, and the patient's stay in the PACU may last several hours. After an initial observation period of about 15 minutes, critical nursing care is no longer essential and vital sign monitoring every 15 minutes is adequate.

Emotional support of all these patients before, during, and after these procedures must be viewed as a major aspect of their care. Although infection control is the responsibility of all medical personnel, the PACU nurse is often the main overseer of this essential aspect of patient care. Ideally a section of the PACU that can be physically isolated should be used for all special procedures. Donning of operating room garb should be required before entering this area. Sterile gloves, masks, caps, and washing facilities should be readily available. Use of disposable equipment is recommended. Frequent hand washing between patient contact and a one-to-one patient/nurse ratio curtails infection transfer.

Electroconvulsive Therapy

Electroconvulsive therapy (ECT) is a form of treatment for many manic-depressive types of psychiatric illnesses. Important considerations in these patients include the following:

History of cardiovascular disease. Hypertension and bradycardia may result from electrically induced convulsions. Before therapy, medical consultation should indicate that any hypertensive state or dysrhythmia is under the best possible control.

Evaluation of musculoskeletal disease. History of osteoporosis, frequent fractures, back pain, or disk disease should be noted because one of the complications of ECT is bony injury caused by muscle contraction.

Careful emotional support. A course of ECT involves usually 5 to 10 applications over a 3- to 5-week period. Moreover, by the nature of the illness, patients are frequently depressed or withdrawn. Special efforts should be made to communicate with the patients and to reassure them.

Oral intake. Two problematic areas may exist. Frequently patients are extremely dehydrated because of disinclination to eat. Preanesthetic preparation may require intravenous infusion of 1 liter or more of dextrose and lactated Ringer's solution. Because patients on the psychiatric service are frequently unreliable, a careful check must be made that a fasting state has been maintained for 6 hours before induction of general anesthesia.

Dentition. Poor attention to physical well-being is often manifest by oral sepsis. Loose teeth should be identified and, if necessary, removed because the induced seizure may cause them to break loose under anesthesia.

These patients are often treated as outpatients either from home or during a short transfer from a nearby psychiatric hospital. The usual preanesthetic checklist prevails and includes the following:

1. Identification.
2. Consent.
3. Nothing orally during the preceding 6 hours.
4. Securing of personal items (jewelry, other

DISCHARGE CRITERIA

1. Vital signs: ☐ Stable ☐ Other _____
2. ☐ Swallow   Cough   ☐ Gag
3. Able to ambulate: ☐ Yes ☐ No
4. Nausea, vomiting, dizziness: ☐ Minimal ☐ Other: _____
5. Absence of respiratory distress: ☐ Yes ☐ No
6. Alert and oriented: ☐ Yes ☐ No
7. Time: _____ Hours
8. Date: _____
9. Discharge note from MD _____
10. RN signature: _____

- -

SHORT STAY UNIT
POSTOPERATIVE PHONE CALL

Date call made: _____ Informant: _____

Procedure: _____ Home phone: _____

CHECK (✓) APPROPRIATE ANSWER and COMMENT IF NECESSARY

Call not completed: ☐ N/A ☐ Busy ☐ Wrong no. ☐ Not in service ☐ Disconnected ☐ Unlisted

☐ Message left with no response from parents   Comment: _____

Any vomiting?   ☐ None ☐ 1 Time ☐ 2 Times ☐ 3 Times ☐ 4 Times ☐ > 4 Times

Comment: _____

If any item below is checked ☑ Yes, describe in COMMENT section.

Sleep extra hours?   ☐ No ☐ Yes   When was child back to normal, alert self? _____

Oozing from suture line/dressing?   ☐ Normal ☐ Excessive

Elevation of temperature?   ☐ < 101° ☐ > 101°

☐ Sore throat (If adenoidectomy, please state "Adenoids" in COMMENT section) ☐ Croupiness ☐ Cough

Bad dreams?   ☐ Yes ☐ No   Muscle pain?   ☐ Yes ☐ No   Loss of appetite?   ☐ Yes ☐ No

Upset stomach?   ☐ Yes ☐ No   Headache?   ☐ Yes ☐ No   Dizziness?   ☐ Yes ☐ No

COMMENTS: _____
_____
_____
_____
_____
_____

Signature: _____

FIGURE 13-3
A sample discharge form.

valuables). Removal of dentures may not be necessary if these are tightly secured within the mouth. Also it may not be necessary and may even be therapeutically detrimental to insist on undressing the patient.

5. History and physical, including careful note of all maintenance medications.
6. Basic laboratory tests: serum chemistries, Hb, white cell count, urinalysis, ECG, and chest x-ray film. These tests need not be repeated before every treatment if no new disease processes have developed. Individual local and hospital requirements vary, but laboratory findings are generally valid for 2 to 3 weeks.

ECT should be administered in a section of the PACU that can be curtained off to provide privacy and space for treatment and recovery.

The necessary medications and equipment are listed in the box below. The patient is prepared in bed by monitoring the blood pressure, electrocardiogram, and oxygen saturation. A peripheral vein is cannulated. After preoxygenation, atropine (0.4 mg) and a barbiturate are given. Before injection of the short-acting muscle relaxant, the blood pressure cuff is inflated to prevent flow of blood to one arm. Should frequent premature ventricular contractions develop, lidocaine 1 to 2 mg/kg is given. As soon as the patient loses consciousness, ventilation must be supported. When muscle relaxation is complete, a bite block is inserted in the mouth. Electrodes that are coated with sufficient paste are applied bilaterally or unilaterally to the head. A single shock is administered. An attenuated seizure or downward toe movement may be observed, which lasts 1 to 2 minutes. The seizure can usually be followed more accurately by observing the nonparalyzed arm.

Hypertension and either bradycardia or tachycardia occur almost immediately after the treatment. These effects are usually transient (lasting 1 to 15 minutes) and rarely require treatment. However, careful monitoring is essential. The patient should be responsive and awake within 10 minutes.

Record keeping of the vital signs, amounts of medication given, and the shock strength is very important because individual variation is commonly seen in these patients because of interaction with other long-acting drugs (such as tranquilizers, sedatives, and antidepressants). Appropriate modification of drug dose can then be made during subsequent treatments.

Cardioversion

Cardioversion is a simple, safe, and usually effective means of converting cardiac dysrhythmias to sinus rhythm. The main indications, atrial flutter and fibrillation, are usually not life-threatening situations and may be treated electively. Other dysrhythmias that respond to cardioversion include ventricular tachycardia and ventricular fibrillation. These are emergency situations and are considered more fully in Chapter 4.

Because elective cardioversion is usually preceded by a trial of drug therapy, these patients are generally already in the hospital. Patients with a history of atrial fibrillation are frequently receiving anticoagulant medication both before and after cardioversion to avoid postconversion embolization. Quinidine is often given to patients for at least 24 hours before therapy because approximately 10% of cases may be converted by this drug alone. Digitalis and β-adrenergic blocking agents are generally discontinued on the day before cardioversion because

---

Equipment and medications necessary for ECT

Medications	Equipment
Atropine 0.4 mg	Anesthetic machine or Ambu bag
Pentothal 3-5 mg/kg	
Succinylcholine 1 mg/kg	ECG
Lidocaine 1-2 mg/kg	Suction apparatus
O$_2$ supply	Sphygmomanometer
Intravenous solutions	Electrodes delivering shock
	Conductive paste
	Artificial airways
	Equipment for endotracheal intubation
	Intravenous cannulation equipment
	Pulse oximeter

overdose of these medications may make the procedure ineffective. Hypokalemia must also be corrected.

After the patient is comfortably settled in bed, essential monitoring equipment (ECG, blood pressure, oximeter) is applied. Supportive and resuscitative equipment as outlined for ECT must be readily available. A peripheral vein is cannulated, and adequate pulmonary ventilation is maintained with an enriched oxygen supply.

Before application, it is important to clean the paddles and check for formation of oxide on the surface, which may impede the delivery of adequate energy. Light anesthesia or sedation, which should be managed by an anesthesiologist, is induced with small doses of sodium pentothal (2 to 3 mg/kg), diazepam (5 to 10 mg), or midazolam (2 to 5 mg). Muscular contractions may be caused by cardioversion but are much less severe than during ECT. However, cases have been reported of torn spinous processes, and it is therefore our routine to use small doses (0.3 to 0.5 mg/kg) of succinylcholine chloride and support ventilation. Deep general anesthesia is not required if energies of 100 watt-sec or less are employed. The duration of shock is 2.5 msec, and pain is not generally severe. The unanesthetized patient may complain of a sensation of touching an exposed electrical outlet. However, repeated conversion at higher output levels in apprehensive, elderly patients requires more sedation.

The paddles of the cardiovertor are applied over the precordium and on the patient's back (anterolateral positions may be used but these require slightly higher energy outputs). Cardioversion can be successful only when adequate amounts of conductive paste are used, the paddles are far enough apart with no bridge of gel or sweat between them, and firm contact is applied.

Initial treatment for dysrhythmias of recent onset should start with low-energy current (about 20 to 40 watt-sec). If the first discharge is not successful, successive shocks of 50 to 100 watt-sec, followed by increments of 100 watt-sec are given until the dysrhythmia converts. Final discharge is 400 watt-sec.

Although slight, there is a risk of electrocution, and therefore the patient is not touched when the shock is delivered. The complications and treatment of problems that may be related to cardioversion are listed in Table 13-1.

Diagnostic Nerve Blocks

The ability to provide a sterile environment and skilled monitoring makes the PACU a suitable area for performing many types of blocks. Some of the more commonly administered nerve blocks are listed in Table 13-2.

Epidural injection, either as a single shot or as a continuous technique through a catheter, affords

---

TABLE 13-1

Complications and treatment of problems related to or caused by cardioversion

Complication	Precipitating factors	Therapy
A-V nodal dysrhythmias	Cardioversion	None—usually resolve spontaneously
Ventricular dysrhythmias	Digitalis, quinidine, hypokalemia, hypoventilation, metabolic acidosis	Lidocaine 1 to 2 mg/kg; correct cause
Cardiac arrest	Any of above	Closed chest massage; cardiac pacing
Hypotension	Multiple shocks High energy levels	Vasopressors, (norepinephrine, dopamine), cardiac pacing
Pulmonary edema	Myocardial damage	Sedation, digitalis, diuretics
Burn injuries	Inadequate gel application	Local treatment

TABLE 13-2	
Blocks administered in the PACU	
Block	**Indication**
Epidural	Pain relief; sympatholytic effect
Intercostal nerves	Postoperative pain relief; Herpes zoster
Subarachnoid	Intractable pain
Brachial plexus	Preoperative—anesthetic technique; severe angina
Stellate ganglion	Sympatholytic effect; Raynaud's disease
Celiac plexus	Chronic pain

good postoperative pain relief, particularly valuable in addicted patients in whom avoidance of narcotics is preferable. It may also be used as a diagnostic tool to assess the effect of pharmacological (and therefore temporary) interruption of pain pathways before permanent surgical or chemical section. A marked sympatholytic effect, as evidenced by increase in temperature of the lower extremities, not only indicates the benefits of surgical sympathectomy in the ischemic limb but ensures maximal blood flow to reattached tissue.

The technique involves insertion of a large-bore needle (16-gauge) into the epidural space at the appropriate level. A catheter is threaded into position and the needle withdrawn. Solutions of local anesthetic agents may then be infused as necessary, and the block may be maintained for hours or even days. When therapy is discontinued, the catheter should be carefully inspected to ensure its intactness and this finding noted in the patient's record.

Intercostal nerve blocks are given to relieve the pain of rib fractures and to provide analgesia after abdominal surgery and thus facilitate deep breathing and coughing. Because of overlapping of the distribution of nerves, three nerves must be injected to provide complete anesthesia for one dermatome.

Subarachnoid block is usually done for relief of chronic pain associated with cancer. In the terminal stages of this illness, subarachnoid alcohol block is used to cause a chemical posterior rhizotomy. Other techniques include the use of cold, hypertonic saline injections into the subarachnoid space. Pain relief has also been reported after barbotage of cerebrospinal fluid. Injection of local anesthetic agent combined with steroids, such as methylprednisolone or dexamethasone, may be effective in decreasing pain by an antiinflammatory effect. Injection is made adjacent to the suspected site of the lesion.

A small-gauge needle (22- or 25-gauge) is inserted under sterile conditions into the subarachnoid space at the appropriate level, and a local anesthetic solution (usually tetracaine, which may be combined with epinephrine for longer action) is injected.

Operations involving the hands and arms are frequently performed after block of the brachial plexus, which may be done by either a supraclavicular or axillary approach. Because this anesthetic technique has a relatively slow onset of action (about 20 to 30 minutes until total blockade), the procedure may be performed in a holding area or in the PACU. The technique involves placement of a small-gauge needle within the sheath of the brachial plexus and injection of about 20 to 40 ml of local anesthetic solution. Brachial plexus block has also been used successfully in the therapy of angina pectoris involving pain in the left arm.

Stellate ganglion block is used in the treatment of peripheral vascular disease. By abolishing sympathetic supply to the upper extremity, maximal vasodilation is achieved, which is advantageous for preserving blood supply in newly anastomosed vessels or in the treatment of Reynaud's disease. It is performed by direct injection of small volumes of anesthetic solution around the stellate ganglion in the neck.

Celiac plexus block is used in the management of chronic pain from upper abdominal viscera (usually cancer pain). If several control blocks indicate good effect, the plexus may be destroyed by injection of 25 ml of 50% alcohol.

Before performing a nerve block, which is usually done by an anesthesiologist or neurosurgeon, an intravenous route must be secured. Baseline vital signs should be recorded and appropriate monitoring (ECG, blood pressure) established. Equipment for emergency resuscitation should be available.

Other requirements include the following:
1. Well-lit area
2. Sterile field
3. Block sets as indicated
4. Local anesthetic solutions—usually lidocaine 0.5%; tetracaine 1%; or chloroprocaine 0.5% to 3%
5. Epinephrine 1 ml 1:1000 (to retard absorption of local anesthetics)

Reactions and complications after blocks are rare and are listed in Table 13-3. Local effects may be caused by direct puncture of the nerve or nearby blood vessels, or inadequate sterility. Systemic reactions are directly related to the concentration of the anesthetic in the blood, which is determined by the absorption, distribution, and metabolism of the agents. Injection into highly vascular areas or direct intravascular infusion will result in high blood concentrations. Complications usually involve the cardiovascular and central nervous systems. Myocardial depression, bradycardia, and severe hypotension may occur. Although local anesthetic agents have a sedative effect on the central nervous system at low blood levels, at higher levels, excitation and frank seizures may develop with respiratory impairment.

True allergy is extremely rare and limited mainly to ester type of drugs, such as procaine. Again cardiovascular collapse and respiratory dysfunction (especially bronchospasm) may occur. Therapy includes cardiorespiratory support, sedation, and vasopressor infusions (for example, neosynephrine 0.02% infusion, ephedrine 12.5 mg) as indicated.

More commonly, reaction may result from overdose of added vasoconstrictor substances. Treatment includes administration of α- and β-adrenergic blocking drugs (such as phentolamine and propranolol), sedation, and constant reassurance.

Blood Patches

A distressing complication of subarachnoid puncture is headache. Although this symptom usually resolves with bed rest, analgesics, and adequate hydration, occasionally the pain may be incapacitating. An epidural injection of normal saline (30 to 50 ml) or of the patient's own blood may be beneficial. A catheter is inserted into the same interspace at which the subarachnoid puncture was performed, and fluid is injected slowly until the headache abates. Adequate hydration must be maintained, and the patient should be cared for supine for 24 to 48 hours.

Blood Transfusions

Again for reasons of sterility, appropriate monitoring, and availability of skilled personnel, the PACU may be used as a convenient location to admit patients who require frequent and repeated blood transfusions. These patients are often debilitated with other severe medical problems, such as renal failure, metastatic carcinoma, leukemia, and hemophilia.

Requirements for blood transfusion include the following:
1. Warm, quiet area—preferably with a view through a window

TABLE 13-3	
Reactions and complications after nerve blocks	
Local effect in the immediate area of the block	Pain Hematoma Paresthesias Infection
Systemic reaction affecting the body as a whole	Local anesthetic action Cardiovascular collapse Seizures Allergic phenomenon Vasopressor action Tachycardia Hypertension Sweating Apprehension

2. ECG and blood pressure monitoring
3. Facilities for hand washing
4. Intravenous trays
5. Equipment for warming blood

Occasionally patients prefer some light sedation before receiving blood. If a television set or radio is available, this provides excellent diversion. Warming blood before infusion decreases the incidence of cardiac dysrhythmias and patient discomfort from cooling. Some filtration system in the administration set is also essential. However, platelets should not be given through a blood filter.

During transfusions, patients should be kept warm, the electrocardiogram monitored for dysrhythmias caused by cold or hyperkalemia, and the infusion site frequently inspected for infiltration or other reactions.

Hemolytic reaction, an immediate complication of blood transfusion, is caused by incompatibility between antibodies in the recipient's plasma and antigen contained in the donor erythrocytes (Table 13-4). General hemolysis follows. The commonest causes of this reaction are mistakes in typing, cross matching, initial sampling, or unit administration. The hemolytic process may rapidly progress to disseminated intravascular coagulopathy (DIC). Signs and symptoms include fever, shivering, chills, apprehension, hypotension, tachycardia, and hemoglobinuria.

Treatment, which is aimed at control of bleeding and prevention of renal damage, is along these lines:

1. Stop the transfusion; return the blood to the bank.
2. Describe the patient's symptoms to the bank technician or supervisor and physician of record.
3. Support the cardiovascular system; give fluids including protein and hetastarch until compatible blood is available; administer vasopressors as necessary.
4. Monitor the blood and urine for free hemoglobin.
5. Give mannitol (0.5 to 1 g/kg intravenously) and follow with furosemide 40 to 80 mg

TABLE 13-4	
Common complications associated with blood transfusions	
Disease transmission	Hepatitis (serum, infectious)
	Malaria
	AIDS
	Syphilis
	Brucellosis
Hemolytic transfusion reaction	Shivering
	Apprehension
	Hypotension
	Hemoglobinuria
	DIC
Cardiac failure	Hypotension
	Tachycardia
	Pulmonary edema
Bacteremia	Fever
	Chills
Allergic reactions	Urticaria
	Flushing
	Tachycardia
	Fever
	Bronchospasm

intravenously to ensure renal output of at least 100 ml per hour.
6. An arterial cannula should be placed and blood gases monitored.
7. Acidosis and hyperkalemia should be corrected.
8. Steroids may be given to modify the antigen antibody reaction; antihistamines may also be used (diphenhydramine 50 mg).
9. Platelet count, partial thromboplastin time, and complete blood counts should be followed hourly; hematological consultation should be sought early.
10. Should DIC develop, supportive therapy must be maintained.
11. All steps must be carefully documented on the hospital record.

If blood is transfused too rapidly, especially if there is preexistent cardiac disease, circulatory overload may develop. Useful drugs that improve cardiac function and allow the vascular system to better tolerate expansion include calcium chloride, dopamine, and digitalis preparations. Diuretics, such as furosemide, may be necessary. Occasionally ventilatory support is indicated.

By-products of bacteria that persist after sterilization are termed *pyrogens*. Use of disposable equipment has essentially eliminated this problem. However, errors in technique of blood collection may result in contamination, especially with gram-negative bacteria and their endotoxins. If septicemia develops, the outcome is usually fatal despite vigorous therapy. Prevention includes adequate refrigeration, dating procedures, careful biological control, and discarding of open bottles.

Allergic reactions caused by the presence in the donor blood of an antigen or antibody whose immunological counterpart is present in the recipient occurs during about 1% of transfusions. The reactions are usually transient, and the transfusion may be continued. Rarely angioneurotic edema or bronchospasm may require emergency therapy with epinephrine, steroids, and respiratory support.

Preoperative Placement of Invasive Monitoring Systems

Monitoring during anesthesia frequently involves measurements from catheters in veins and arteries. In the interest of efficient use of time, these cannulas may be inserted preoperatively under sterile conditions in the PACU. Although emotional support of the patients is necessary, general anesthesia is usually not required. Central venous, Swan-Ganz, and arterial catheters may all be conveniently placed. Requirements include sterile techniques, cardiovascular monitoring, and suitable transducers and other recording apparatus.

LEGAL ISSUES

All procedures performed in the PACU must be outlined in the hospital's manual. Although the physician performing the procedure (for example, the psychiatrist for ECT, the cardiologist for cardioversion) assumes medical responsibility for the patient in the PACU, the department of anesthesiology is in charge of the PACU in many hospitals. Therefore all such therapies should be scheduled with the anesthesiologist, who usually will either perform the test (for example, blocks, cannula insertion) or be in attendance (for example, ECT, cardioversion).

All procedures (except blood transfusion) require a signed and witnessed surgical consent. It is the PACU nurse's responsibility to verify the consent form.

SUGGESTIONS FOR FURTHER READING

Dunbar BS: Anesthesia for the outpatient, Amer Soc Anes Refresher Courses, San Francisco, 1988, no 214.

Korttila K: How to assess recovery from anesthesia, Amer Soc Anes Refresher Courses, Atlanta, 1987, no 224.

Lichtiger M and Moya F: Introduction to the practice of anesthesia, ed 2, New York, 1978, Harper & Row Publishers, Inc.

Ogg TW et al: Day care anesthesia and memory, Anaesthesia 34:784, 1979.

Stark DCC: Practical points in anesthesiology, ed 2, New York, 1980, Medical Exam Publishing.

CHAPTER 14

Postanesthetic Care of the Burned Patient

Gerald Scheinman

Recent surveys have found that more than 2 million people each year seek medical care secondary to burns and 100,000 of them are hospitalized. Despite improvements in both acute and chronic care of these patients, there are more than 10,000 deaths annually. It is estimated that there is a 1 in 70 chance that a resident of the United States will be hospitalized because of a burn injury.

There are two phases in the care of the burn patient: acute and chronic. The initial care centers around resuscitation and stabilization of the cardiovascular and pulmonary systems. The chronic aspect of the care of the burn patient involves treatment of the cosmetic and functional abnormalities that have resulted, as well as meeting the patient's nutritional and metabolic requirements. There has been a trend recently toward early operative procedures to excise dead tissue and apply skin grafts. This is based on findings that support an improved survival rate and cosmetic result and decreased length of hospitalization.

Because the skin is the largest organ in the body, a severe burn imposes a tremendous physiological stress on the patient. The two layers, the epidermis and dermis, have different functions. The outermost part of the epidermis is dead but provides a mechanical barrier against the environment. Within the dermis are the nerves and blood vessels to the skin. Thus a partial-thickness burn that leaves parts of the dermis intact is painful, whereas a full-thickness burn is totally anesthetic. The skin plays an important role as a barrier against bacterial invasion, as well as regulating the loss of heat and fluids.

CLASSIFICATION OF BURNS

Age, preexisting disease, and severity of burn all have a major role in determining outcome. Mortality tends to be higher at either end of the age spectrum. The severity of burn relates both to the depth of skin and the amount of body surface area involved.

First-degree burns involve minimal damage to the epidermis and are characterized by pain and erythema. Treatment is symptomatic and directed toward relief of the discomfort and fever. The wounds usually heal within 5 to 10 days.

Second-degree burns involve the entire epidermis and extend partially into the dermis. Because of exposure to the nerve endings, this type of wound is very painful. If the damage to the dermis is superficial, the wound heals rapidly because of the presence of epidermal elements in the surviving sweat glands and hair follicles. There tends to be minimal scarring. A deep burn occurs when the majority of the epidermal cells are damaged. Scarring tends to be common, and functional and cosmetic problems occur.

Third-degree burns result in total destruction of the dermis and epidermis. As a result, they are vascular and anesthetic. This type of burn will not heal spontaneously and requires skin grafting. There is a zone of ischemia present beneath these burns that is composed of injured but viable tissue. Further hypoxia, ischemia, or the development of infection makes this tissue nonviable and increases the size of the third-degree burn area. Aggressive resuscitation and management from the beginning of the patient's hospital stay is necessary to salvage this potentially viable tissue.

The percentage of the total body surface area (BSA) damaged by the burn can be calculated by several methods. The rule of nines, which divides the body into areas of 9% or multiples of 9% is probably the simplest (Figure 14-1). The total BSA

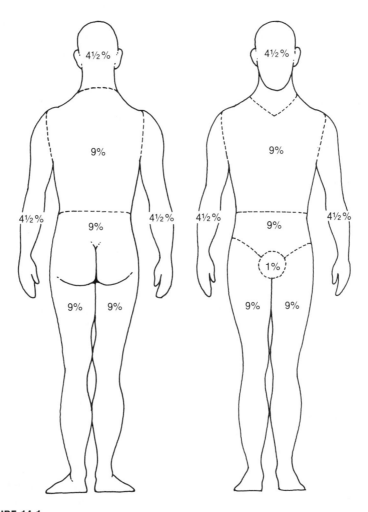

FIGURE 14-1

Multiples of 9% currently are used in assessing the amount of burned surface area.

From Parcel G: Basic Emergency Care of the Sick and Injured, ed 4, St Louis, 1990, The CV Mosby Co.

involved and the severity of the burns are important in calculating the fluid requirements necessary for resuscitation.

During the burn victim's stay in the PACU, certain aspects of his overall care are especially important. Maintenance of stability of the cardiovascular, pulmonary, and metabolic/thermoregulatory systems is the primary postoperative concern, as well as ensuring adequate pain relief and reassurance.

HEMODYNAMIC CONTROL

Primary management of the changes in the cardiovascular system that result after a severe burn is very important to good outcome. These changes may persist for as long as 48 hours after the initial injury. The leading causes of death before routine use of current treatment protocols were hypovolemic shock and/or subsequent renal failure. The loss of plasma in patients with burns that involve more than 30% of their BSA may exceed 4 ml/kg per hour.

The hypovolemia that results is caused by several factors:
- Increased microvascular permeability that occurs at the burn site
- A generalized cell membrane defect that shifts large volumes of extracellular fluid into the cell with further exacerbation of the intravascular volume depletion
- Increased interstitial oncotic pressure relative to intravascular pressure caused by an increase in vascular permeability and the evaporation of fluid as a result of the loss of the protective skin layers
- Vasoactive mediators that are released from the burned tissues

Fluid replacement can increase or decrease morbidity. Inadequate replacement can increase the amount of third-degree burn by allowing the transition of a viable but ischemic deep burn to a nonviable, full-thickness burn. Also, fluid replacement leads to generalized edema, which can also increase morbidity. Tissue edema in burned areas can result in a decreased O_2 tension as a result of an increased diffusion distance and can cause further insult to

cells already ischemic. Moreover, edema increases tissue pressure and may increase ischemia by compromising blood flow to damaged areas. This is especially important in the extremities, where circumferential burns may increase tissue pressure under the deep fascia and totally occlude the vascular supply to the limb. An immediate fasciotomy may be necessary to reestablish blood flow.

Thermal injury to tissues results in an initial decrease in blood flow. Edema begins through the heat-damaged vessels. The rate at which the edema develops and its severity depend on the amount of flow through the microcirculation and therefore the adequacy of fluid resuscitation. Systemic hypovolemia that results after a large injury may delay the rate of edema formation, which may not peak until 18 to 24 hours after the injury. In smaller burns, large gaps between endothelial cells occur in vessels in burned areas. These histological changes occur minutes after the injury and may persist from several days to weeks in those vessels that remain patent. The microvasculature becomes permeable to macromolecules the size of fibrinogen and larger. Vasoactive agents that are released from the burned tissue, leukotrienes, O_2 radicals, and prostaglandin are also thought to be responsible for the vascular changes that occur. Fluid resuscitation has to be undertaken carefully because increases in the hydrostatic pressure can markedly increase the fluid losses to the interstitial compartment because of these vascular changes. Tissues that are distant from the immediate burn site also become edematous during fluid resuscitation. The severe hypoproteinemia that results from the burn and fluid resuscitation alters the Starling forces, favoring an outward shift of the intravascular fluid. There also appears to be a loosening of the interstitial matrix, facilitating the movement of the intravascular fluid into the interstitial space. Burns that involve greater than 30% of the BSA (combined deep, partial thickness and full thickness) cause a generalized decrease in the cellular transmembrane potential that is especially prominent in muscle. This allows a shift of extracellular sodium and water into the intracellular space and generalized cellular swelling, thus increasing the volume needed for adequate resuscitation. If the fluid replacement is adequate, the membrane changes resolve after 24 to 36 hours; if not, cell death may ensue.

The burn patient's stay in the PACU may be short, but it is essential to understand the physiology of injury to continue care. Certain parameters guide hemodynamic management. As mentioned, the volume necessary for resuscitation depends on the age of the patient and BSA and on depth of burn. Several formulas help to calculate the volumes necessary for fluid replacement, but they serve only as general guidelines to be used while monitoring hemodynamic status and urine output (Table 14-1). The presence of inhalational injury markedly increases fluid requirements because the

TABLE 14-1

Commonly used formulas for estimating fluid needs of adult burn patients

Formula	Crystalloid fluid	Colloid fluid	Glucose in water
First 24 hours			
"Burn budget" of Cope and Moore	Lactated Ringer's: 1000-4000 ml 0.5 Normal saline: 1200 ml	7.5% of body weight	1500-5000 ml
Evans	Normal saline: 1.0 ml/kg/% burn	1.0 ml/kg/% burn	2000 ml
Brooke	Lactated Ringer's: 1.5 ml/kg/% burn	0.5 ml/kg/% burn	2000 ml
Parkland	Lactated Ringer's: 4 ml/kg/% burn		
"Hypertonic saline" (250 mEq Na/L)	Volume to maintain urine output of 30 ml/hr		
Modified Brooke	Lactated Ringer's: 2 ml/kg/% burn*		
Second 24 hours			
"Burn budget" of Cope and Moore	Lactated Ringer's: 1000-4000 ml 0.5 Normal saline: 1200 ml	2.5% of body weight	1500-5000 ml
Evans	½ of first 24-hour requirement	½ of first 24-hour requirement	2000 ml
Brooke	½ to ¾ of first 24-hour requirement	½ to ¾ of first 24-hour requirement	2000 ml
Parkland		20% to 60% of calculated plasma volume	To maintain adequate urinary output
"Hypertonic saline"	Up to 3500 ml of ⅓ isotonic salt solution		
Modified Brooke		0.3 to 0.5 ml/kg/% burn†	To maintain adequate urinary output

From Trauma: emergency surgery and critical care, p 72, New York, 1987, Churchill Livingstone, Inc.
*3 ml/kg/% burn in pediatric age group.
†Albumin diluted to physiological concentration in normal saline.

injured lung acts as an additional fluid reservoir. With the trend toward earlier operative procedures, it is possible that a patient presents in the PACU during the period when major fluid shifts still are occurring. Careful monitoring is essential.

The blood pressure is not a reliable parameter of the adequacy of fluid replacement because of the marked increase in catecholamine release that occurs. The maintenance of a heart rate less than 110 beats per minute usually indicates adequate fluid resuscitation except in the older patient in whom the heart may not respond appropriately to hypovolemic stress. In these patients, urine output is a more valuable guide to the degree of fluid replacement because it reflects the maintenance of renal blood flow. Indirectly, urine output may also be used to gauge the degree of perfusion of other organs. Because of the high levels of circulating catecholamines, the adult burn patient tends to be glucose intolerant. The fluid used for resuscitation should be glucose free, or an osmotic diuresis may result, which would eliminate an important indicator of the appropriateness of fluid replacement. Children differ from adults in that they lack equivalent glycogen stores or the ability to convert fats or protein to glucose. Therefore resuscitation fluid in the pediatric patient should contain glucose, and if glycosuria occurs, the glucose concentration should be decreased. The urine output in adults should be maintained at 0.5 to 1.0 ml/kg per hour and 1.0 ml/kg per hour in children. Children have a greater fluid requirement than adults for the same degree of burn and require formal fluid resuscitation at lesser percentages of BSA burns than adults. Some of the commonly used resuscitation formulas in the first 24 hours after a burn injury are listed in Table 14-1.

The use of central venous or pulmonary artery catheter monitoring in burned patients has a higher risk of complications than in other patients. During the phase of increased capillary permeability, the central venous pressure may not provide an accurate assessment of the intravascular volume. Invasive monitoring devices should probably be reserved for patients who do not respond as expected despite large volumes of resuscitative fluids.

Adequate perfusion may be accomplished with low filling pressures; the risks of empirically increasing the pressures must be weighed against those of overhydration and edema. Along with the severe hypovolemia that occurs secondary to fluid shifts, cardiac output is also decreased by a myocardial depressant factor present in plasma. It is most apparent in patients with severe burns involving BSA greater than 40%. The cardiovascular system becomes hyperdynamic, and cardiac output increases twofold to threefold. This effect may continue for several months after the injury and is the result of an increase in catecholamine and renin activity.

The use of arterial blood gases analyses to measure acid-base balance provides valuable information about the adequacy of perfusion. A persistent base deficit indicates inadequate perfusion. However, in circumstances where there has been inhalation of either carbon monoxide or cyanide, there may be inhibition of mitochondrial enzymes, leading to anaerobic glycolysis and a persistent base deficit.

AIRWAY MANAGEMENT

Pulmonary injury is the leading cause of death in patients who have suffered a major thermal burn, with a 45% to 78% mortality. The most immediate cause of death is from carbon monoxide poisoning. Management of those survivors presenting to the emergency room is based on both history and clinical examination. The history of (1) involvement in a closed-space fire or (2) impaired sensorium should increase suspicion of an inhalational injury. The presence on phyical inspection of facial or neck burns, singed eyebrows or nasal hairs, carbon deposits on the mucosa, hoarseness, a change in voice, or carbonaceous sputum is further indication of injury to the respiratory system. Fiberoptic bronchoscopy is the standard technique of diagnosis of upper airway injury. Serial examinations may be necessary because of the progressive changes that can occur over the first 18 to 36 hours. Positive findings include airway edema or inflammation, mucosal necrosis, presence of soot, or charring of the airway. Pulmonary function tests can be helpful in identifying patients with inhalational injury. The most useful is the maximum expiratory flow volume loop because it allows verification of the depression of the peak flow rate. Injury to the distal airways can be determined by performing a xenon-133 ventilation/perfusion scan. An unequal retention of the radioactive gas within the lung parenchyma beyond 90 seconds after injection constitutes a positive examination.

The patient with a major thermal burn that includes injury to the airway often has damage limited to the upper airway and larynx because of the efficiency with which the nose and mouth absorb heat. Any suspicion of an upper airway burn necessitates early intubation, because the airway may become increasingly edematous, making intubation more difficult. Airway edema may take as long as 24 hours to develop. Performing a tracheostomy after edema is established has a significantly increased risk of morbidity and mortality. The presence of thermal damage to the airway increases pulmonary lymph flow and microvascular permeability, which leads to edema formation. Pulmonary blood flow is also increased as a result of an increased metabolic rate with a high cardiac output. The net result is that the lungs are more sensitive to fluid overload and it is necessary to balance adequate perfusion against excess fluid administration. Burns that involve the respiratory tract of young children are more dangerous than similar injuries in adults for the following reasons:

1. The child's airway is smaller in diameter and more prone to become obstructed by edema.
2. Children have less respiratory reserve and fatigue more rapidly with the increased work of breathing in the presence of respiratory burns.
3. Children have increased baseline metabolic demands and O_2 consumption that are compounded by any surface burn.

Many toxic products of combustion may be present at the scene of a fire that cause a chemical burn of the airway. Water-soluble gases, such as chlorine, ammonia, hydrogen chloride, and sulfur dioxide, can damage the upper airways by their ability to react with the aqueous part of the mucous membrane to form strong acids and alkalis that ulcerate the mucous membrane and cause edema.

The lipid-soluble gases tend to travel further down the respiratory tract and cause deep burns. Soot and carbon particles may absorb these gases and help carry them down to the lower respiratory tract. All of these agents tend to impair the function of the respiratory cilia, which normally act to clear mucus and debris. This results in small airway obstruction and exacerbation of respiratory dysfunction. Proliferation of bacteria is favored in a host that is already immunocompromised.

Severe diffuse bronchoconstriction can result from direct chemical stimulation of the airways by the toxic gases and stimulation of neural reflexes. This can result in atelectasis, ventilation/perfusion (V/Q) mismatch, increased shunting, and decreased compliance. The surfactant activity of the lung also tends to be reduced, resulting in further congestion and atelectasis.

The burn patient in the PACU requires careful respiratory management. If surgery has occurred soon after the initial injury, extubation may not be possible, especially if there was any question of an inhalation burn. He is also at increased risk for hypoxemia because of increased O_2v consumption and atelectasis with V/Q mismatch. The latter results from the following:

- Decreased ciliary function with impaired mucus clearance
- Mucosal sloughing
- Release of chemotactic factors that cause an increase in white blood cell sequestration in the lung and inflammatory response
- Decreased surfactant activity

All of these combine to yield casts that obstruct and can create a ball valve effect, resulting in areas of hyperinflation and atelectasis, thus increasing $\dot{V}/\dot{Q}$ mismatch. The work of breathing is increased from the loss of surfacant activity and decreased chest wall compliance.

During recovery from anesthesia, inhalation of increased inspired concentrations of humidified, warmed oxygen is necessary for all the reasons mentioned. If the endotracheal tube is to be maintained, application of positive airway pressure may be beneficial by increasing functional residual capacity and decreasing $\dot{V}/\dot{Q}$ mismatch. In operations where large volumes of fluids have been administered secondary to blood loss, continued intubation is indicated. Vigorous pulmonary toilet is often necessary to help clear secretions, although these maneuvers may be limited by pain and by the need to keep newly grafted areas immobile.

If the decision is made to attempt a trial of extubation in a patient with suspected inhalation injury, very careful monitoring is required. Any increase in respiratory rate above 25% or decrease in oxygen saturation of 5% to 10% requires reevaluation by the anesthesiologist with a view to reintubation.

TEMPERATURE REGULATION

The burned patient is at risk of hypothermia because of the loss of the protective skin layer and the development of a hypermetabolic state. Increased evaporative and convective heat losses result from the destruction of the skin layer. These patients are at further risk in the operating room because of the following:

Large areas are exposed during the operative procedure.

Large volumes of cold or room temperature blood and crystalloid are frequently administered.

The operating suite is cold.

The patient's thermoregulatory control mechanism is disrupted by anesthesia.

A patient's normal response to hypothermia is to shiver, which increases the total oxygen consumption by 400% to 500%. The burn patient is already hypermetabolic and may not be able to meet this additional metabolic stress. It is important therefore to take appropriate measures to prevent unnecessary heat loss by the following:

• Warming the recovery area
• Warming all intravenous solutions
• Covering as much of the patient as possible
• Humidifying and warming all inspired gases
• Using a radiant heater near the patient
• Wrapping the patient in aluminum foil

Humidification is important in preventing the loss of heat because of evaporation from the lung. It also helps to protect lungs that have suffered thermal injuries and have an impaired ability to eliminate secretions.

MONITORING

During the recovery period, essential monitoring includes vital signs (heart rate, blood pressure, respiratory rate, and temperature). Urine output and arterial blood gas analyses can also supply valuable information about the adequacy of intravascular volume and perfusion.

In all patients suspected of an inhalational injury, continuous monitoring of pulse oximetry is indicated. Capnography recording should be available for patients in whom intubation is maintained.

Blood loss during surgical débridement and grafting can be extensive and can continue as oozing into the postoperative period. Measurement of the following laboratory tests and appropriate correction is important:

1. Hemoglobin and hematocrit
2. Platelet count
3. Serum electrolytes including glucose
4. Ionized calcium
5. Coagulation profile

Blood products should be given as indicated to maintain an adequate oxygen-carrying capacity and correct any coagulopathies.

INFECTION CONTROL

Burns quickly become colonized with microorganisms because they are filled with necrotic cellular material and function as excellent culture media. Any organism may be a pathogen in the burn patient, and it is usually one that is already present. Potential sources are the gastrointestinal tract, nonburned skin, or the vaginal flora. Early closure of a large burn wound by excision and grafting decreases the chance of infectious wound complications. Major excisions of infected wounds can shower the circulation with toxic by-products and cause septicemia. Tachycardia, tachypnea, an increase in temperature, and a decrease in blood pressure are signs of developing sepsis. Supportive measures should be instituted to stabilize the patient, and appropriate antibiotics should be administered.

The burn patient should be cared for in an isolated, sterile area. All attempts must be made to minimize spread of infection to the patient from other patients, visitors, or staff.

PAIN MANAGEMENT

As has been noted, full-thickness burns are not painful. However, donor areas of skin from which split-thickness grafts have been taken may be extremely painful. Also, the patient may have already undergone several procedures and been subjected to varying degrees of pain for days or weeks. Prolonged narcotic administration combined with fear and other neurobehavorial disturbances as a result, in part, of a chemical toxic effect combine to make adequate pain control very difficult.

If the trachea is still intubated and ventilatory support is provided, there should be no hesitation in administering adequate doses of narcotics. If the patient is breathing spontaneously, careful assessment of respiratory function is essential after narcotic administration. In this setting, pulse oximetry is invaluable. Wherever feasible, epidural narcotics should be used.

Often ketamine is used for dressing changes or short procedures. On emergence, patients may hallucinate. Before the patient regains consciousness, administration of small doses of diazepam or droperidol may be beneficial in reducing the severity of this complication. Grafting and resuscitative procedures require delicate surgery, and movement of the repaired area must often be strictly limited. It is of great value if the PACU nurse had been able to establish rapport with the patient preoperatively—especially if the patient is a child. Cooperation can more easily be obtained, and it may not be necessary to restrict movement. The presence of a parent or close friend beside the patient may also help to ensure a smooth emergence.

DISCHARGE

Discharge from the PACU should not occur until all changes of the recovery phase have stabilized. The patient should also have regained his prior level of consciousness and be free of pain.

SUGGESTIONS FOR FURTHER READING

Cahalane M and Demling RH: Early respiratory abnormalities from smoke inhalation, JAMA 251(6):771, 1984.

Cote CJ: Burn debridement. In Stehling, LC, editor: Common problems in pediatric anesthesia, Chicago, 1982, Year Book Medical Publishers, Inc.

Dasco CC, Luterman A, and Curreri PW: Systemic antibiotic treatment in burned patients, Burns Surg Clin North Am 67(1)57, 1987.

Demling RH: Burns, N Engl J Med 313(22):1389, 1985.

Demling RH: Fluid replacement in burned patients, Burns Surg Clin North Am 67(1):15, 1987.

Demling RH: Pathophysiology of burn injury. In: Richardson JD, Polk HC, Jr, and Flint LM, editors: Trauma: clinical care and pathophysiology, Chicago, 1987, Year Book Medical Publishers, Inc.

Formosa PJ and Waxman K: Inhalation injuries in burn patients, Hospital Physician p. 69 July 1986.

Hammond JS and Ward CG: Complications of the burn injury, Burns Crit Care Clin 1(1):175, 1985.

Haponik EF and Summer WR: Respiratory complications in burned patients: pathogenesis and spectrum of inhalation injury, J Crit Care 2(1):49, 1987.

Heimbach D: Inhalation injury. In Wachtel TL and Frank DH, editors: Burns of the head and neck, Philadelphia, 1984, WB Saunders Co.

Herdon DN et al: Pulmonary injury in burned patients, Burns, Surg Clin North Am 67(1):31, 1987.

Lamb JD: Anesthetic considerations for the major thermal injury, Can Anaesth Soc J 32(1)84, 1985.

Lund CC and Browder NC: The estimation of areas of burns, Surg Gynecol Obstet 79:352, 1944.

Luterman A, Dasco CC, and Curreri PW: Infections in burn patients, Am J Med 81(1A):45, 1986.

Merrell SW et al: Fluid resuscitation in thermally injured children, Am J Surg 152:664, 1986.

Monafo WW and Freedman B: Topical therapy for burns, Burns, Surg Clin North Am 67(1):133, 1987.

Moran K and Munster AM: Alterations of the host defense mechanism in burned patients, Burns, Surg Clin North Am 67(1):47, 1987.

Solomon JR: Pediatric Burns, Burns, Crit Care Clin 1(1):159, 1985.

Wachtel TL, Long WB, and Frank HA: Thermal injuries of the upper respiratory tract. In Wachtel TL & Frank DH, editors: Burns of the head and neck, Philadelphia, 1984, W.B. Sanders Co.

Ward CF: Anesthesia for head and neck burn surgery. In Wachtel TL & Frank DH, editors: Burns Philadelphia, 1984, W.B. Saunders Co.

CHAPTER 15

Cardiopulmonary Arrest

Marcelle M. Willock

Cardiac arrest is not a common complication in the PACU, although other life-threatening emergencies occur there. These are mostly respiratory or cardiovascular events, but surgical, neurological, metabolic, and pharmacological reasons may abound and earlier recognition and treatment of these problems may avoid more serious sequelae. Training for nurses and physicians in PACU management has always addressed these emergencies.

Standards and Guidelines for Cardiopulmonary Resuscitation (CPR) and Emergency Cardiac Care (ECC) was first published by the American Heart Association (AHA) in 1974, in the Journal of the American Medical Association and was updated in 1980 and substantially revised in 1986 (Table 15-1). These guidelines are divided into two components: basic life support (BLS) and advanced cardiac life support (ACLS). BLS covers airway maintenance, breathing, and circulation at a minimum level; ACLS covers the use of adjunctive equipment and drugs to improve ventilation and the cardiovascular and metabolic consequences of the initial problem. All physicians and nurses should be certified in basic CPR skills. It is highly recommended that all anesthesiologists be certified also in ACLS and that the course be given to PACU nursing staff, with or without a requirement for certification. When ACLS follows BLS promptly, the outcome of patients is significantly improved. Because the necessary equipment and drugs, as well as staff knowledgable in their use, are always available in the PACU, BLS and ACLS are integrated here for PACU care.

CODE DIRECTOR

For ACLS to be effective, there must be a code director, that is *one* person in charge to direct and coordinate all aspects of patient care in a logical and authoritative manner. This person should be a qualified ACLS provider. If a PACU nurse initiates the code, a qualified physician, as designated by hospital protocol, should assume the role of code director as soon as possible. The physician should elicit the patient's history, especially the anesthetics received, the surgical procedure performed, and what transpired during surgery. If the patient fails to respond to the resuscitation, the physician team leader should decide if and when to terminate resuscitative efforts. The chapter on medicolegal aspects in the *Textbook of Advanced Cardiac Life Support* presents an excellent overview of the topic. The code director should review the documentation of the resuscitation and sign it. The code sheet should contain the following: (1) time of arrest; (2) ECG rhythms, pulse, and BP; (3) drugs—time, dose, and route of administration; (4) countershocks— time and energy used; (5) other procedures—such

TABLE 15-1

Principles for the management of cardiac arrest

Priorities	Equipment from cart	Intervention
1. Recognition of arrest		1. Initiate CPR and call for help
2. Arrival of resuscitation team, emergency cart, monitor/defibrillator	2 a. Cardiac board b. Mouth-to-mask or bag-valve-mask unit with O_2 tubing c. Oral airway d. Oxygen and regulator if not already at bedside	2 a. Place patient on cardiac board b. Ventilate with 100% O_2 with oral airway and mouth-to mask or bag-valve-mask device c. Continue chest compressions
3. Identification of team leader		3 a. Assess patient b. Direct and supervise team members c. Solve problems d. Obtain patient history and events leading up to the code
4. Rhythm diagnosis	4. Cardiac monitor with quick-look paddles—defibrillator (limb leads, ECG machine—12 lead)	4 a. Apply quick-look paddles first b. Apply limb leads, but do not interrupt CPR
5. Prompt defibrillation if indicated		5. Use correct algorithm
6. Venous access	6 a. Peripheral or central IV materials b. IV tubing, infusion fluid	6 a. Peripheral: antecubital b. Central: internal jugular or subclavian
7. Drug administration	7. Drugs as ordered (and in anticipation, based on algorithms) for bolus and continuous infusion	7 a. Use correct algorithm b. Bolus or infusion
8. Intubation	8 a. Suction equipment b. Laryngoscope c. Endotracheal tube and other intubation equipment d. Stethoscope	8 a. Connect suction equipment b. Intubate patient (interrupt CPR no more than 30 seconds) c. Check tube position (listen for bilateral breath sounds) d. Hyperventilate and oxygenate
9. Ongoing assessment of the patient's response to therapy during resuscitation		9. Assess frequently: a. Pulse generated with CPR (IS THERE A PULSE?) b. Adequacy of artificial ventilation c. Spontaneous pulse after any intervention/rhythm change (IS THERE A PULSE?) d. Spontaneous breathing with return of pulse (IS THERE BREATHING?) e. Blood pressure if pulse is present f. Decision to stop if no response to therapy
10. Documentation	10. Resuscitation record	10. Accurately record events while resuscitation is in progress
11. Drawing arterial and venous blood specimens	11. Arterial puncture and venipuncture equipment	11 a. Draw specimens b. Treat as needed, based on results
12. Controlling or limiting crowd		12. Dismiss those not required for bedside tasks

Many of these activities will be enacted simultaneously; their order in this table does not mandate their exact sequence of occurrence in the code setting.

as intubations, lines, and pacemakers, including time and by whom performed; and (6) time resuscitative efforts were stopped. At regular intervals the CPR or code committee should review all resuscitation efforts.

AIRWAY

The tongue is the most common cause of upper airway obstruction in unconscious patients in the supine position. The causes of loss of tone and airway obstruction in the PACU are myriad and include (1) unconsciousness secondary to residual anesthetic agents, either inhalational or intravenous, (2) residual muscle relaxant effect, (3) preoperative condition of the patient, (4) intraoperative events, (5) shock, (6) medications given in the PACU, and (7) surgical causes, for example, type of operation, hemorrhage, and edema. With loss of time, the tongue falls back against the posterior pharyngeal wall and obstructs free passage of air into and out of the lungs.

Extending the head and lifting the chin (head tilt–chin lift) is the simplest method to open the airway. Alternatively, extending the head and thrusting the mandible forward (head tilt–jaw thrust) by placing the thumb or third fingers behind the angles of the mandible or lifting the chin can accomplish the same goal. For patients who have cervical spine injuries, the jaw thrust without head tilt is preferred. In the PACU it is common to nurse patients in the lateral position, which allows the tongue to fall forward. If the patient suffers a cardiopulmonary arrest, he should be turned supine, for it is easier for the rescuer to perform the above maneuvers with the patient in the supine position, and the patient must be supine for effective external cardiac compression. Should there be surgical causes of airway obstruction, for example, hemorrhage into the neck or airway, evacuation of blood is mandatory.

If the tilting, lifting, or thrusting maneuvers fail to relieve the obstruction or do so only temporarily, it is necessary to use adjuncts, that is, nasopharyngeal or oropharyngeal airways, or endotracheal tubes. The nasopharyngeal airway is usually better tolerated by semiconscious patients. If the oropharyngeal or nasopharyngeal airway is insufficient to relieve the obstruction, as may be the case in epiglottic obstruction, endotracheal intubation is indicated. In cases of cardiac arrest, orotracheal intubation is indicated, for it is usually easier and quicker than nasotracheal intubation. If orotracheal intubation is difficult, cricothyrotomy should be considered. The esophageal obturator airway (EOA) and the esophageal gastric tube airway (EGTA) are devices designed for out-of-hospital use and have no place in the PACU.

BREATHING

Once the airway is patent, the adequacy of breathing must be ascertained. Adequacy is defined as normal alveolar ventilation for each patient in terms of rate and tidal volume and, as sometimes measured, by blood gases. Many of the causes of airway obstruction will also depress respiration and reduce alveolar ventilation. Allied to the mechanical ability to maintain an adequate minute ventilation is the lung's ability to oxygenate the blood. Patients in the PACU receive supplemental oxygen and occasionally mechanical ventilation with varying concentrations of oxygen. Given by nasal prongs, oxygen enriches the air by 4% for each liter of oxygen. When a patient in the PACU develops cardiac or respiratory arrest, (1) immediate ventilation must be instituted, using resuscitation ventilation bags, and (2) a tidal volume of 10ml/kg must be given or a volume sufficient to raise the chest and delivered in 1 to 1.5 seconds. These bags are designed to fit onto masks or endotracheal tubes, to self-inflate, and when squeezed to deliver varying amounts of gas into the lungs. There is a one-way valve at the mask or tube end so that the patient's expired gas passes to the atmosphere and there is no rebreathing. If a patient arrests while on a ventilator, manual ventilation should be instituted because the pressure generated by external cardiac compression will exceed the pressure limit of the ventilator and abort the breathing cycle.

These bags are commonly known by their trade names, for example, Ambu, Hope. The oxygen concentration can be increased to 50% to 60% by adding oxygen at a flow rate of 10 to 15 L per minute through tubing attached to the inflow nipple. If a reservoir (either a bag or length of tubing equal in volume to the bag) is also added, the oxygen concentration in the bag may be increased to almost 100%. In cases of cardiopulmonary arrest, a bag configured to deliver 100% oxygen must be used to achieve the highest PaO_2 possible. Thus adjuncts for ventilation include the following:

- Oxygen
- Oral airways
- Nasal airways
- Endotracheal tubes
- Masks
- Ambu bags

CIRCULATION

Support of depressed circulation is usually achieved by pharmacological means except in early hypovolemic shock, in which care fluids, Trendelenburg position, or antishock garments are used, and in cardiogenic shock, when an intraaortic balloon for counterpulsation is used. When the circulation stops, as in cardiac arrest, compression of the sternum or open chest massage of the heart is mandatory to provide an instant cardiac output. The algorithms for reestablishment of circulatory function are illustrated in Figures 15-1-15-6. Adjuncts for artificial circulation include the following:

- Bed board
- Manual chest compressor
- Automatic chest compressor
- Antishock garments
- Intraaortic balloon

The technique of cardiac compression is described in the AHA guidelines and should be perfected by practice on mannequins. CORRECT HAND POSITION IS ESSENTIAL. The heel of one hand is put on the lower long axis of the sternum, and the heel of the second hand is put on top of the first; the elbows are locked, the arms straight, and the shoulders directly above the hands, so that the force of compression is straight down. Recommended cardiac compression rate is 80 to 100 per minute in the adult with sufficient force to depress the adult sternum 1½ to 2 inches, and this may generate a peak systolic pressure of 100 mm Hg, but a low diastolic pressure. A breath is interspersed on the upstroke of every fifth compression. A compression/relaxation ratio of 50:50 is recommended.

CPR should not be interrupted for longer than 30 seconds for any manuevers, such as intubation or defibrillation. A bed board should be placed under the patient's back, because the mattress pads on stretchers or beds are too soft. Manual or automatic mechanical compressors can be purchased. The cardiac press is manual and consists of a back board attached to a compressor that is manually adjustable to compress the sternum 1½ to 2 inches. This device relieves the staff of the exhausting task of compression but has a tendency to slip from its initial position and the tightening screw to loosen, resulting in less excursion and inadequate compression. The automatic chest compressor has a back board, but its plunger is powered by compressed gas. In addition, it can be set to ventilate the lungs in relation to cardiac compression. Recent data seem to indicate that a slightly longer compression/relaxation ratio and compression with the lungs inflated result in better blood flow and blood pressure.

Closed-chest massage is the preferred method of cardiac resuscitation. However, in the PACU, surgical procedures in the thoracic cavity may result in conditions such as cardiac tamponade that are best treated by opening the chest and directly compressing the heart. Open-chest massage of the heart provides better cardiac index and coronary perfusion pressure. If the patient has anatomical deformities of the chest that interfere with effective closed-chest compression, and if certain other conditions are present, such as abdominal hemorrhage, pulmonary embolus, or severe hypothermia, open-chest massage should be considered. Open-chest massage has other advantages, especially in hypovolemic shock, for it facilitates the diagnosis of an empty heart, for example, severe hypovolemia.

The pneumatic antishock garment (PASG) or military antishock trousers (MAST) is a device to

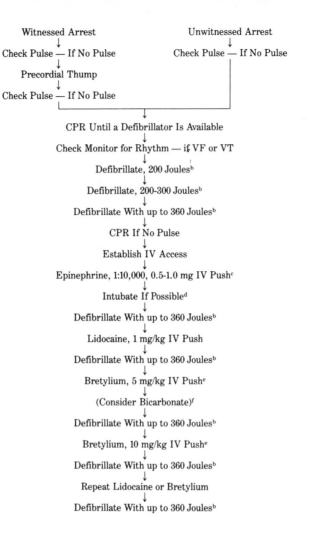

FIGURE 15-1

Ventricular fibrillation (and pulseless ventricular tachycardia). This sequence was developed to assist in teaching how to treat a broad range of patients with ventricular fibrillation (VF) or pulseless ventricular tachycardia (VT). Some patients may require care not specified herein. This algorithm should not be construed as prohibiting such flexibility. Flow of algorithm presumes that VF is continuing. *CPR,* cardiopulmonary resuscitation.

[a]Pulseless VT should be treated identically to VF.

[b]Check pulse and rhythm after each shock. If VF recurs after transiently converting (rather than persists without ever converting), use whatever energy level has previously been successful for defibrillation.

[c]Epinephrine should be repeated every 5 minutes.

[d]Intubation is preferable; if it can be accompanied simultaneously with other techniques, then the earlier the better. However, difibrillation and epinephrine are more important initially if the patient can be ventilated without intubation.

[e]Some may prefer repeated doses of lidocaine, which may be given in 0.5 mg/kg boluses every 8 minutes to a total dose of 3 mg/kg.

[f]Value of sodium bicarbonate is questionable during cardiac arrest, and it is not recommended for routine cardiac arrest sequence. Consideration of its use in a dose of 1 mEq/kg is appropriate at this point. Half of original dose may be repeated every 10 minutes if it is used.

Reproduced with permission, © *Textbook of Advanced Cardiac Life Support,* 1987, American Heart Association.

If Rhythm Is Unclear and Possibly Ventricular
Fibrillation, Defibrillate as for VF. If Asystole is Present[a]

↓

Continue CPR

↓

Establish IV Access

↓

Epinephrine, 1:10,000, 0.5 - 1.0 mg IV Push[b]

↓

Intubate When Possible[c]

↓

Atropine, 1.0 mg IV Push (Repeated in 5 min)

↓

(Consider Bicarbonate)[d]

↓

Consider Pacing

FIGURE 15-2

Asystole (cardiac standstill). This sequence was developed to assist in teaching how to treat a broad range of patients with asystole. Some patients may require care not specified herein. This algorithm should not be construed to prohibit such flexibility. Flow of algorithm presumes asystole is continuing. *VF,* ventricular fibrillation; *IV,* intravenous.
[a]Asystole should be confirmed in two leads.
[b]Epinephrine should be repeated every 5 minutes.
[c]Intubation is preferable; if it can be accomplished simultaneously with other techniques, then the earlier the better. However, CPR and use of epinephrine are more important initially if patient can be ventilated without intubation. (Endotracheal epinephrine may be used.)
[d]Value of sodium bicarbonate is questionable during cardiac arrest, and it is not recommended for the routine cardiac arrest sequence. Consideration of its use in a dose of 1 mEq/kg is appropriate at this point. Half of original dose may be repeated every 10 minutes if it is used.
Reproduced with permission, © *Textbook of Advanced Cardiac Life Support,* 1987, American Heart Association.

raise arterial pressure by increasing peripheral resistance in the lower part of the body. It is a one-piece outfit with separate compartments for the legs and abdomen and can be inflated to a maximum internal pressure greater than 100 mm Hg. The legs should always be inflated before the abdominal section, and the thoracic cage should never be encircled by the garment. Inflated, the garment increases venous return and cardiac output. If this autotransfusion results in hemodynamic and clinical improvement, there is reasonable certainty of hypovolemia. The garment should be deflated slowly in the reverse order, that is, abdomen first and legs last. The patient's blood pressure should be continually mon-

itored; a fall in pressure means more fluid is needed, and it may be necessary to reinflate the garment in the interim. If inflation of the antishock garment does not result in hemodynamic and clinical improvement, other causes of shock should be sought. The use of this device is contraindicated in cardiogenic shock, for the autotransfusion will only augment pulmonary congestion.

For those patients with cardiogenic shock refractory to fluid and pharmacological therapy, an intraaortic balloon may be helpful. This device must be inserted surgically after the patient has been heparinized. It consists of a catheter with an elongated balloon that is placed in the descending aorta. Posi-

FIGURE 15-3

Electromechanical dissociation. This sequence was developed to assist in teaching how to treat a broad range of patients with electromechanical dissociation. Some patients may require care not specified herein. This algorithm should not be construed to prohibit such flexibility. Flow of algorithm presumes that electromechanical dissociation is continuing. *CPR,* cardiopulmonary resuscitation; *IV,* intravenous.

[a]Epineprine should be repeated every 5 minutes.

[b]Intubation is preferable; if it can be accomplished simultaneously with other techniques, then the earlier the better. However, epinephrine is more important initially if the patient can be ventilated without intubation.

[c]Value of sodium bicarbonate is questionable during cardiac arrest, and it is not recommended for routine cardiac arrest sequence. Consideration of its use in a dose of 1 mEq/kg is appropriate at this point. Half of original dose may be repeated every 10 minutes if it is used.

Reproduced with permission, © *Textbook of Advanced Cardiac Life Support,* 1987, American Heart Association.

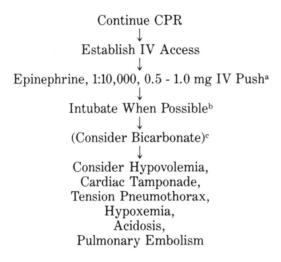

Continue CPR
↓
Establish IV Access
↓
Epinephrine, 1:10,000, 0.5 - 1.0 mg IV Push[a]
↓
Intubate When Possible[b]
↓
(Consider Bicarbonate)[c]
↓
Consider Hypovolemia,
Cardiac Tamponade,
Tension Pneumothorax,
Hypoxemia,
Acidosis,
Pulmonary Embolism

tion is checked by x-ray or fluoroscopy examination. The balloon is mechanically and automatically operated. A sensor reads the ECG, and the balloon is inflated, occluding the distal aorta right after closure of the aortic valve and improving coronary perfusion. At the onset of ventricular systole, the balloon is deflated, lessening impediment to left ventricular ejection and reducing left ventricular stroke work. If the use of the balloon results in hemodynamic and clinical improvement, duration of full counterpulsation is variable before weaning from and eventual withdrawal of this mechanical support to the circulation. Surgical closure of the arteriotomy is necessary, as is checking the distal pulses, either by palpation or Doppler, to ascertain good distal perfusion.

INTRAVENOUS FLUIDS

Every patient in the PACU should have at least one patent, free-flowing intravenous cannula in place. Fluid balance is part of the admission history, and thus if a cardiac arrest occurs, the staff will have a fair estimate of the fluid state. If hypovolemia is present, one or more routes are needed for volume expansion with one or more of the following: crystalloids, colloids, and/or blood. Central lines, for example, jugular, subclavian, or femoral, may be

FIGURE 15-4

Sustained ventricular tachycardia (VT). This sequence was developed to assist in teaching how to treat a broad range of patients with sustained VT. Some patients may require care not specified herein. This algorithm should not be construed as prohibiting such flexibility. Flow of algorithm presumes that VT is continuing. *VF,* ventricular fibrillation.

[a]If patient becomes unstable (see footnote b for definition) at any time, move to "Unstable" arm of algorithm.

[b]Unstable indicates symptoms (for example, chest pain or dyspnea), hypotension (systolic blood pressure <90 mm Hg), congestive heart failure, ischemia, or infarction.

[c]Sedation should be considered for all patients, including those defined as unstable, except those who are hemodynamically unstable (for example, hypotensive, in pulmonary edema, or unconscious).

[d]If hypotension, pulmonary edema, or unconsciousness is present, unsynchronized cardioversion should be done to avoid delay associated with synchronization.

[e]In the absence of hypotension, pulmonary edema, or unconsciousness, a precordial thump may be employed before cardioversion.

[f]Once VT has resolved, begin intravenous (IV) infusion of antidysrhythmic agent that has aided resolution of VT. If hypotension, pulmonary edema, or unconsciousness is present, use lidocaine if cardioversion alone is unsuccessful, followed by bretylium. In all other patients, recommended order of therapy is lidocaine, procainamide, and then bretylium.

Reproduced with permission, © *Textbook of Advanced Cardiac Life Support,* 1987, American Heart Association.

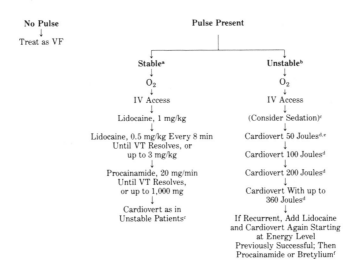

needed for certain drugs. If the arrest is not associated with hypovolemia, fluids should be given with caution. If the patient has only a peripheral IV, after delivery of the drug, a bolus of 50 ml fluid should be given to facilitate delivery of the drug to the central circulation.

DEFIBRILLATORS

The many different defibrillators on the market all operate on the same principles. They may be electrically or battery operated, but are all DC defibrillators. The energy is stored in capacitors and passes through current-limited inductors to the paddles.

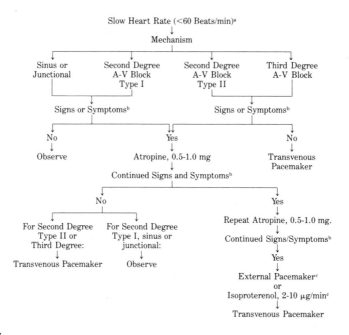

FIGURE 15-5

Bradycardia. This sequence was developed to assist in teaching how to treat a broad range of patients with bradycardia. Some patients may require care not specified herein. This algorithm should not be construed to prohibit such flexibility. *AV,* atrioventricular.
[a] A solitary chest thump or cough may stimulate cardiac electrical activity and result in improved cardiac output and may be used at this point.
[b] Hypotension (blood pressure <90 mm Hg), premature ventricular contractions, altered mental status or symptoms (for example, chest pain or dyspnea), ischemia, or infarction.
[c] Temporizing therapy.

Reproduced with permission, © *Textbook of Advanced Cardiac Life Support,* 1987, American Heart Association.

The optimal paddle shape and size for adults seem to be a round shape of 13 cm diameter. For infants 4.5 cm diameter paddles are used, and for children 8 cm paddles.

For external defibrillation there is a choice of paddle placement: standard and anterior/posterior. In standard placement, one paddle is to the right of the sternum and below the clavicle, and the other is at the apex of the heart. In the anterior/posterior placement, one paddle is over the precordium and the other is under the back directly behind the heart. This requires a flat paddle for the posterior position. For open-chest defibrillation, one paddle is placed over the right atrium and the other at the apex of the heart. If the patient has a pacemaker, the paddles should be at least 5 cm from the pulse generator. Recently, automatic implantable cardioverter-defibrillators (AICD) have been inserted in patients who are at high risk for ventricular fibrillation (VF). These patients may safely be given external defibrillation shocks at standard energies.

The skin poses resistance to the current reaching the heart, and therefore some means of reducing the resistance is necessary. This may be accomplished by using commercial defibrillator pads, saline-moistened sponges, or electrode paste between the paddles and the patient's skin. The sponges should be moistened but not so wet that the saline flows all over the chest. Similarly, the electrode paste should be only under the paddles; if not, when the current

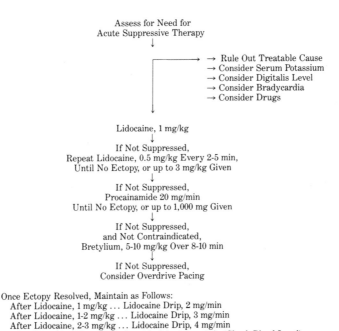

Assess for Need for
Acute Suppressive Therapy
↓

→ Rule Out Treatable Cause
→ Consider Serum Potassium
→ Consider Digitalis Level
→ Consider Bradycardia
→ Consider Drugs

Lidocaine, 1 mg/kg
↓
If Not Suppressed,
Repeat Lidocaine, 0.5 mg/kg Every 2-5 min,
Until No Ectopy, or up to 3 mg/kg Given
↓
If Not Suppressed,
Procainamide 20 mg/min
Until No Ectopy, or up to 1,000 mg Given
↓
If Not Suppressed,
and Not Contraindicated,
Bretylium, 5-10 mg/kg Over 8-10 min
↓
If Not Suppressed,
Consider Overdrive Pacing

Once Ectopy Resolved, Maintain as Follows:
After Lidocaine, 1 mg/kg ... Lidocaine Drip, 2 mg/min
After Lidocaine, 1-2 mg/kg ... Lidocaine Drip, 3 mg/min
After Lidocaine, 2-3 mg/kg ... Lidocaine Drip, 4 mg/min
After Procainamide ... Procainamide drip, 1-4 mg/min (Check Blood Level)
After Bretylium .... Bretylium Drip, 2 mg/min

FIGURE 15-6

Ventricular ectopy: acute suppressive therapy. This sequence was developed to assist in teaching how to treat a broad range of patients with ventricular ectopy. Some patients may require therapy not specified herein. This algorithm should not be construed as prohibiting such flexibility.

Reproduced with permission, © *Textbook of Advanced Cardiac Life Support*, 1987, American Heart Association.

is applied, it may bridge over rather than transverse the chest. In open-heart defibrillation, saline-moistened sponges are placed on the right atrium and apex of the heart under the paddles.

Operating the defibrillator is relatively easy after it is switched on. Some have "quick-look" paddles, that is, the ECG can be picked up via the paddles and displayed on the defibrillator screen. The energy is selected, and the capacitor switch is activated to charge it to the preselected level.

Once the desired energy level is achieved, the paddles are placed with firm pressure (25 lbs) on the patient's chest and the ECG rechecked for VF. The operator should ensure that every one is clear of the patient and then depress both buttons simultaneously, discharging the energy into the patient. After defibrillation, the ECG and pulse are checked. If

fibrillation is still present, the defibrillator must be recharged to discharge another shock. If the fibrillation is successfully terminated, the defibrillator should be turned off.

Steps in defibrillation are the following:

1. Identify VF on ECG monitor.
2. Turn defibrillator on.
3. Select energy level (200 joules, first shock) (260 joules, second shock) (360 joules, third shock)
4. Charge capacitor.
5. Apply defibrillator pads, saline-soaked sponges, or electrode jelly to patient's chest.
6. Place paddles on patient's chest in proper

position with firm pressure.

7. Recheck rhythm on ECG monitor.
8. Check that everyone is clear of patient.
9. Call out "All clear".
10. Defibrillate by depressing both buttons on paddles simultaneously.
11. Recheck rhythm on EGC.
12. Feel for carotid pulse.

In cases of ventricular and supraventricular tachydysrhythmias, a synchronized cardioversion is indicated, in which case the operation of the defibrillator is slightly different. The synchronizing switch is activated, which prohibits the operator from discharging the energy. Instead, the defibrillator is programmed to be activated by the R wave of the ECG. The energy level is selected at 50 joules, the capacitor charged to that level, and the paddles applied firmly on the patient over an appropriate skin-resistant reducing substance. The ECG on the defibrillator is checked to ensure that a prominent R wave is visible, and both buttons are depressed and kept depressed on the defibrillator. The defibrillator will discharge on being activated by the R wave. After the shock is given, the ECG should be checked for rhythm and the pulse palpated. It may be necessary to repeat the synchronized cardioversion, in which case all the steps must be followed again. Should ventricular fibrillation occur after a synchronized cardioversion, *the synchronizer switch must be turned off,* and the process for defibrillation followed.

Steps in synchronized cardioversion are the following:

1. Identify VT or supraventricular tachycardia (SVT) on ECG monitor.
2. Turn defibrillator on.
3. Activate synchronizer switch.
4. Select energy level.
5. Charge capacitor.
6. Apply defibrillator pads, saline-soaked sponges, or electrode jelly to patient's chest.
7. Place paddles on patient's chest in proper position with firm pressure.
8. Recheck rhythm on ECG monitor; look for R wave.

9. Check that everyone is clear of patient.
10. Cardiovert by depressing and holding down both buttons on paddles until discharge occurs.
11. Recheck rhythm on ECG.
12. Feel for carotid pulse.

DRUG THERAPY

Several first-line drugs must be immediately available (Table 15-2). The aims of drug therapy are as follows:

1. Correct hypoxemia
2. Reestablish spontaneous circulation
3. Increase myocardial contractility
4. Control ventricular ectopy
5. Correct acidosis
6. Treat pulmonary edema
7. Alleviate pain

Of major importance is the correction of hypoxemia by adjunctive airway equipment, administration of 100% oxygen, and measurement of arterial blood gases to determine adequacy of oxygenation and ventilation and the extent of metabolic and respiratory acidosis. With FiO_2 1.0, PaO_2 should be at least 80 mm Hg. If it is less, the endotracheal tube, oxygen flow rate, and resuscitation bag must be checked to determine that the tube is properly located and that oxygen is flowing and is connected to the resuscitation bag. If hypercapnia is present, the patient's minute ventilation must be increased. Repeated blood gas determinations are necessary.

Inadequate perfusion and inadequate ventilation lead to metabolic and respiratory acidosis. When resuscitation is begun promptly in a previously normal patient, acidosis will not be present initially. Acidosis will ensue with time even when cardiac compression is carried out according to AHA protocol, because a low-flow state exists because it is estimated that cardiac output is only about 25% to 30% of normal with external chest compressions. Both left and right ventricular outputs are depressed. Problems in oxygenation and CO_2 elimination may occur, and there is a buildup of carbonic and lactic acids. Providing 100% oxygen and adequate minute ventilation is essential to correct the respiratory component of acidosis associated with

TABLE 15-2

First-line drugs: their dosages and actions

Drug	Bolus dose	Action
Oxygen	15 L/min	Correct hypoxia
Epinephrine	0.5-1.0 mg	Increase perfusion pressure; enhance myocardial contractility; promote coarse fibrillation; increase myocardial automaticity
Lidocaine	1 mg/kg (maximum 225 mg)	Suppress ventricular ectopy
Procainamide	100 mg q 5 min (maximum 1 g)	Suppress ventricular ectopy
Bretylium	5-10 mg/kg (maximum 20 mg/kg in 2 hrs)	Elevate fibrillation threshold
Atropine	0.5-2.0 mg (maximum 2.0 mg)	Reduce vagal tone
Verapamil	0.075-0.15 mg/kg	Block slow calcium channels
Morphine	2-5 mg q 5-30 min	Relieve pain; increase venous pooling; decrease systemic vascular resistance
Sodium bicarbonate	1 mEq/kg	Correct acidosis

cardiac arrest and to alleviate the metabolic components.

Sodium bicarbonate ($NaHCO_3$) should be administered promptly *only* if the patient is known to have been in metabolic acidosis before the arrest. Establishing an effective circulation with adequate oxygenation is the best way to correct the metabolic acidosis initially, and efforts should be directed thusly; but if after 10 minutes, there is *not* an effective circulation, $NaHCO_3$ 1 mEq/kg should be given and subsequent doses of 0.5 mEq/kg every 10 minutes, or as indicated by blood gases. In the past, higher doses of $NaHCO_3$ were recommended, but it is now known that it yields a high CO_2 that enters the cells, thus aggravating the intracellular acidosis and hypercarbia.

Epinephrine is the drug of choice to improve perfusion pressure and promote spontaneous or better myocardial contractility. It is given in large doses, 1 mg every 5 minutes, at which dosage the α- effect predominates. If an intravenous route is not available, the same dose, 1 mg in 10 ml, should be given via the trachea. The intratracheal route results in a lower but longer sustained blood level. The intra-

cardiac route is the least preferred and generally not recommended because it takes time to perform and is associated with complications, such as failed administration, lung puncture, and myocardial damage.

Epinephrine will also convert fine fibrillation to coarse fibrillation, which is more amenable to defibrillation. In asystole, epinephrine has been found to initiate electrical and mechanical activity; in other pulseless rhythms, such as electromechanical dissociation (EMD), it can augment myocardial contractility.

Oxygen and epinephrine are the two first-line drugs that can be administered after a cardiac arrest without awaiting a more specific diagnosis. Other first-line drugs—atropine, lidocaine, procainamide, bretylium, verapamil, and morphine—are targeted to a diagnosis.

Atropine is indicated in bradycardia with hypotension, asystole, or pulseless idioventricular dysrhythmias. Lidocaine is given to suppress ventricular ectopy. If it is not effective, procainamide is the next choice, for it also suppresses ventricular dysrhythmias. Bretylium is useful in patients with malignant or refractory ventricular tachycardia and fibrillation. When paroxysmal supraventricular tachycardia presents, the drug of choice is verapamil. If patients are experiencing pain or acute pulmonary edema, morphine is the drug of choice.

DYSRHYTHMIAS

All patients in the PACU should be monitored by ECG, preferably lead II or a modified V_5. The common dysrhythmias are discussed in Chapter 4, and it is expected that all PACU staff can recognize them. Immediate life-threatening dysrhythmias—ventricular tachycardia, ventricular fibrillation, ventricular asystole, and electromechanical dissociation—are discussed here.

By definition, ventricular tachycardia (VT) is three or more sequential ventricular complexes occurring at a rate greater than 100 per minute but usually less than 220 (Figure 15-7). The rhythm may be regular or irregular and may or may not generate a pulse. Normal sinoatrial (SA) node activity may continue and can result in a variety of pictures on the ECG screen. P waves may occur but show no relationship to the QRS complex. SA node discharge may be received by the AV node, and by the HIS-Purkinje system when these are nonrefractory, and therefore a "normal" QRS complex (a capture beat) may occur. It is also possible that the ventricle will be depolarized from an aberrant focus at the same time, resulting in a fusion beat. Last,

the ventricles may depolarize the atria by retrograde conduction, and in this case there may be a constant relationship between the QRS and P waves.

When a patient with VT by monitor has a pulse and is hemodynamically stable, intravenous lidocaine is the drug of choice. Initial dose is 1 mg/kg, followed immediately with an infusion at the rate of 1 mg per minute. If the dysrhythmia is not terminated by the first bolus, repeated 50 mg boluses can be given every 5 minutes, up to 225 mg total. If the patient does not respond to lidocaine, procainamide is the next drug of choice. The dosage is 100 mg every 5 minutes given at a rate of 20 mg per minute. The endpoint of this medication is any of the following: (1) the dysrhythmia ceases, (2) hypotension, (3) QRS increase by 50% of original width, or (4) total of 1 g given. If the VT is refractory to both lidocaine and procainamide, bretylium is indicated. The dosage is 5 to 10 mg/kg over 8 to 10 minutes. If the abnormality persists, the dose can be repeated an hour later.

When the patient with VT is pulseless or otherwise hemodynamically unstable (hypotension or pulmonary edema), immediate DC-synchronized cardioversion is indicated. Initial dosage is 50 joules. If the first shock is unsuccessful, repeated shocks should be given, the energy increased incrementally 100, 200, up to 300 joules. In cases of recurring VT or VT refractory to drug therapy, an external or a transvenous pacemaker, set for overdrive pacing, may relieve the dysrhythmia. A rare

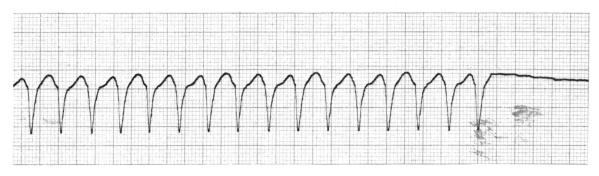

FIGURE 15-7
Ventricular tachycardia.

form of VT is torsade de pointes, in which the QRS complex appears to be constantly changing in amplitude and direction, and is usually a manifestation of toxicity to Type 1A antidysrhythmic drug. Electrical pacing is the treatment.

Ventricular fibrillation (VF) is a dire, life-threatening complication (Figure 15-8). Depolarization of the ventricles is random, resulting in chaotic contraction of the myocardial fibers and no stroke volume ejected. The ECG may show small wave amplitude (fine VF) or large wave amplitude (coarse VF). When VF or pulseless VT appears in a patient being monitored and someone is at the bedside, one precordial thump should be given immediately and the defibrillator brought into the room immediately. If the thump is not successful in stopping the dysrhythmia, defibrillation should be instituted immediately, *before* starting basic life support, with an initial energy setting of 200 joules. If the first shock is unsuccessful, another should be given immediately, with a setting of 200 to 300 joules. If this is also unsuccessful, a third shock at 360 joules is given. If this is unsuccessful, cardiac compression and ventilation with 100% oxygen should be started, epinephrine 1 mg given, and countershocks at a maximum 360 joules applied. If the chest is open and the paddles applied directly on the heart, the initial dose is 5 joules and is incrementally increased to a maximum of 40 joules if repeated shocks are needed.

Ventricular asystole means cardiac standstill. There is neither electrical nor mechanical activity in the heart, although P waves may rarely be seen. Asystole may occur spontaneously or may follow VF. Basic CPR should be started, the patient intubated quickly and ventilated with 100% oxygen, and epinephrine 0.5 to 1.0 mg given intravenously. This may initiate cardiac action, and if metabolic

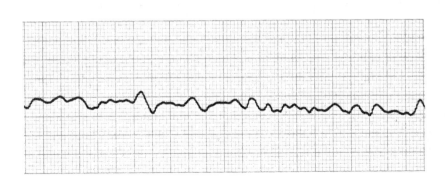

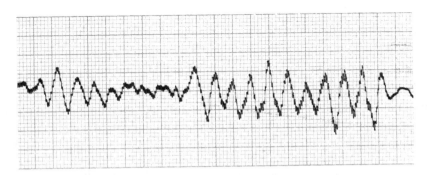

FIGURE 15-8
Ventricular fibrillation.

acidosis is present, sodium bicarbonate 1mEq/kg should be given. Atropine 1 to 2 mg intravenously similarly may cause spontaneous cardiac action. Cardiac compression must be continued throughout the resuscitation to provide an effective circulation. Defibrillation may be tried, for it is sometimes difficult to distinguish fine fibrillation from asystole on the ECG.

Cardiac standstill may follow ventricular defibrillation. First, adequacy of ventilation should be ascertained and acidosis corrected, then the usual procedures for asystole followed. Ventricular fibrillation may recur after a successful defibrillation. Oxygenation and acid-base balance must be checked and corrections made as needed, and cardiac compressions should be reinstituted. Epinephrine 0.5 to 1.0 mg is given, and defibrillation is again attempted at 200 joules. If fibrillation persists, bretylium 5 to 10 mg/kg is given.

Electromechanical dissociation (EMD) is a condition whereby the electrical depolarization of the heart is not followed by mechanical contraction. Once it is diagnosed, basic CPR with intubation and administration of 100% oxygen are followed by epinephrine 0.5 to 1.0 mg. Should no change result, acidosis should be corrected and further doses of epinephrine given. Isoproterenol may be helpful. In the PACU especially, other causes of pulselessness should be considered, such as cardiac tamponade, myocardial rupture, or ruptured aneurysm.

POSTRESUSCITATION MANAGEMENT

What happens after resuscitation and the patient's outcome depend on (1) the patient's prearrest status, (2) the duration of the resuscitative effort, and (3) the patient's immediate response.

After successful defibrillation, the carotid pulse should immediately be palpated and a blood pressure taken to determine the adequacy of the circulation. An artery should be cannulated to allow continuous monitoring of systemic arterial pressure, and frequent blood gases and electrolytes should be measured. The patient should continue to receive 100% oxygen.

Assuming the patient (1) is a previously healthy individual with a short period of resuscitation who awakens rapidly, (2) is appropriately responsive, (3) has stable hemodynamic values, and (4) breathes spontaneously, normal PACU care (that is, monitoring of vital signs and the ECG and administration of oxygen) should be continued while a diligent search for the cause of the arrest is made.

A number of dysrhythmias may occur. There may be a supraventricular rhythm, sinus or otherwise, with a normal or fast rate. A lidocaine bolus 1mg/kg followed by a continuous infusion of lidocaine 1 to 4 mg per minute should be administered. There may be bradycardia with junctional escape or atrioventricular dsyrhythmia. Adequacy of oxygenation should be checked and acidosis corrected if present. Should these measures fail to result in a rate greater than 50 beats per minute and a stable blood pressure, atropine 0.5 mg intravenously should be given to a maximum of four doses, or 2.0 mg. Isoproterenol may be effective, and other drugs, such as epinephrine, norepinephrine, dopamine, or dobutamine, may be needed to raise arterial blood pressure. A pacemaker may also be needed for overdrive pacing or complete heartblock.

A complete neurological examination should be performed to assess the patient's status and to compare it with the prearrest or preoperative state. A chest x-ray should be done and the film reviewed to rule out any pulmonary problems and to confirm placement of any central cannulas. A 12-lead ECG should be recorded, dated, and timed for a comparison with previous and subsequent strips. Blood for serum electrolytes, arterial blood gases, and cardiac enzymes should be drawn. The patient should be closely watched in the PACU for some time, and the decision to transfer him from the PACU to another unit should be made after reassessing his status through multidisciplinary consultation.

Patients may manifest single-system or multisystem failure after resuscitation. The baseline PACU care remains the same, but these patients may require continued endotracheal intubation with any of the various modalities of mechanical ventilation and varying concentrations of oxygen. Close monitoring of arterial blood gases is needed, and appropriate changes in ventilation should be made to correct respiratory acidosis or akalosis. If metabolic acidosis is present, $NaHCO_3$ may be indicated. Support of the circulation may call for vasoactive, cardiotonic, or diuretic drugs (Table 15-3). Measures to forestall occurrence of dysrhythmias should be started. A lidocaine infusion (1 to 4 mg/minute) should be considered in patients with continued ventricular ectopy. Caution is advised in the elderly and in those with congestive heart failure and shock, for toxic levels are quickly reached. Needless to say, lidocaine infusions should not be given to those patients where the cause of the arrest was an overdose of local anesthetic agent. Patients who manifest A-V nodal reentrant tachydysrhythmias

may benefit from verapamil. Arterial and pulmonary artery pressures should be monitored and cardiac output determined. A transvenous pacemaker may also be needed. A Foley catheter in the bladder provides a means of assessing renal function and fluid balance.

The central nervous system will have suffered a great insult by the cardiopulmonary arrest. After 2 to 4 minutes of arrest, brain glucose and glycogen stores fall, and after 5 minutes, adenosine triphosphate (ATP) is gone, resulting in inactivation of the intracellular sodium pump mechanism and increase in intracellular water. Not only does intracellular edema occur, but there are also changes in cellular and vascular permeability, and autoregulation of the cerebral circulation is lost. Blood flow to the brain will depend on an effective perfusion pres-

TABLE 15-3

Second-line drugs: their dosages and actions

Drug	Infusion dose	Action
Amrinone	2-20 µg/kg/min	Increase cardiac output; decrease preload
Dobutamine	2.5-20 µg/kg/min tritrated	Increase myocardial contractility
Dopamine	2-20 µg/kg/min tritrated	Increase cardiac output; increase blood pressure
Epinephrine	1-4 µg/min tritrated	Increase myocardial contractility; increase perfusion pressure
Isoproterenol	2-10 µg/min tritrated	Increase heart rate; increase myocardial contractility; decrease systemic vascular resistance
Lidocaine	1-4 mg/min	Suppress ventricular ectopy
Metaraminol	0.4 mg/ml tritrated	Increase blood pressure
Nitroglycerin	10-50 µg/min tritrated	Dilate coronary arteries; decrease blood pressure
Nitroprusside	0.5-8 µg/kg/min tritrated	Decrease blood pressure
Norepinephrine	2-12 µg/ml	Increase myocardial contractility
Propranolol	1-5 mg tritrated	Decrease heart rate; suppress dysrhythmias

sure, that is, mean arterial pressure minus intracranial pressure (ICP). It may be necessary to monitor ICP directly. Therapy is aimed at maintaining adequate cerebal perfusion pressure (CPP) at 80 to 100 mm Hg with well-oxygenated blood PaO_2 greater than 80 mm Hg and a $PaCO_2$ between 28 and 32 mm Hg. Elevating the head 30 degrees promotes venous drainage and decreases cerebral edema. Osmotic and loop diuretics are given to reduce cerebral edema. A number of other drugs—prostaglandin inhibitors, benzodiazepines, high-dose thiopental, steroids calcium-channel blockers—have been used to improve neurological outcome, but no one drug has emerged definitively as the one best, and research continues.

If coma persists, other causes should be sought, for example, hyperosmolar state, diabetes, severe electrolyte imbalance, and catastrophic intracranial events, and appropriate therapy should be instituted. Fever must be controlled, but although hypothermia is theoretically beneficial, it is not routinely used. Should convulsions occur, these must be controlled with barbiturates, diphenylhydantoin, or diazepam.

General supportive care is important. The eyes should be coated with methylcellulose and protective measures taken to avoid corneal abrasions or ulceration. Tracheal suctioning should be done quickly, for ICP rises with each suction. The hands and feet should be supported in functional positions. A nasogastric tube should be inserted and its output checked for volume and signs of bleeding. An H2 blocker may be indicated because of the high incidence of gastric stress ulceration.

EQUIPMENT

Every PACU should have a defibrillator and a crash cart. The cart should be stocked with airway equipment, as well as minor surgical trays and thorocotomy trays. The numbers of each item must be adjusted to meet the size and needs of the unit.

First-line drugs should be stocked on the crash cart in easily opened and administered packages and in standard doses. Second-line drugs are commonly found in the medicine cabinet, and it may not be necessary to have these on the cart.

The crash cart and defibrillator should be checked at least once daily and on every shift in those units open 24 hours. Once a month the bioengineering department should check the accuracy of the output of the defibrillator through a resistance of 50 ohms and record on the defibrillator the date of the test and accurate output.

SUMMARY

The guidelines of the American Heart Association for BLS and ACLS are presented, tailored to the specific problems of the PACU. It is highly recommended that all anesthesiologists and PACU nursing personnel take a full course in ACLS. The textbook on ACLS should be a standard text in the PACU.

SUGGESTIONS FOR FURTHER READING

American Heart Association Subcommittee on Emergency Cardiac Care: Standards and guidelines for cardiopulmonary resuscitation (CPR) and emergency cardiac care (ECC), JAMA 255: 2905, 1986.

American Heart Association: Textbook of advanced cardiac life support, Dallas, 1987, AHA.

CHAPTER 16

Criteria for Establishment of Brain Death

David Myland Kaufman

The concept that brain death means that the person has died has expanded our traditional determination of death, which had been based exclusively on loss of the heart beat. The brain death concept has been accepted not only by the medical community, but by the general public, most religious groups, and the federal and most state governments. As stated in the report of the President's Commission after the concept had been evolving within the medical community for two decades, "an individual with irreversible cessation of all functions of the entire brain, including the brainstem, is dead."

The staff of any PACU should be familiar with the concept and criteria of brain death. A PACU staff might receive patients in several of the following conditions that involve brain death:

- Potential donors of vital organs, such as the heart, liver, or kidney. Transplantation, which was the impetus for the development of the brain death concept, remains its most important application. Sometimes the bodies of individuals who have been declared brain dead are cared for by the PACU staff in anticipation of transplantation of those individuals' organs. Occasionally, people who are expected to become brain dead are cared for with the expectation that they will imminently become organ

donors. Until the criteria are met and the protocols are complete, their organs must remain in the body so that they are perfused by the normal circulation. Vital functions must be maintained, which often requires tremendous effort on the part of the PACU staff.

- Patients who, despite surgery, during surgery, or perhaps because of surgery, have suffered massive brain damage. While in the PACU, a surgical patient may be declared brain dead. In that case, the usual procedures for a postoperative death may be followed or, if the patient had been a potential transplant donor, respirators and other devices may be left in place until the organs are harvested.

- Potential murder cases in which the victim was shot or otherwise suffered a serious head injury. In some states, the declaration of death and the subsequent legal course may be affected by the finding that although there was no neurological activity, there was cardiac activity. In this situation, the legal issues may take precedence over the medical criteria. In any case, adherence to protocols and documentation must be meticulous.

- Cases where the PACU staff should discontinue support systems because the patient is brain dead. Application of standard for brain death will permit the staff to act with a clear conscience, conserve its resources, and apply its efforts more fruitfully to other cases.

- Cases, on the other hand, that involve severe but not fatal brain injury. In particular, anesthetic accidents that have caused extensive cerebral hypoxia sometimes cause cerebral dysfunction that is entirely reversible. At other times, anoxic damage may be extensive and permanent but not to the degree that it merits the determination of brain death. In any case, the brain death criteria in cases of cerebral hypoxia are slightly different from those instances when death occurs from other causes.

THE CRITERIA SET BY THE PRESIDENT'S COMMISSION

Many respected bodies, including Harvard Medical School, a presidential commission, and the National Institutes of Health, have set forth criteria for brain death. Although conservative by today's practice standards, the President's Commission guidelines, published in 1981, have been the most widely accepted *in toto* or are the most often used as the basis for other, usually local criteria. Its criteria for death require complete and irreversible loss of brain functions as an alternative to irreversible cessation of circulatory function (see box on right). The clinical diagnosis of brain death, which is subject to confirmation by an electroencephalogram (EEG) or other laboratory tests, rests on the following determinations by an experienced physician.

Absence of Cerebral and Brainstem Function

To establish that cerebral function is absent, the examiner must demonstrate that the individual is in deep coma, unresponsive to stimulation by noise, light, or touch. Although the individual must not display decerebrate or decorticate posturing, noxious stimulation of the limbs may elicit a withdrawal movement and reflexes in the legs may be preserved. These movements, called *spinal reflexes,*

may be present in individuals with brain death because they are modulated by spinal reflex arcs that are independent of the brain. Only some stringent criteria, such as the original Harvard criteria, would exclude individuals with spinal reflexes from the diagnosis of brain death.

To establish that brainstem function is absent, the examiner must find that the individual has lost all reflexes that are mediated by the brainstem, called *cephalic reflexes*. The examination includes the following:

- Pupillary light reflexes are tested in the standard manner by shining a bright light directly into each pupil and noting any constriction.
- Corneal reflexes are tested by touching each

The President's Commission guidelines for the determination of brain death

Cerebral function is absent.
  Deep coma must be present.

Brainstem functions are absent.
  Cephalic reflexes are absent.
    Pupillary light
    Corneal
    Oculocephalic
    Oculovestibular (cold calorics)
  Apnea must be present.
    Apnea testing* must not elicit respirations.

The cause of coma is identified, sufficient, and irreversible.
  Exclusion of correctable causes must include testing for:
    Sedative drug intoxication†
    Hypothermia (temperatures below 90° F [32.2° C])
    Hypotension (but blood pressure not specified)
    Neuromuscular blocking agents

Cessation of all brain function is persistent.
  Appropriate period of observation
    With a confirmatory test, 6 hours
    Without a confirmatory test, 12 hours
    Following cerebral hypoxia, 24 hours

Confirmatory testing is "desirable".
  EEG, under strict standards, is isoelectric*
  Four-vessel angiogram shows no circulation

Exclusion of children younger than 5 years‡

*See text for details.
†Tested as serum barbiturate level; result must be <10 µg/ml (1 mg%).
‡See text for criteria for infants and children.

cornea with a cotton swab or similar instrument in an attempt to elicit reflex eyelid closure.

- Oculocephalic reflexes are tested by rotating the individual's head and noting any compensatory reflex movement of the eyes. (Because the term *doll's eyes* is confusing, the examiner should discuss only the presence or absence of oculocephalic reflexes.)
- Oculovestibular reflexes, which are essentially the popular *cold caloric reflexes,* are tested by instilling 50 ml of ice water directly into one otic canal and after 5 minutes the other canal, using the tubing from an ''Angiocath'' or ''scalp vein needle.'' Assuming that no obstruction, such as blood or cerumen, blocks the water, the irrigation would normally produce a slow, tonic movement of both eyes toward the side of the water.
- Oropharyngeal reflexes include the common gag and cough reflexes. They are difficult to assess in the PACU, where patients are usually intubated; however, some indication might be achieved by stimulating the trachea with a suction catheter inserted through the endotracheal tube. A reaction to the catheter, such as a cough or gag, is evidence of brainstem function and precludes the diagnosis of brain death.

To demonstrate that the individual has lost brainstem function, the examiner must also show that apnea is present. The respirator is disconnected for a period of observation during which time the individual must not breathe. The President's Commission states that apnea testing should begin by ventilating the individual with pure oxygen or a mixture of oxygen and carbon dioxide for 10 minutes before withdrawal of the respirator. Oxygen is then supplied through a tracheal cannula or by other passive means, during which time blood gas determinations should confirm that $PaCO_2$ rises. (Some authors suggest that blood gas analysis be obtained to document that the $PaCO_2$ is at least 60 mm Hg.) If no spontaneous breathing occurs in 10 minutes, the individual is said to be apneic. The theory is that because 30 seconds of a $PaCO_2$ greater than 60 mm Hg would induce breathing, this procedure induces

hypercarbia sufficient to trigger respirations if the brainstem respiratory centers were functional. In the interim, the passive administration of oxygen should maintain the PaO_2 to prevent hypoxic damage to the brain (if viable) and other organs.

Irreversibility

The cause of coma should be established by the history, physical examination, and, if necessary, laboratory testing. Moreover, it must be sufficient to account for the loss of brain function. Investigations must exclude potentially correctable causes, particularly overdose with barbiturates or other sedative drugs, hypothermia, neuromuscular blockade, and cardiovascular collapse. When a cause cannot be determined, irreversibility can be inferred after an extensive evaluation, including a sufficiently long observation period or a four-vessel intracranial angiography demonstrating absent blood flow to the brain.

The duration of observation, as the President's Commission concedes, is a matter of clinical judgment. It suggests longer periods of observation than are generally practiced, especially when the cause is an obvious massive head injury, the EEG shows no electrical activity (see below), or angiography shows no blood flow. Although most medical centers seem to make a declaration of brain death as soon as an acceptable test confirms the clinical determination, the Commission has suggested a 6-hour period of observation when the clinical diagnosis is confirmed by an EEG, 12 hours in the absence of a confirmatory test, and 24 hours if the cause is cerebral hypoxia, as might pertain to anesthetic accidents, ventilatory problems, and intraoperative cardiac arrests.

Confirmatory Tests

The confirmatory tests provide reliable, objective, and permanent records of brain death. Moreover, they each entail another physician who must interpret the test and thereby double-check the diagnosis. The tests are of two types: EEG and methods to demonstrate blood flow in the brain.

The Commission states that EEG confirmation is "desirable;" however, most medical centers are more rigorous in this regard, and their standard practice is always to obtain one. The EEG recording must be performed and read under the strict criteria established by the American Electroencephalographic Society, which include eight scalp electrodes, tests for artifacts, high gain, special qualifications for the EEG technician, 30 minutes of recording, no transmission of the recording over telephone lines, and exclusion in the presence of barbiturates or hypothermia. If the EEG shows *electrocerebral silence* or is considered *isoelectric* if the body is not hypothermic and no significant amounts of barbiturates are detectable (see Complicating Conditions), it confirms the diagnosis of brain death. EEG records are rarely perfectly "flat" because they contain artifacts from numerous sources, such as cardiac activity, ventilators, intravenous fluid dripping, movement of the body by examiners, or even people walking nearby. The physician interpreting the EEG must distinguish these artifacts from genuine electrocerebral activity.

As an alternative confirmatory test to the EEG, four-vessel intracranial angiography can be performed. If it shows no blood flow in the brain, the individual can be considered brain dead. Although this study requires special equipment and moving the individual, respirator, and probably other equipment to an x-ray department, it is definitive and obviates the technical errors that can affect the EEG. Moreover, unlike the EEG, angiography is reliable in the setting of drug overdose or hypothermia. Similar tests, which can also demonstrate absent blood flow in the brain, fall within the guidelines of the President's Commission and the practice of many medical centers. The most common test in this category is radioisotope bolus cerebral angiography, a technique that is as cumbersome as the others because it requires isotopes, gamma camera imaging, and different technical problems. In the future, digital venous angiography (DIVA), which is less technically difficult than four-vessel angiography, might be accepted as an alternative.

Complicating Conditions

Because strict precautions were imposed to prevent the misdiagnosis of brain death in cases where brain injury may be partly reversible or at least not fatal, the preliminary clinical criteria and confirmatory tests may not be applicable or definitive in certain situations. Patients should have determinations of serum concentrations of barbiturates or other sedatives because an overdose could mimic brain death clinically and electroencephalographically, although not angiographically. In cases where an intoxicant is found in a patient who fulfills the clinical criteria for brain death, serial determinations must be obtained until the intoxicant is cleared from the circulation. Alternatively, angiography may be performed and the usual radiographical criteria applied. Neuromuscular blocking agents and narcotics might create a clinical picture that mimics brain death, but in these cases, subtle clinical signs and a relatively normal EEG would prevent misdiagnosis.

Another condition that would preclude a diagnosis of brain death is hypothermia. For the clinical and EEG evaluations to be valid, the core body temperature must be above 90° F (32.2° C). A permissible maneuver is to warm the individual with electric blankets so that the clinical and EEG examinations may be performed within the permissible temperature range.

The clinical criteria are also not valid when shock is present. Unlike the situation in other complicating conditions, angiography is not valid because decreased blood pressure might not perfuse the brain with sufficient force to reveal blood flow.

Although the President's Commission guidelines excluded persons younger than 5 years, brain death can now be diagnosed in infants and children by applying newly published criteria.

Guidelines for Determining Brain Death in Infants and Children

The President's Commission did not speak to the relatively common clinical problem of declaring an infant or child, younger than 5 years, brain dead. In

1987 a task force, endorsed by the preeminent neurological and pediatric societies, published guidelines that have been generally accepted. The task force's criteria may be applied only to full-term newborns older than 7 days and specifically exclude premature infants. Compared with criteria for adults, those for infants and young children are more rigorous, require more confirmatory testing, and stipulate longer observation periods. For older children, the criteria are more similar to those for adults.

History

The routine history and physical examination of the infant or child should, as for adults, indicate the cause of brain injury and, most important, exclude potentially correctable causes of coma, such as medications and drugs, neuromuscular blocking agents, shock, and hypothermia. This guideline differs from the comparable one for adults, which indicates that under certain circumstances a cause need not be established before brain death can be determined.

Physical Examination Criteria

As for adults, the primary physical neurological criteria are coma and apnea. Likewise, cephalic reflexes must be tested and found to be absent, after which tests for apnea "using standard methods *can* be performed" (italics added). Although spinal reflexes may persist, muscles must be flaccid and there must be no consciousness, spontaneous movement, or vocalization. Blood pressure and body temperature must be normal for the age. The neurological abnormalities should remain throughout the observation and testing.

Observation Periods

As noted, the guidelines are applicable neither to full-term newborns younger than 1 week nor to premature infants. With these exceptions, the recommended lengths of observation, which depend on the age of the patient, are the following:

- During the period of 7 days to 2 months, two clinical and EEG examinations at least 48 hours apart.
- During the period of 2 months to 1 year, two clinical and EEG examinations at least 24 hours apart. However, if a concomitant radionuclide angiographic study (CRAG) demonstrates no visualization of cerebral arteries, the second set of examinations is unnecessary.
- After 1 year, two clinical and EEG examinations 12 hours apart.

When an irreversible cause exists, laboratory testing is not required except in cases of cerebral hypoxia, for which longer periods of observation, for example, 24 hours, and confirmatory testing are recommended. (This is the criteria that might have to be applied in the PACU.)

Laboratory Testing

The same standards for EEG confirmation of electrocerebral silence for adults are applied to infants older than 2 months and to children, except, because of smaller head size, for shorter distances between electrodes. In these infants and children, the task force recommends CRAG as an alternative to traditional contrast angiography. Several techniques, such as DIVA, xenon computed tomography, and Doppler determinations of cerebral blood flow, are described as being "under investigation."

CRITERIA IN OTHER COUNTRIES

The criteria suggested in Canada are based on a committee composed of that country's own neuroscientists rather than simply an adoption of either the United States' or United Kingdom's criteria. Nevertheless, they are similar and compatible. Their primary requirements, which are also felt to be a clinical decision, are cessation of brain function and irreversibility. Minor differences include the need for the $PaCO_2$ to rise only as high as 50 to 55 mm Hg (rather than 60 mm Hg) when testing for apnea, an observation period "as short as 2 hours," and the specification that mean arterial blood pressure be greater than 80 mm Hg when cerebral perfusion is assessed. The Canadian criteria, which were published in 1986, do not pertain to infants and children.

The British criteria, published 5 years before the President's Commission's guidelines, were written more stringently, in a different format, and with different wording. However, they are somewhat more streamlined regarding the technical aspects but more rigorous regarding the professional staff. The requirement for complete and irreversible cessation of all brain function is implicit. Differences in criteria include the following: a $PaCO_2$ must be 50 mm Hg when testing for apnea; the body temperature must only be greater than 35° C; and an EEG is "not necessary," except in the initial stages of cases where the diagnosis is in doubt. Repeat testing is unnecessary when brain death is "obvious." Two physicians, a specialist and another doctor, are required to concur with the diagnosis.

The criteria in Japan are similar to those in Western countries: irreparable brain damage, apnea, and absent cephalic reflexes. Cases that occur in children younger than 6 years or that involve intoxications, metabolic aberrations, or hypothermia were excluded. An isoelectric EEG and at least a 6-hour period of observation are required.

CONDITIONS THAT CAN MIMIC BRAIN DEATH

The most important condition that must not be confused with brain death is cerebral hypoxia, which is sometimes called *anoxic encephalopathy*. A patient might suffer such an injury because of intraoperative or postoperative cardiac or respiratory arrest, any other ventilation or perfusion problem, or an anesthetic accident. Because the cerebral cortex is exquisitely vulnerable to inadequate perfusion by oxygenated blood, patients with cerebral hypoxia are typically initially unconscious or comatose, areflexic, and quadriplegic. Although their unresponsiveness may superficially resemble brain death, since the brainstem is relatively resistant to hypoxia, their pupils react to light and they have intact oculocephalic reflexes. Also, depending on their neurological and pulmonary status, they may be able to breathe. Within 48 hours, most patients who have suffered cerebral cortical injuries regain consciousness. Depending largely on the duration of the hypoxic episode and a fall in blood pressure, they may have permanent mental impairments. Regardless of the severity of mental impairment, however, these patients do not fulfill the criteria for brain death (see discussion on persistent vegetative state, next page).

A more serious situation occurs when patients sustain hypotension with hypoxia, as occurs during cardiac arrests for more than 3 to 5 minutes. In these cases, patients usually have damage to the brainstem, as well as the cerebral cortex, and their cephalic reflexes including their respiratory drive are impaired. Some patients recover brainstem function after 6 hours, but if they have no demonstrable brainstem function at that time, a diagnosis of brain death might be considered. This is probably the greatest dilemma for PACU personnel. In cases of cerebral hypoxia, unlike in most other cases, the criteria for diagnosing brain death require an observation period of 24 hours in both children and adults and a confirmatory test.

Barbiturates and similar sedatives, which are commonly used in committing suicide, impair cerebral and brainstem function so much so that they can abolish consciousness, cephalic reflexes, and the respiratory drive, and render the EEG isoelectric. Although a barbiturate overdose can mimic the clinical and EEG criteria of brain death, patients with barbiturate overdose can be rescued and their cerebral function restored almost regardless of the depth of coma and loss of EEG activity. A justifiably standard guideline in determining brain death is that a serum barbiturate concentration or "toxicology screen" be obtained before either the clinical evaluation is concluded or the EEG is interpreted: the barbiturate concentration must be less than 10 μg/ml (1 mg%). Similar tests for other drugs and alcohol intoxication are sometimes suggested. Likewise, neuromuscular blocking agents are described as being substances that can create an illusion of brain death; however, a history of their use would be available in a PACU and they would not affect either the EEG or angiogram.

The *persistent vegetative state* is a chronic condition that usually evolves from a state of coma and results from damage to the entire cerebral cortex or the vital, immediate subcortical structures, such as the thalamus. It often follows anoxic encephalopathy. Patients are immobile, mute, and severely impaired in all their mental functions. Although they are alert and have relatively normal breathing and other brainstem functions, and their EEG shows cerebral activity, patients fully depend on mechanical devices and nursing personnel for feeding and total bodily care. This condition's resemblance to brain death is superficial. Although it is unlikely to evolve in a PACU, the persistent vegetative state has become a timely PACU subject because it does result from cerebral cortex hypoxia from cardiac arrests, anesthetic accidents, carbon monoxide poisoning, and similar insults.

Another condition in which the brain is injured to a nonfatal but otherwise devastating extent is the *locked-in syndrome*. This condition is usually caused by a lesion at the base of the pons, most often a basilar artery thrombosis, that has severed the neurological tracts coming and going from the cerebral hemispheres to the body. A similar clinical state results from severe Guillain-Barré syndrome, which essentially interrupts all the cranial and peripheral nerves. As in the vegetative state and brain death, in the locked-in syndrome, patients are mute and immobile, and they depend on respirators and mechanical feeding devices. However, because the lesion is usually caudal to the oculomotor nerves, patients are conscious and alert, and they may have pupillary and some extraocular movements through which they can communicate. Most important, because the cerebral hemispheres are not damaged, patients with the locked-in syndrome have normal mentation and a relatively normal EEG.

THE PROTOCOL FOR DETERMINING BRAIN DEATH

In the PACU, as elsewhere, the form in which the determination of brain death is made, the *protocol,* may be as important as the actual criteria. Without a

protocol to ensure full acceptance by the family, hospital administration, legal authorities, and PACU personnel, serious repercussions may follow. A protocol must be published in a readily accessible hospital manual and approved by the administrative, legal, and medical staffs. The following protocol is an example:

- Two physicians, who must be licensed, are required to determine brain death. One physician may be a member of the patient's primary medical care givers, but the other must be a board-certified neurologist or neurosurgeon who is known to be familiar with the current criteria for determining brain death. In cases of transplantation, these two physicians must be disinterested: they should not be either a member of the transplantation team or physicians for the intended transplant recipient.
- Routine medical procedures, such as the history and physical examination, must be reviewed, dated, timed, and signed by the primary physician. If that physician makes a diagnosis of brain death, based on the President's Commission criteria for adults or the criteria for children and infants, an EEG, four-vessel angiography, or other confirmatory test is performed. Then the second physician consults. Depending on the clinical situation, clinical and confirmatory tests may be repeated after an appropriate period of observation. If the physicians' diagnosis of brain death is confirmed, the patient is pronounced dead and life-support systems are disconnected.
- In cases of transplantation, which must be documented in advance, the systems are left in place until after the organs are harvested.
- Although the determination of death is a medical decision and the family's consent is not legally required, at least in New York State, the staff should consult with the family before removing the systems, especially if they might be familiar only with the classic definitions of death. The staff might also request a review from the hospital administration before acting, especially in cases that might have legal repercussions.

• The medical examiner's or coroner's office must be notified, as usual, in cases of known or suspicious death from homicide, suicide, or accident, and in deaths after abortions, diagnostic procedures, surgery, or anesthetic procedures—all cases that might be seen in the PACU. Of course, in cases of brain death from natural causes, these authorities need not necessarily be notified.

Although the medical aspects of the criteria and protocol can be codified, the special difficulties facing the nursing staff itself have not been recognized until recently. Davis and Lemke have confronted the problems that the nursing staff face. Nurses, who typically have the responsibility of dealing with the family, as well as the individual, could feel that they have been relegated, as these authors say, ''to caring for a corpse on a respirator.'' They suggest that nurses acknowledge their feelings about death and dying, be kept as part of a team, and formulate a care plan that includes physiological stabilization of patient while maintaining privacy and dignity.

The entire staff should make a serious commitment to transplantation because of the tremendous shortage of organs and, in many cases, the psychological benefit to the family in feeling that something was salvaged. Overall, the concept of brain death has long been proven valid, accepted by almost all concerned groups, and, when properly administered, humane in its application.

SUGGESTIONS FOR FURTHER READING

American Electroencephalographic Society: Guidelines in EEG 1-7 (revised 1985), J Clin Neurophysiol 3: 131, 1986.

Davis KM and Lemke DM: Brain death: nursing roles and responsibilities, J Neurosci Nurs 19: 36, 1987.

Guidelines for the determination of death: report of the medical consultants on the diagnosis of death to the President's Commission for the Study of Ethical Problems in Medicine and Biomedical and Behavioral Research, JAMA 246: 2184, 1981.

Kaufman HH and Lynn J: Brain death, Neurosurgery 19: 850, 1986.

Lamb D: Death, brain death and ethics. Albany, NY, 1985, State University of New York Press.

Nelson RF: Determination of brain death. Can J Neurol Sci 13: 355, 1986.

Takeuchi K et al: Evolution of criteria for determination of brain death in Japan. Acta Neurochir (Wien) 87: 93, 1987.

Task Force for the Determination of Brain Death in Children: Guidelines for the determination of brain death in children, Neurology 37: 1077, 1987.

The diagnosis of brain death, Lancet 2: 1069, 1976.

PART III

ADMINISTRATION

CHAPTER 17

Planning the Physical Structure of the PACU

Margaret DeFranco

The fundamental purpose of the PACU, or post anesthesia care unit, is to provide direct and continuous patient observation during emergence from general or regional anesthesia. During this period the PACU nurse is responsible for the constant monitoring of the patient's vital functions, including cardiovascular, respiratory, and neurological status. Administration of oxygen therapy, intravenous fluids, and blood, and inspection of tubes, drains, and dressings are also performed simultaneously. Prevention or prompt recognition and treatment of postoperative complications are also objectives during this phase of the surgical experience. In addition to the specific nursing actions unique to the PACU, nurses in this critical care unit must provide for the care of the patient requiring advanced life support measures after surgery. In this situation, mechanical ventilation, invasive pressure monitoring (systemic arterial, pulmonary artery, intracranial), cardiac dysrhythmia detection and treatment, administration of intravenous vasoactive medications, peritoneal dialysis, intraaortic balloon counterpulsation, or cardiopulmonary resuscitation may be indicated.

The dynamic and critical environment of the PACU necessitates that the structural format facilitate the demanding nature of patient care. To meet the primary objective, that of continuous observation of the post anesthesia patient, guidelines for the design and furnishing of a PACU are provided.

GENERAL PHYSICAL CONSIDERATIONS

The available floor space, location of support services and facilities, financial status of the institution, building and fire codes, and anticipated surgical patient volume and population determine the structure and function of the individual PACU. It is essential that medical and nursing personnel who are experts in the care of the postanesthetic patient collaborate with the architect when planning the design of this area. This ensures a unit that is architecturally acceptable and optimally functional.

Structural Configuration of the Unit

The four geometrical considerations involved in the layout, or floor plan, of the PACU are the circle, semicircle, square, and rectangle. Each has its advantages and disadvantages. All are capable of providing space for efficient and functional patient care environment.

Circle

The circular configuration (Figure 17-1) is a completely round unit, usually with the nurses' station in the center. The nurses' station in the core provides complete visual surveillance of all patients. The distance from this central station to any one patient is equal and usually minimal, allowing immediate access to the patient's bedside when necessary.

Often with the circular design, storage space is limited or is physically removed from the main area. Thus the nurse cannot watch the patient when retrieving supplies. The circular setup is not recommended for a unit that requires more than a six- to eight-bed capacity, because this would decrease efficient space use. The central nurses' station is a potential source of noise and excess activity. This problem may be avoided by enclosing the station within a glass partition.

Semicircle

The semicircle (Figure 17-2) is similar in form to the circle except that the nurses' station is along the straight wall of the half-circle. The supply area can be along this wall on either side of the nurses' station, providing the nurse with access to supplies and equipment while observing the patient.

If the nurses' station also conforms to the semicircle, it has the same patient observation advantages as the circular plan. If it is along the wall, the distance between the station and each patient varies. The semicircle also is not intended for a unit requiring a large bed capacity.

Square

A square unit (Figure 17-3) can provide efficient patient visualization and adequate storage space. If

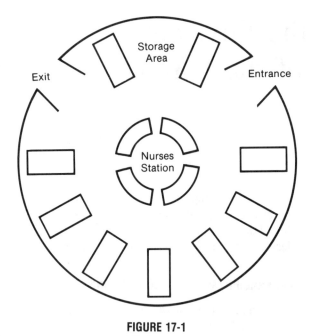

FIGURE 17-1
Circle.

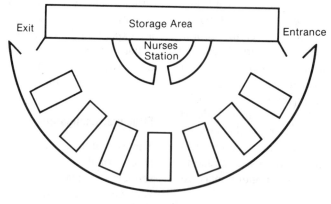

FIGURE 17-2
Semicircle.

the nurses' station is in the center of the square, the advantages are comparable to the circular plan. If the station is along one wall of the square, the disadvantages are similar to those of the semicircle. Often the supply area in this format is behind the nurses' station, requiring the nurse to lose sight of the patients when obtaining equipment and supplies. Bed capacity with the square configuration depends on location of the nurses' station.

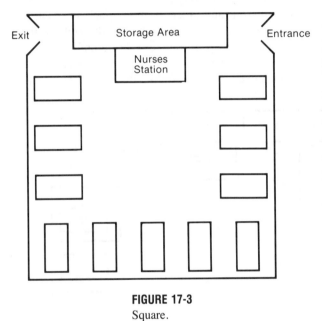

FIGURE 17-3
Square.

Rectangle

The rectangular floor plan (Figure 17-4) provides adequate storage space and can accommodate a large bed capacity, often 20 beds or more. Depending on the size of the room, two nurses' stations (one at either end) may be advisable to provide the necessary patient observation requirements. If one central nurses' station is used, patient visualization, as well as the distance between nurses' station and the patient, will vary.

Patient Observation

Bed placement in the patient care station has historically been controversial. The head of the bed may be proximal to the nurses' station, allowing the nurse immediate access to the patient, as well as visualization of all patients while at the bedside. This placement, however, may be cumbersome when working with suction, oxygen, and x-ray equipment. These obstacles may be avoided if preplanning of the unit involves placement of oxygen, suction, and electrical outlets on ceiling-suspended columns, which are raised and lowered as needed.

The alternative bed position is with the head distal to the nurses' station. If equipment and supplies are along the wall, this placement is more practical for the administration of nursing care. Complete visualization of the patient's head and chest from the nurses' station is not always possible, particularly if the patient is lying down.

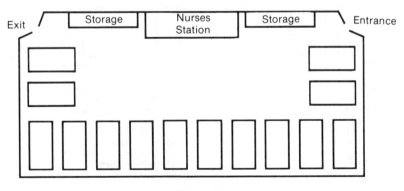

FIGURE 17-4
Rectangle.

Support Structures

Pillars and support columns should not interfere with the visualization of or access to patients. As mentioned, ceiling-suspended equipment columns are often desirable, especially where space is limited, because they can be raised out of the way when not in use.

Central Nurses' Station

The main nurses' station should be located in an area of the unit that is equidistant from all patients to assure adequate visualization. This will vary according to the geometrical shape of the unit. The high activity level that occurs at the nurses' station is a constant source of noise pollution in the PACU.

This area may be enclosed in a glass barrier to reduce the noise level; however, this may also result in the loss of vital auditory cues from the patient in actual or potential distress. The top of the nurses' station desk should allow an unobstructed view of the entire patient unit. Chairs should be mobile and adjusted to a height that allows the nurse to see over the desk.

The majority of the PACU nurse's time is spent at the patient bedside rendering direct patient care; complete patient observation cannot be accomplished from any other location. Each staff nurse should be provided with a chair at the bedside for physical relief from routine walking and standing, as well as to avoid congregating of the staff at the main nurses' station. The chairs should be at the

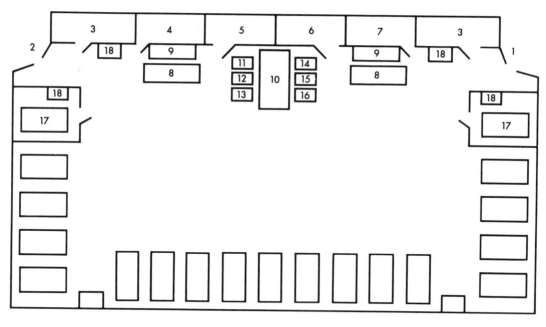

1. Entrance
2. Exit
3. Storage area
4. Office space
5. Clean utility room
6. Dirty utility room
7. Staff lounge/conference area/toilet
8. Nurses stations
9. Medication areas
10. Supply and linen exchange cart
11. Blanket warmer
12. Emergency medication trays
13. Intubation cart
14. ECG machine
15. Defibrillator
16. Emergency "crash" cart
17. Isolation rooms
18. Sinks

FIGURE 17-5
Schematic representation of PACU.

Recommended PACU stock medications

Acetaminophen suppositories
Aminophylline suppositories
Apresoline hydrochloride (Hydralazine)
Aminophylline
Aspirin suppositories
Atropine sulfate
AquaMEPHYTON (vitamin K)
Calcium chloride
Calcium gluconate
d-Tubocurarine chloride (Curare)
Dexamethasone (Decadron)
Dextran (low molecular weight)
Dextrose 50%
Digoxin
Diazoxide (Hyperstat)
Diphenylhydramine hydrochloride (Benadryl)
Dopamine
Doxapram hydrochloride (Dopram)
Droperidol (Inapsine)
Edrophonium chloride (Tensilon)
Ephedrine sulfate
Fentanyl (Sublimaze)
Furosemide (Lasix)
Glycopyrrolate (Robinul)
Hydrocortisone
Hydroxyzine (Vistaril)
Insulin (regular)
Mephentermine sulfate (Wyamine)
Naloxone hydrochloride (Narcan)
Neostigmine (Prostigmine)
Nitroglycerin—sublingual, paste, Transderm
Oxytocin (Pitocin)
Pancuronium bromide (Pavulon)
Phenylephrine hydrochloride (Neo-Synephrine)
Phenytoin sodium (Dilantin)
Physostigmine (Antilirium)
Procainamide hydrochloride (Pronestyl)
Prochlorperazine (Compazine)
Promethazine hydrochloride (Phenergan)
Propranolol (Inderal)
Protamine sulfate
Sodium heparin
Succinylchloline chloride (Anectine)
Trimethobenzamide hydrochloride (Tigan)

Parenteral narcotics and controlled substances:

Codeine
Diazepam (Valium)
Hydromorphone hydrochloride (Dilaudid)
Meperidine hydrochloride (Demerol)
Methyldopa (Aldomet)
Midazolam (Versed)
Morphine sulfate
Phenobarbital
Nifedipine
Ranitidine (Zantac)
Verapamil

patient's bed level and freely mobile. This type of chair, with the addition of a small connected desk, provides the additional advantage of a flat surface for documentation of patient observations.

Dividing Walls

Dividing walls between patient units provide privacy, prevent cross contamination, and control noise. It is recommended that the upper portions of these partitions be glass to allow observation of other patients. Dividing walls, especially if solid, often require an increase in the number of staff necessary for optimum patient care. Often glass walls are used to divide the unit into halves or thirds. Any type of dividing wall, however, will reduce critical auditory patient observations.

LOCATION OF EQUIPMENT AND SUPPLIES (FIGURE 17-5)
Nurses' Station

Ideally the nurses' station should contain a central electrocardiogram (ECG) monitoring console with readout capabilities. Clinical supplies, phones (at least two per desk), and an addressograph machine are required items. Adequate desk space for physicians' and nurses' documentation is also necessary.

Medications

A medication storage and preparation area should be close to the nurses' station. Provision must be made for a single- or double-locked cabinet for storage of controlled substances. Some hospital pharmacies can provide unit-dose medications on an immediate demand basis. If this is not possible, a stock medication inventory should include commonly used analgesics, corticosteroids, diuretics, antibiotics, anesthesia reversal agents, antidysrhythmics, antiemetics, cardiotonics, antihypertensives, and a surplus of emergency drugs. In addition to the above categories of drugs, the medications listed in the box on the left are highly recommended stock items for the PACU.

Emergency Equipment

An adult emergency "crash" cart should always be available for immediate use. The medications listed in the box below should be on the cart or be immediately available on the unit. It is also suggested that an extra supply of these medications be stored in the PACU.

The emergency cart should also contain equipment necessary for endotracheal intubation, and central venous, systemic arterial, and pulmonary artery catheter insertion. The adult emergency cart is acceptable for use in pediatric emergencies; however, a list of pediatric drug dosages and specific pediatric intubation equipment should be readily available.

A portable defibrillator with adult and pediatric paddles and a 12-lead ECG machine should be in the PACU.

Because of the comparatively high incidence of respiratory emergencies in the PACU, it is advisable to have a separate intubation cart or tray for adults and children. This eliminates use of the entire emergency "crash" cart for respiratory emergencies. The contents of the adult intubation tray are listed in the box to the right (middle).

The pediatric intubation cart or tray should contain the same equipment as the adult tray but should be slightly modified for pediatric use. Suggested guidelines are listed in the box to the right (lower).

A malignant hyperthermia crisis tray should be available for immediate use. The contents are listed in the box on p. 193.

It may be advantageous to have a separate procedure cart on wheels for specialized equipment used in the PACU. The contents vary, depending on need. Examples of equiment and materials for

---

Adult intubation tray

Laryngoscope handle
Extra laryngoscope batteries
Laryngoscope blades: sizes medium and large; example: Miller, nos. 2 and 3 straight; Macintosh, nos. 3 and 4 curved
Extra blade lamps
Stylette or guidewire (malleable metal or plastic)
Water-soluble lubricant
Lidocaine ointment
Oropharyngeal airways: sizes small, medium, large; example: Guedel, nos. 3, 4, 5, 6
Nasopharyngeal airways: sizes small, medium, large; example: Guedel, nos. 28, 30, 32 French
Manual resuscitator bag (preferably capable of administering 100% oxygen); example: PMR 2 manual resuscitator
Manual resuscitator bag masks: sizes small, medium, large; example: B.O.C., Foregger, nos. 3, 4, 5
Cuffed endotracheal tubes: sizes 6.5 to 10.0 mm I.D.
Syringe
Tongue blade
Succinylcholine: 10 ml vial
Two 20 ml syringes of sodium pentothal 2.5% (replaced daily)

Emergency medications

Atropine sulfate
Bretylium tosylate (Bretylol)
Calcium chloride
Dobutamine hydrochloride (Dobutrex)
Dopamine hydrochloride
Epinephrine, intravenous and intracardiac
Isoproterenol hydrochloride (Isuprel)
Lidocaine, single intravenous dose and intravenous infusion
Nitroglycerin, intravenous drip infusion
Sodium bicarbonate
Procainamide hydrochloride (Pronestyl)
Sodium nitroprusside (Nipride)

Pediatric intubation tray

Laryngoscope blades; examples: premature newborn, no. 0 Miller (straight); full-term newborn, no. 1 straight; 3 to 5 years, no. 2 curved; over 5 years, no. 3 curved
Uncuffed endotracheal tubes: sizes 2.5 to 6 mm I.D.
Oral airways: sizes premature to small adult; examples: Guedel nos. 000 to 3
Manual resuscitator bag: sizes baby, adult
Manual resuscitator bag masks: sizes premature, infant, child; examples: Rendell-Baker Soucek, B.O.C., Ambu type—sizes nos. 0 (premature newborn), 1, 2
Suction catheters: sizes 6 to 12 French
Nasopharyngeal airways: sizes 26 to 30 French

Malignant hyperthermia crisis tray

Drugs

Sodium bicarbonate
Furosemide
Mannitol
Dantrolene sodium
Procainamide hydrochloride
Regular insulin
Dextrose 50%

Equipment and solutions

Foley catheter insertion equipment
Nasogastric tube
Electronic temperature recorder and probe
Cooling blanket
Iced normal saline solution for infusion and irrigation
Iced lactated Ringer's solution for infusion
Rectal tube
IV insertion equipment; central venous catheter
Blood study equipment (blood chemistries, gases, enzymes)
100% oxygen source

---

dressings, arterial line, pacemaker, Swan-Ganz, intravenous, and tonsil emergencies are given in the box on p. 194.

In addition to this emergency equipment, at least one ventilator (preferably volume cycle) should be in the PACU at all times. If this is not possible, mechanical ventilators should be immediately available from the respiratory therapy department. A portable ECG monitor/defibrillator unit must be available for the transport of critically ill patients who require continuous monitoring.

Supply Cabinets

Storage areas for supplies should be situated to allow the nurse to obtain needed supplies or equipment without losing sight of the patient. Equipment that may be housed in these areas includes intravenous solutions and tubings, oxygen therapy supplies, dressings, tapes, monitoring equipment, drainage tubes and bags, irrigation kits, and monitoring transducers. Exchange carts that are centrally supplied and restocked daily are ideal for the PACU. They are mobile, may be approached from

either side, and may be placed anywhere in the unit where space permits. Linens may also be stored and stocked in the same fashion.

Plumbing

All plumbing systems are subject to the *National Standard Plumbing Code,* Chapter 14, "Medical Care Facility Plumbing Equipment."

A staff toilet located within the PACU is necessary and contributes to the continuous immediate availability of PACU personnel.

There should be a clinical sink with elbow or foot controls for every three to four patient units. An automatic, wall-mounted soap dispenser of approved germicidal soap and disposable towels and waste receptacles for each sink are also necessary.

A "dirty" utility room for disposal of wastes and testing of specimens must be provided. This room contains the flushable bedpan hopper, receptacles for measurement of drainages, and materials for specimen testing.

Electrical Safety

In the event of interruption of normal electric power supply, the emergency generator must be brought to full voltage and frequency within 10 seconds.

Miscellaneous

Because of the particular susceptibility of the post anesthesia patient to hypothermia, a blanket-warming machine is a necessity. An automatic ice machine is also desirable for local cold applications.

Tympanic membrane temperature probes are now being used in the PACU. They are accurate and reliable. One unit for every two patients is usually sufficient. An electric hypothermia/hyperthermia blanket unit is also desirable for treatment of extremes in core temperature.

An x-ray film illuminator unit facilitates viewing of postoperative x-ray films.

The ambient temperature in the PACU should be maintained at 23°C (75°F), with a relative humidity of 50% to 60%. A minimum of two air changes of

---

Equipment and materials for special procedures

Dressings

Sterile gloves
Syringes (3 ml and 10 ml)
Needles
Antibiotic ointment
Betadine
Packages of sterile gauzes

Arterial line

Arterial line flush kit with heparinized saline (500 ml)
High pressure tubing
Transducer domes
Male Luer-Lok plugs
Short armboard
Kerlix
Arterial blood gas sampling sets
Heparin (10 ml:1000 u/ml)—if preassembled set not available
Syringes (3 ml and 5 ml)

Central venous pressure

Central venous pressure set (preassembled)
Water manometer
Buretrol with minidrip
Intracath (no. 16, 8 inch)
D_5W (500 ml)
Triple-lumen catheter

Pacemaker

Transmyocardial pacing kit
Arrow introducer kit (size 8 or 8.5)
Medtronic pacer wire (no. 5)
Disilet-Hoffman percutaneous introducer
Cournand style 18-gauge needle
Torkfloat Cordis pacer wire (no. 5)
Battery and generator
Alligator clamps (sterile and unsterile)

Swan-Ganz

Flow-directed thermodilution catheter (size 7 French)
Arrow percutaneous sheath introducer kit with side-port adapter (size 8 French)
Flush kit with transducer dome
Color-coded pressure lines
Male Luer-Lok plugs
Heparinized saline (500 ml)
Disposable sterile gowns, drapes, towels, gloves

Intravenous insertion

Betadine
Alcohol
Armboards
Intravenous catheters (sizes nos. 22 to 14 gauge)
Tape
Syringes
Sterile gauze sponges
Tourniquet
Lidocaine (for infiltration)
Band-Aids

Tonsil tray

Silver nitrate sticks
Tongue blades
Sterile Q-tips
Sponge stick
Tonsil clamp
Mouth gag
2-0 plain suture
Lidocaine 1% plain
Spinal needles (nos. 18, 20, 22, 25)
Yankauer suction tip
Allis clamp
Needle holder

---

outdoor air per hour is required to be supplied to the room.

SENSORY DEPRIVATION

If possible, the construction of the PACU should include windows that allow daylight to be visible. This provides a natural source of visual relief for the PACU personnel. It also provides a day/night orientation for the awakening patient or the patient who must remain in the PACU for an extended period, either for physical or logistic reasons.

Because of the relative geographical isolation of the unit, PACU personnel are continuously subject to a lack of environmental diversion. The confinement of the self-contained unit, the close working relationships of the relatively small staff, the critical level of nursing care delivered, and the limited opportunities to leave the unit all contribute to a heightened anxiety atmosphere. It is thus essential that, when feasible, the physical environment be manipulated to reduce physical and psychological stressors.

A lounge or conference area physically removed from the PACU but close to the unit is recommended for relaxation, stress reduction, and classes.

SENSORY BOMBARDMENT

Noise pollution is inherent to the nature of the PACU environment. Mechanical devices, excessive personnel and patient traffic, and the acute nature of the medical and nursing care delivered all contribute to the increased noise level. To reduce sensory stimulation for both staff and patients, lighting, whenever possible, should be soft and diffuse. If fluorescent overhead lighting is used, it should be a shade that closely simulates daylight to assure accurate clinical observations. Colors of walls, wallpaper, and draperies should be pastels or beige. Ceiling patterns should be simple and of shapes that do not resemble twisting or complex configurations that could contribute to visual distortions by the patient emerging from anesthesia.

INDIVIDUAL PATIENT CARE UNITS
Stretchers (Beds)

Each patient care unit should have one stretcher. These should be stored in an area out of the direct line of traffice flow but accessible to the operating room. Pneumatically controlled stretchers provide ease of use and relatively low maintenance requirements. The stretcher must be capable of being maneuvered into several positions, including (1) elevation of head, knees, and feet, (2) total elevation, (3) Trendelenburg, and (4) reverse Trendelenburg. A chart rack or foot board provides convenience for the nurse, as well as patient safety. If a head board is a component of the stretcher, it should be capable of easy and rapid removal in emergency situations. The mattress should be of firm, durable, and washable material. Stretchers with many crevices and intricate lines are not easily cleaned or disinfected and pose a threat to infection control.

Size and Number

Each patient care unit should be at least 10 feet long to allow maneuverability of the bed in and out of the unit. There should be 4 feet of space between each unit to accommodate personnel and equipment necessary to render total patient care.

The PACU should contain at least 1½ to 2 patient care units for every surgical suite.

Equipment and Supplies
Mandatory

The articles and equipment in the box below are required for any size PACU. These items ideally are wall mounted to prevent excess congestion of supplies and equipment at the bedside.

Monitors should be capable of continuous ECG monitoring, with readout capabilities. At least half of the monitors should contain one or two additional monitoring modes and transducer equipment for pulmonary artery, systemic arterial, right atrial, apnea, or intracranial pressure monitoring.

The following items may be in individual unit cabinets or on counter tops and shelves:

- Suction catheters: (no. 14 French, whistle tip and straight designs)
- Yankauer suction tip (tonsil suction)
- Oxygen delivery system: cannula or prongs; nebulizer (cool and heated) with face tent or mask; masks (nonrebreathing), adult and pediatric; and tracheostomy collars
- Tongue blades
- Water-soluble lubricant
- Emesis basins
- Sterile water: individual 50 to 100 ml containers for rinsing suction catheters
- Syringe (10 ml)
- Sterile disposable gloves

Required equipment and supplies for PACUs

Sphygmomanometer: one per unit
Vacuum/suction outlets: at least three per unit (nasogastric, endotracheal, chest)
Oxygen source: at least two per unit (oxygen administration for the nonintubated patient, mechanical ventilation)
Compressed air outlet: one per unit
X-ray receptable: one per two units
Emergency call button: one per unit
Monitors (hemodynamic): one per unit

- Unsterile disposable gloves

The following are ideally ceiling mounted or suspended:
- Overhead surgical lamp: one per unit
- Dividing drapes or curtains
- IV pole: one per unit

Highly recommended are the following:
- Sterile dressing supplies
- Washcloths, facial tissues, plastic disposable bed pads (Chux)
- Noninvasive blood pressure monitoring machine (Dinamap): one per patient
- Volumetric infusion pump: one or more per PACU

Pulse oxymetry is recommended for routine use in the PACU for noninvasive monitoring of the arterial oxygen saturation. One unit per patient is ideal; one unit for every two patients may suffice.

PROXIMITY OF SUPPORT SERVICES AND FACILITIES

Operating Room

Ideally, the operating room (OR) corridors should communicate directly with the entrance to the PACU. The critical period involving transfer of the patient from the OR to the PACU should be accomplished within minutes. This decreases the incidence of post anesthesia complications that must be managed during transit when vital supplies, equipment, and personnel are not readily available. The proximity of the OR to the PACU allows the PACU nurse to physically enter the OR for consultation with the OR nurse, anesthesiologist, or surgeon when indicated.

A communication system (telephone, intercom) to allow the PACU nurse to contact OR personnel is essential. This system should allow communication with each OR suite, as well as with a central OR control office. An overhead page system that is audible in the OR corridors is also necessary.

Anesthesia Services

Access to the anesthesia office and lounge should also be available through a verbal communication system. These areas should also be within a reasonable distance (seconds) to the PACU to enable prompt response from the anesthesiologist in an emergency and for direct communication between the PACU nurse and anesthesiologist concerning specific patient management.

Blood Bank and Clinical Laboratories

The blood bank should be adjacent to the OR for immediate retrieval of blood products. If this is not possible, an acceptable blood storage refrigerator containing blood products for the day's surgical case load should be located within the OR. Dispensing of the blood in this case should be monitored by a designated staff member.

Facilities for blood gas determinations and hematocrit estimation should be in the immediate vicinity of the OR or PACU. Laboratories for blood chemistry, hematology, microbiology, and urinalysis are ideally located on the same floor as the PACU. If this is not possible, ancillary personnel should be available to expedite delivery of laboratory specimens to the appropriate areas.

Surgical Intensive Care Unit

To minimize transfer-induced patient trauma and postoperative complications, the surgical intensive care unit (SICU) should be on the same floor as the OR and PACU. Equipment and personnel necessary to continuously monitor cardiac status, blood pressure, and ventilatory support during transport of the patient to the SICU must be readily available.

Elevators

Specific patient elevators should be designated for transporting patients from the PACU to the patient care areas. They should be equipped with a device that permits the cars to bypass all landing button calls and be dispatched directly to any floor. The PACU nurse should have a key to operate these elevators.

Entrances and Exits

All PACU doors should be wide enough to accommodate the widest bed used in the hospital (with the siderails in the raised position) and the tallest traction or orthopedic bed. The size of other mechanical-assist devices (mechanical ventilators, intraaortic balloon pumps) should also be considered when determining door width and height. Ideally, doors leading to and from the PACU should be double width with an electronic switch for automatic operation.

To decrease traffic congestion, it is recommended that traffic flow in one direction. This would require that the entrance and exit doors be at opposite ends of the PACU.

INFECTION CONTROL
Isolation Rooms

At least one isolation room for every 10 to 12 beds is recommended:

Patients requiring isolation (as detailed by the Infection Control Committee or Department) will be cared for in a designated area in the PAR (preferably a separate room), apart from other patients. If such an area is not available, continuous nursing care will be provided elsewhere in the hospital. The quality of care in this situation will be equal to that available in the PAR.

Those patients requiring strict or respiratory isolation must be housed in a private room. (ASPAN Guidelines for Standards of Care, Section IV, G,H.)

Alternative isolation locations in the absence of a PACU isolation room include an operating room suite, a surgical intensive care unit room, or the patient's own private room. It is essential that if an area other than the PACU is used for isolation of a patient, postanesthetic care be rendered by a qualified PACU nurse. Another alternative is to use the PACU and confine the patient to an area that is not in the direct line of traffic. Portable screens or barriers may be used to confine the patient. The nearest patient should be at least two patient units away.

General Guidelines

Additional infection control guidelines are given below. For information regarding specific infection control parameters (hemodynamic monitoring, intravascular, oxygen and suction equipment), the individual hospital infection control department and the Center for Disease Control should be consulted.

1. Personnel with active infections (eye, skin, respiratory, gastrointestinal) should not work in the area.
2. Eating, drinking, and smoking must be restricted to a designated area.
3. Hospital-furnished uniforms must be worn by those giving direct patient care; these are worn once only and then laundered or discarded.
4. Shoes that are worn exclusively in the hospital are allowed in the PACU without shoe covers.
5. When leaving the PACU area, personnel should wear a buttoned lab coat or cover gown; these should promptly be removed upon return to the PACU.
6. Whenever possible, disposable equipment should be used.
7. PACU beds or stretchers must be stripped of linen between each patient use; mattress and bed frame must be wiped down with an approved detergent germicide immediately after use.
8. All horizontal surfaces and equipment are cleaned daily.
9. Floors should be of a smooth surface and cleaned with an approved detergent germicide by the wet vacuum system; carpeting is not recommended for the PACU.

FIRE REGULATIONS AND CODES

Recommended basic fire prevention methods and codes are presented below. For specific minimum standards, the National Fire Protection Association should be consulted.

Walls

All walls that enclose the PACU should be smoke-stop partitions. These walls provide a 90-minute smoke delay.

Doors

Doors leading to and from the PACU, utility rooms, locker rooms, offices, or lounges within the

PACU should be B rated. These provide a 60-minute smoke delay. In the event of a fire emergency, the PACU entrance and exit doors should close automatically. Doors leading to other rooms within the unit should remain closed at all times. Red exit signs must be posted.

Fire Extinguishers

There are four types of fire extinguishers that may be used in the PACU. These extinguishers are type A (water), types B, C (carbon dioxide), and Halon. If the type A and types B, C extinguishers are chosen to supply the area, the following guidelines must be followed:

Type A: One extinguisher is required every 200 square meters (2200 square feet); a staff member should always be within 25 meters (82 feet) of the device.

Types B, C: One is required every 200 square meters (2200 square feet); a staff member must be within 15 meters (50 feet) of the device.

Recently the trend has been toward the use of the Halon fire extinguisher. This device is highly recommended when considering the furnishing of a contemporary PACU. A 14-pound Halon fire extinguisher replaces one type A and four types B,C extinguishers. An added advantage is the provision of one extinguisher that is appropriate for use on any type of fire. The Halon extinguisher also has the advantage of a 30-foot stand-off distance, the distance between user and fire source required to effectively extinguish the fire. In comparison, the stand-off distance for a carbon dioxide extinguisher is 3 meters (10 feet).

Fire Blankets

Fire blankets for fires involving an individual patient are not required to date. However, it is suggested that for future planning, each PACU have one fire blanket per two to four patients.

Sprinkler Systems

Automatic sprinkler systems are presently not required in the PACU. It is anticipated that revision of fire codes in the near future will result in sprinkler system requirements. This should be considered when planning a new unit. However, it is recommended that sprinkler devices be located in storage areas, janitor closets, and utility rooms.

CONCLUSION

When planning the physical environment of the PACU, it is essential that the personnel who will be caring for the post anesthesia patient have input into the decision-making process. Experts in each related field should be consulted for the most current information. The nature and volume of surgery will determine the specific needs of the PACU. To achieve the primary goals of the PACU, that is, scrupulous patient observation and prevention, early recognition, and treatment of complications in the postanesthetic period, basic minimum standards must be met.

SUGGESTIONS FOR FURTHER READING

Britt BA, editor: Malignant hyperthermia, Int Anesthesiol Clin 17(4), 1979.

Cook KG: Assessment and management of anxiety in recovery room patients, Curr Rev Recov Room Nurses 5(7), 1983.

Drain CB, and Shipley SB: The recovery room, Philadelphia, 1979, WB Saunders Co.

Dripps RD, Eckenhoff JE, and Vandam LD: Introduction of anesthesia: the principles of safe practice, ed 6, Philadelphia, 1982, WB Saunders Co.

Levin RN: Pediatric anesthesia handbook, ed 2, New York, 1980, Medical Examination Publishing Co.

National Fire Protection Association, Code 101: Life Safety, 1982.

Roizen MF, editor: Chemonucleolysis anaphylaxis: recognition and treatment, Chicago, 1983, Smith Laboratories.

Snow JC: Manual of anesthesia, ed 2, Boston, 1982, Little, Brown and Co. Inc.

CHAPTER 18

Nursing Requirements in the Post Anesthesia Care Unit

Karen D. Spadaccia

This chapter delineates the nursing responsibilities of patient care and the measures for achieving them. The purpose of PACU nursing is to provide skilled individualized care to the patient in the immediate postoperative period. The post anesthesia nurse is an integral member of the health team who communicates and collaborates with other team members to deliver safe, effective care.

POSITION REQUIREMENTS
Head Nurse/Manager

The head nurse has a dual role—that of clinician and manager. The head nurse must be knowledgeable in medical and surgical nursing, as well as proficient in the practice of post anesthesia nursing. This proficiency must include an appropriate knowledge of human physiology and the effects on it of surgical intervention, anesthetic agents, and related drugs.

In addition to this clinical base, the head nurse must also have managerial skills that allow for appropriate staff assignments, counseling of subordinates, appropriate rapport with other departments, and the ability to function within the chain of command (Figure 18-1). The role responsibilities

continue to evolve and expand and now must include budgeting and fiscal monitoring, quality assurance, and equipment review. Additionally, it is recommended that formal liaisons with the physicians be established via the OR/anesthesia hospital committees.

The suggested qualifications for the head nurse are the following:
- Minimum of 5 years of medical/surgical post anesthesia nursing
- Minimum of 2 years of management experience
- Involvement in professional organization—American Society of Post Anesthesia Nurses
- Bachelor of science in nursing
- Basic life support certification
- Coronary care certification
- Demonstrated competence with budgeting
- Certified Post Anesthesia Nurse (CPAN)

The Joint Commission on Accreditation of Healthcare Organizations (JCAHO) requires written performance appraisals of all nursing personnel at the end of their probationary period and at least annually. These appraisals must be criteria based and individualized. They must directly reflect particular performance and be stated in measurable

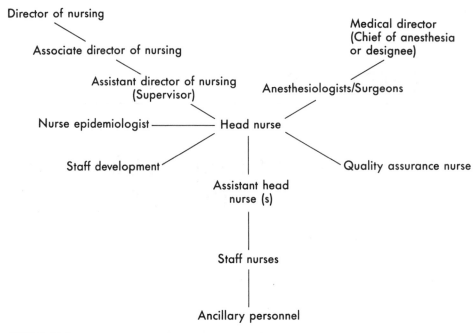

FIGURE 18-1
Chain of command.

goals and objectives. The responsibility of these appraisals falls to the head nurse. To facilitate the completion of these appraisals, professional credential files must be maintained on each staff nurse. The files should reflect staff development and continuing education activities, involvement in professional organizations, and communication and interpersonal skills. The most efficacious means of maintaining these files is through anecdotal records (Figure 18-2) and submission of monthly goals and objectives by staff (Figure 18-3). These goals and objectives are discussed at monthly meetings held with the manager and staff nurse. These activities assure a more complete appraisal and one that reflects a broad spectrum of events and issues.

Nursing Staff

The PACU is a critical care area and as such should be staffed by professional nurses whose qualifications are appropriate for the acuity level of PACU patients. The ability to use the nursing process is essential in this setting (Figure 18-4).

Because of the short-term relationships between nurses and patients and the continually changing needs of these patients, the nurse must be flexible and able to adapt easily to changes. Therefore the suggested requirements for staff nurse are the following:

- Registered professional nurse
- Minimum of 3 years of medical/surgical nursing
- Basic life support certification
- Coronary care certification
- Ability to function as a team member

The role of licensed practical nurses (LPNs) in the PACU is limited by their training. They can play an important part in data collection and in direct patient care. However, it falls to the professional nurse to make assessments and plan intervention. Therefore constant supervision is mandatory should LPNs be employed in a PACU.

Nursing assistants, orderlies, and clerks can play a vital role in this area as they can perform nonnurs-

Nursing: Anecdotal Records

Employee Name ______________________ Month/Year ______________________

Unit ______________________ Position ______________________ Length of Time in Position ______________________

AREAS FOR CONSIDERATION	COMMENTS
1. Clinical Performance—i.e., handles heavy assignment well, works extra shift, organization skills and ability to set priorities appropriately.	
2. Professional Development—i.e., pursuing degrees, national certification, involvement in professional organizations, Nursing Grand Rounds, attends inservices and conferences.	
3. Interpersonal Relationships—i.e., interactions with families and patients, MDs, ancillary personnel, and coworkers—particularly in stressful situations.	
4. Communications Skills—i.e., written and verbal, develops a standard of care, procedure, or nursing care plan, telephone manners.	
5. Role Model and Leadership Skills—i.e., acts as resource person for new personnel and other staff, serves on hospital committees, assumes charge in absence of HN and AHN.	

Evaluator's Signature ______________________ Date ______________________

Employee's Signature ______________________ Date ______________________

COMMENTS:

FIGURE 18-2
Anecdotal nursing record.

Staff Goals and Objectives

Name:_____

Date: _____

General Headings and Goals	Objectives	Proj. Date of Achievement
Communications:		
Clinical:		
Professional:		
Education:		
Committee Work:		

FIGURE 18-3
Staff goals and objectives.

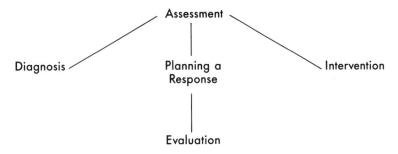

FIGURE 18-4
Steps of nursing process.

ing functions and thereby allow the nurse to function in her expected role. Responsibilities falling to these personnel include the following:

- Assisting with transport
- Maintaining equipment
- Stocking
- Keeping of logs
- Telephoning
- Cleaning
- Communicating with family members
- Writing requisitions

All staff assigned to this area must have a comprehensive orientation program and ongoing education to update their skills and knowledge on all levels. An in-depth approach to this is discussed in Chapter 19.

STAFFING PATTERNS

Staffing needs will vary from institution to institution, because they are based on size, census, and hours of operation. Perhaps of most importance is the type of patients receiving care. It would be ideal to staff based on acuity level; however, most institutions would not lend themselves to this type of staffing. It would require advanced knowledge of the operative schedule, as well as a medical history of each patient. This is not always feasible and would not lend itself to projected long-term staff scheduling.

Before determining staffing needs for a unit, certain criteria and parameters must be established. First, a classification system for all patients must be designed to determine the acuity level of the patient (Table 18-1). This system can also be used to make

TABLE 18-1		
Classification system		
Classification I **(1:1 nurse-patient ratio)**	**Classification II** **(1:2 nurse-patient ratio)**	**Classification III** **(1:3 nurse-patient ratio)**
1. All pediatric patients 2. All patients on admission 3. Mechanical ventilation 4. Presence of ET tube 5. Continual ECG or hemodynamic monitoring 6. Frequent medications 7. Frequent assessment 8. Constant nursing intervention 9. Admission score of 1 to 4	1. Frequent vital signs 2. ECG monitoring 3. Confusion and/or restlessness 4. Obtundation of gag reflex 5. Periodic medications 6. Frequent nursing intervention 7. Admission score of 5 to 8	1. Vital signs q 15 minutes 2. Evaluation periodically 3. Admission score of 9 or 10

assignments. A log should be maintained documenting (1) acuity levels of patients on admission and discharge and (2) length of stay. This keeps an ongoing record, and staffing patterns can be adjusted accordingly. A smaller unit requires that a policy be established whereby patients requiring long-term intensive care nursing may be transferred directly to the intensive care unit from the operating room, thus eliminating the possibility of one staff member being involved in the care of one patient for an entire shift.

Staffing according to census appears to be the most plausible in this setting. It allows for coverage during peak hours and can lend itself to the use of alternative methods of staffing, that is, per diem pool, staggered shifts, and "on call." A good rule of thumb to follow is one nurse for each two beds in use (Figure 18-5).

Unless direct access to emergency assistance is available, there should be two personnel in the PACU when there is a patient. One of these staff members must be an RN. This may mean that smaller institutions must develop an on-call system. The personnel involved may not work regularly in the PACU. Therefore teaching sessions must be provided for these other nurses.

DOCUMENTATION
The Record

The PACU record is sole documentation of the care a patient has received during this phase of the perioperative period. Therefore it should reflect accurately and completely what has occurred. It is a nursing record and so should indicate all phases of the nursing process. The record should lend itself to ease of documentation, as well as ease in discerning data collected.

A flow sheet is mandatory, because time for documentation is limited. The use of admission and discharge checklists is advisable (Figures 18-6 and 18-7). This gives a concise picture of the patient's

	Monday to Friday			Weekends and Holidays	
7 am to 3 pm	3 RNs	1 aide		2 RNs	1 aide
10 am to 6 pm	3 RNs	1 aide		—	—
3 pm to 11 pm	2 RNs	1 aide		1 RN	1 aide
11 pm to 7 am	1 RN	1 aide		1 RN	1 aide

Type of unit: 16-bed unit; average weekday census 48; average of 9.4 classification 1 patients; OR schedule 7–4 pm, but often runs until 7 or 8 pm. Used as overflow for ICU; average overnight stays 2.3. Emergency cases only after 5 pm and weekends.

	Monday to Friday			Weekends and Holidays	
7 am to 3 pm	1 RN			1 RN	1 aide
8 am to 4 pm	2 RNs			—	
9 am to 5 pm	1 RN	1 aide		—	
or					
10 am to 2 pm	1 RN				
10 am to 6 pm	1 RN			—	

Type of unit: 8-bed unit; average week day census 22; average of 2.3 classification 1 patients; OR schedule 7–3 pm, but often runs until 5 pm. ICU used on evenings, nights, and weekends other than Saturdays 7–3.

FIGURE 18-5

Examples of staffing pattern using census.

status. The record itself can be designed in any fashion to meet the needs of the institution (Figure 18-8). Preestablished criteria for categories on these checklists and the use of scoring systems eliminate a good portion of the subjectivity of these records, thus making them a more universal reflection of patient status (see Appendixes 1, 2, and 9).

A carbonized record is advisable, and this copy should be kept with a copy of the anesthesia record. JCAHO requires a minimum of six staff meetings per year to evaluate care given in the PACU. Retaining a copy of both records allows for accurate auditing and the isolation of problems or potential problems.

Sole responsibility of documentation on this record falls to nursing personnel. However, the anesthesiologist must make use of this record, his or her own observations, and verbal input from the staff when he or she evaluates patient status and records this in the progress notes.

It is not possible in every institution to have a physician or a nurse anesthetist assigned to the PACU. Therefore it is essential to establish standing orders and protocols by which the nursing staff

---

```
Preoperative diagnosis_____
Procedure  _____
Anesthetic:     General _____  Spinal _____  Local _____  Sedation _____
Preoperative vital signs: T _____  BP _____  P _____  R _____
Initial assessment:                          Activity                    Score
                                             LOC              _____
                                             Respirations     _____
                                             Color            _____
                                             Movement         _____
                                             Circulation      _____
                                                   Total      _____

EBL _____
Intraoperative Fluids:                       Type             Amount
                              Solutes    _____         _____
                                         _____         _____
                              Colloids   _____         _____
                                         _____         _____
                                         _____         _____

Dressing:              Type _____      Status _____
Drains:                Type _____      Status _____
                            _____           _____
                            _____           _____

O₂ therapy:            Type _____      FiO₂ _____
Monitoring equipment:  ECG _____
                       Arterial line  _____
                       SG _____
                       ICP _____
```

FIGURE 18-6
Admission checklist. *LOC,* level of consciousness; *EBL,* estimated blood loss; *ECG,* electrocardiogram; *SG,* Swan-Ganz; *ICP,* intracranial pressure.

Discharge vital signs: T ＿＿＿＿ BP ＿＿＿＿ P ＿＿＿＿ R ＿＿＿＿

Final assessment:

	Score
Activity	＿＿＿＿
LOC	＿＿＿＿
Respirations	＿＿＿＿
Color	＿＿＿＿
Movement	＿＿＿＿
Circulation	＿＿＿＿
Total	＿＿＿＿

Fluid therapy in PACU:

	Type	Amount
Solutes	＿＿＿＿	＿＿＿＿
	＿＿＿＿	＿＿＿＿
Colloids	＿＿＿＿	＿＿＿＿
	＿＿＿＿	＿＿＿＿

Dressing: Status ＿＿＿＿

Drains: Type ＿＿＿＿   Status ＿＿＿＿
＿＿＿＿   ＿＿＿＿

Medicated: Drug ＿＿＿＿ Dose ＿＿＿＿ Time ＿＿＿＿
and
Route ＿＿＿＿   ＿＿＿＿   ＿＿＿＿

O_2 therapy: Type ＿＿＿＿ FiO_2 ＿＿＿＿

FIGURE 18-7
Discharge checklist.

can function. These should include the following areas:

1. Oxygen therapy
2. Medications
   Intravenous or intramuscular
   Reversal agents
   Split doses
3. Weaning criteria
4. Extubation
5. Fluid management
6. Emergency measures
   Cardiac arrest protocols: adult and pediatric
   Malignant hyperthermia
7. Discharge criteria
8. Verbal orders

These protocols should be documented in the policy manual and reviewed periodically by the head nurse and the medical director of the unit. In this fashion, care given and recorded on the record is legally covered by these existing policies.

NURSING STANDARDS OF CARE

Guidelines for standards of practice are currently in existence. It is advisable to be conversant with these and have copies in the policy manual. These guidelines have all been published with a statement saying that these are only guidelines and must be adjusted to meet the needs of each institution. However, in spite of this disclaimer, it is very possible, given the professional nature of the organizations that have published them, that they will be interpreted as standards. Therefore deviations may be considered unacceptable by a jury of lay persons. A list of some of the current guidelines is given under ''further readings'' at the end of the chapter. It is advisable to check with state or national post anesthesia associations for the existence of such guidelines.

Recognizing that nursing is establishing itself as an accountable profession rather than the historical role of one of delegation, it is apparent that there is a need to define quality nursing care. To this end, each PACU should develop nursing standards of

PACU RECORD

DATE ____________

WRITE OR IMPRINT PATIENT INFORMATION ABOVE

Pre-Op B/P

REMARKS

Name of Operation

Surgeon | Anesthesiologist

Anesthetic

Fluids Given	In Operating Room	In Recovery Room
Lactated Ringer's		
Lactated Ringer's with Dextrose 5%		
Dextrose 5%		
Blood		
Albumin		
Intake Total		
EBL Total		
Urine Output Total		

Medications	Dose	Time	Sig.	Medications	Dose	Time	Sig.
1.				4.			
2.				5.			
3.				6.			

ARRIVAL	DISCHARGE
Dressings	
Urinary	
Lt./Sump	
Other	
Ventilation	
O_2	
Monitor	

TIME:

B.P. V Λ

PULSE •

RESP ○

220 200 180 160 140 120 100 80 60 40 20 0

SYMBOLS

POST ANESTHETIC RECOVERY SCORE

	Norm. Score	Pat. Score Arr.	Pat. Score Disch
Activity	2		
Respiration	2		
Circulation	2		
Consciousness	2		
Color	2		
TOTAL	10		

DISCHARGE NOTE: Time ____________ A.M. P.M.

Signature ____________ M.D.

Signature ____________ R.N.

DeSalvo-Wayne Form No. 31329-B

FIGURE 18-8
Example of PACU record.

Nursing assessment

1. Collecting data or information
2. Using all available sources of information
   a. Primary: patient
   b. Secondary: physician, chart, staff members,
      values from equipment used
3. Identifying problems
4. Establishing priorities
5. Setting goals

care. The standards should follow the nursing process (see Figure 18-4) and establish the minimum level of care that will be allowed for each patient.

Before nursing standards are written, certain criteria must already have been established:

1. Policies and procedures
2. Areas of responsibility: nurse, anesthetist, and surgeon
3. Monitoring criteria: frequency, method, and established parameters

In addition, a working knowledge of the nursing process and a development of assessment skills—observation, palpation, percussion, auscultation, and interviewing—are essential (see box above).

The format used for these standards may vary from institution to institution but should remain constant within one institution. They must also be attainable and reflective of actual care given. When writing these standards, begin with those areas most commonly seen or dealt with in the PACU, that is, admission, discharge, patients who require ventilatory support. Standards can and must reflect universally accepted PACU practice and those established by each institution (See Appendix 1). Based on these established standards, review of care is conducted.

QUALITY ASSURANCE PROGRAMS

It is essential to the proper functioning of a PACU that a quality assurance program be designed. Because the care given in the PACU is jointly one of medical and nursing, the program designed must be multidisciplinary. To further promote the concept of a team approach, the auditing, monitoring, assessment, and actions taken must be a collaborative effort.

The process involved for review can be retrospective or concurrent, but must include each of the following:

1. Established criteria, based on standards of care with no room for individual interpretation. This provides the staff with an expected performance level and the reviewer with tools to evaluate the level of compliance.
2. Method for monitoring. Monitoring can be retrospective or concurrent and should be designed to check on step-by-step compliance with established criteria. An audit is perhaps the easiest method (Figure 18-9).
3. Establishing problems. After collection of data, review and evaluation must take place. Determination of deficiency is made and area of responsibility—nursing or medical—is determined.
4. Action. Problem-solving techniques are designed and action to be taken established. Deadlines for compliance are made, as well as a method for reevaluation.

On completion of an audit, compilation of statistics, and documentation of follow-up, it is essential to integrate this with the institution's quality assurance program.

On January 1, 1981, the JCAH implemented the quality assurance standards and assesses quality assurance programs in the hospitals it surveys based on these standards. They may be found in the *Accreditation Manual for Hospitals* and should be reviewed before setting up programs.

SUMMARY

Written standards of care, job descriptions and delineations, policies and procedures, and documentation of care given are essential to an effective PACU. Without clear definitions of professional practices and compliance, patient care can and will suffer.

Objectives:
1. To evaluate adequacy of present documentation of care given in the PACU.
2. To determine level of compliance with current format.

Criteria: YES   NO   NA

1. Did the patient's name and financial number appear?
2. Type of surgery indicated?
3. Type of anesthesia used indicated?
4. Admission assessment done?

                          LOC
                          Respirations
                          Color
                          Circulatory status
                          Activity

5. Oxygen therapy indicated?
6. Vital signs monitored at least q 15 minutes?
7. Ventilatory status reevaluated?
8. LOC reevaluated?
9. Status of wound indicated?
10. Fluid status indicated?

                          Intraoperative
                          Postoperative

11. Status of drains indicated?
12. Medication administered?

                          Type
                          Dose
                          Route
                          Effect

13. Documentation of anesthesiologist assessment?
14. Nursing discharge assessment done?
15. Record signed—RN?
                      MD?

FIGURE 18-9
Sample audit.

SUGGESTIONS FOR FURTHER READING

American Association of Critical Care Nurses: Standards for nursing care of the critically ill, Reston, Va, 1986, Reston Publishing Co.

American Society of Post Anesthesia Nurses: Guidelines for standards of care, 1986.

DeKornfeld T and Isreal J, editors: Recovery room care, Springfield, Ill, 1986, Charles C. Thomas, Publisher.

Gravenstein JS and Paulus DA: Clinical monitoring practice, ed 2, Philadelphia, 1987, JB Lippincott Co.

Halloran EJ: Staffing assignment: by task or by patient? Nurs Manage 14:16, 1983.

Joint Commission on Accreditation of Healthcare Organizations: Accreditation manual for hospitals. Chicago, 1988.

New York State Society of Anesthesiologists, New York State Association of Nurse Anesthestists, and New York State Recovery Room Nurses Association: Guidelines for recovery room care, 1985.

Pintuton S and Schroeder P: Commitment to excellence developing a professional nursing staff, Rockville, Md, 1988, Aspen Publishers, Inc.

CHAPTER 19

Educational Programs for PACU Personnel

Dorothy M. Williams

The professional nurse should gain clinical skills and knowledge under the direction of the nurse manager, clinical instructor, preceptors, and senior staff nurses through participation in selected progressive clinical experience. This preceptor program is designed to provide a nursing orientation at the unit level that will facilitate (1) the integration of the beginning practitioner into the PACU routines and (2) the assimilation of the unit's philosophy, policies, and procedures into the new nurse's performance. The most important purpose is the development of competence and expertise in post anesthesia nursing.

ROLE AND RESPONSIBILITIES OF THE CLINICAL INSTRUCTOR

The clinical instructor is responsible for facilitating the orientation process of the new staff nurses. This includes planning, coordinating, and evaluating the orientation. She is also responsible for (1) assessing and evaluating the orientee's clinical performance for the first month of employment, in collaboration with the nurse manager and preceptor and (2) participating in the 3-month performance appraisal process of the new staff nurse.

The clinical instructor's responsibilities include the following:

- Participates with the nurse manager in selecting a preceptor for each orientee
- After specific assignment of the preceptor, meets with the nurse manager and preceptor to discuss scheduling of time and areas in which the preceptor will need assistance from the clinical instructor and nurse manager to implement the role
- Facilitates the orientee's assessment of specific learning needs by requesting the orientee to complete the registered nurses's orientation skills checklist (see Appendix 4)

The clinical instructor serves as a behavioral role model for both the orientee and the preceptor. Guidance is provided for the preceptor by the clinical instructor through ongoing feedback, support, and evaluation of the preceptor's role and performance. At the end of the orientation, the clinical instructor meets with the nurse manager and preceptor to discuss positive and negative aspects of the role and to revise implementation of the role as necessary.

PRECEPTOR SELECTION AND EDUCATION

All preceptors involved in the PACU orientation should be selected based on demonstrated proficiency in technical, intellectual, and interpersonal skills. They must also express an interest in teaching and being involved in the appraisal process.

All preceptors should be given inservice and guidance by the nurse manager and clinical instructor in the following:

- Using the orientation checklist
- Assessing the learning needs of new employees
- Giving and receiving feedback
- Developing effective written objectives
- Writing meaningful and objective evaluations

The preceptor should continually collaborate with the clinical instructor and nurse manager during the entire 3-month orientation for the purpose of the following:

- Assessing the learning needs of the orientee
- Planning an orientation specific to the identified learning needs of the orientee
- Implementing the teaching plan by providing the orientee with the necessary supervised clinical experiences, using the checklist as a guide
- Evaluating the nursing care of the orientee, giving constructive feedback and writing a formal appraisal at the conclusion of the orientation

The preceptor's responsibilities include the following:

- Serves as a role model by delivering quality nursing care in accordance with the policies and procedures of the nursing department
- Assists the orientee to integrate socially and professionally into the unit by providing information regarding the roles and responsibilities of all members of the multidisciplinary team while introducing the orientee to the team members
- Assesses the beginning learning needs of the orientee through questioning and observing the orientee during the first few days in the unit
- Schedules weekly meetings with the orientee to review the checklist, develop weekly expectations for the orientee, and discuss problems and concerns—keeps written records of all conferences
- Assists the orientee to identify the orientee's

own learning needs and directs the orientee to the appropriate resource

- Continues to serve as a resource person and evaluator by using the orientation checklist as a guide to experiences pertinent to the orientee's development
- Prepares a written evaluation at the end of the first month; reviews with the nurse manager and participates in oral presentation to the orientee; participates in subsequent advisory and counseling sessions as indicated
- Reviews with the orientee near the conclusion of the day orientation, expectations and available resource personnel on all shifts; supervises the majority of the clinical experiences on the orientation checklist and signs off (with the clinical instructor), while the orientee is on the day shift
- Meets with the assigned preceptor on evenings or nights before the orientee is transferred, to discuss progress and identify future learning needs of the orientee
- The new shift preceptor will fulfill all of the responsibilities of the day preceptor as indicated. The orientee and the new preceptor will be assigned to work in the same zone and on the same evenings or nights during the 1-month orientation to the shift.

WEEKLY ORIENTATION OUTLINE FOR PRECEPTOR PROGRAM
Week 1

Monday, Tuesday, Wednesday:
Orientee in classes with the clinical instructor.
Thursday, Friday:
Preceptor orientation to the unit layout and routines. At the end of these 2 days, the orientee will be responsible for the following:

1. Locating equipment and specific access within the unit
2. Identifying members of the multidisciplinary team
3. Locating and reading reference manuals
4. Reviewing the organization of the patient's chart

5. Understanding the format and use of the anesthesia and post anesthesia record

Weeks 2 to 6

The orientee will shadow the preceptor and will become familiar with unit structure and function and become knowledgeable about the following:

1. Special records and charting. Review and be supervised using the post anesthesia record, the continuous ventilation record, and the standards of charting
2. Review and be supervised using the monitoring systems, defibrillator, electrocardiogram (ECG), and emergency alarm systems
3. Checking equipment. Review and be supervised using the emergency carts and pediatric emergency cart, ordering narcotics and plasma supply, reordering stock supplies and drugs, ventilators, hypothermia machine, portable suctions
4. Arterial lines. Review and be supervised assisting with insertion, the nursing care, and drawing of arterial blood samples from the cannula
5. Central venous pressure (CVP) monitoring. Review and be supervised assisting at insertion of CVP lines, changing CVP dressing, drawing blood samples, and removing CVP lines
6. Swan-Ganz catheters. Review and be supervised assisting at insertion, nursing care, measurement of pulmonary artery pressure and wedge pressure, and troubleshooting
7. Respiratory care. Review and be supervised assisting with intubation, caring for the intubated patient, caring for the patient on the ventilator, intermittent mandatory ventilation (IMV), and positive end-expiratory pressure (PEEP), weaning patients from respirators, use of the Wright respirometer, sterile suctioning procedure, extubating patients, and insertion of airways
8. Blood samples. Review and be supervised obtaining arterial samples that may be used to analyze arterial blood gases; also obtaining blood samples for lactate and pyruvate, ionized calcium, prothrombin time (PT), partial thromboplastin time (PTT), coagulation profile, hematocrit readings, and serum electrolytes.
9. Miscellaneous equipment. Review and be supervised in the use of the IVAC pumps, Venodyne boots, blood warmers, and any other miscellaneous equipment
10. Patient apparatus and equipment. Review and be supervised in the care of patients with chest tubes, total parenteral nutrition (TPN) and TPN catheters, continuous bladder irrigations, administration of blood and blood products.
11. Electrical safety. Review, with clinical instructor, plugs, grounding, beds, and all other pertinent electrical equipment
12. Physiological and anatomical considerations in the PACU. Review with clinical instructor and be responsible for understanding the anatomy and physiology of the respiratory system, cardiovascular system, renal system, gastrointestinal system, and integumentary system
13. Concepts in anesthetic agents. Review with the clinical instructor and be responsible for the postoperative care of patients who have received inhalation anesthetics, intravenous anesthetics, muscle relaxants, and regional anesthetics; also must review drug interactions
14. Postoperative nursing care. Review with the clinical instructor and be responsible for the following:
    - Physical assessment of the post anesthesia patient, airway management, and management of the unconscious patient
    - Standards of care in the post anesthesia care unit
    - Postoperative care after ear, nose, neck, and throat surgery
    - Postoperative care after thoracic surgery

- Postoperative care after vascular surgery
- Postoperative care after orthopedic surgery
- Postoperative care after neurosurgery
- Postoperative care after thyroid and parathyroid surgery
- Postoperative care after gastrointestinal, abdominal, and anorectal surgery
- Postoperative care after genitourinary surgery
- Postoperative care after gynecological surgery
- Postoperative care after breast surgery
- Postoperative care after plastic surgery

15. Special considerations. Review with the clinical instructor and be responsible for the following:
    - The geriatric patient
    - The pediatric patient
    - The immunosuppressed patient
    - Postoperative nausea and vomiting
    - Shock
    - Disseminated intravascular coagulation
    - Cardiopulmonary resuscitation
    - Chemotherapy
    - Radiation therapy
    - Pain medications
    - Anesthetic agents
    - Hypothermia/hyperthermia
    - Care of the patient with invasive monitoring
    - ECG interpretation
    - Acid-base balance and hypoxia
    - Pulmonary edema
    - Congestive heart failure
    - Diabetes

Weeks 6 to 8

Under the guidance of the preceptor, orientees will spend time gaining experience in the organizational skills needed to coordinate their patient care assignments, which will gradually be increased on the day shift. Orientees will continue to expand their knowledge base and expertise in clinical practice.

The following experiences will be provided if they have not already been reviewed:

1. One day in the special care unit to become familiar with any special equipment, for example, mass spectrometer and laminar flow
2. One day following a patient through surgery, including preoperative visit, anesthesia holding area, operating room, and PACU
3. One day with the surgical nurse coordinators, observing the preoperative and postoperative patient and family educators
4. One day shadowing the respiratory therapist to learn chest physiotherapy

Weeks 8 to 10

Upon transfer to an assigned shift, another preceptor will be assigned to the orientee. To assure continuity in the orientation process, the original preceptor will meet with the newly assigned preceptor, the orientee, clinical instructor, and nurse manager. The progress of the orientee and the checklist will be reviewed. The orientee will be assigned to work the same nights or evenings with the preceptor for 1 month. The orientee's patient assignment will be determined by the preceptor in collaboration with the charge nurse. During this time, the orientee will do the following:

1. Meet the nursing and medical personnel on an assigned shift
2. Become familiar with the shift routines
3. Become familiar with the expectations of the registered nurse in post anesthesia care on an assigned shift
4. Observe the preceptor's clinical and organizational skills in delivering patient care to one to five patients
5. Deliver safe, quality patient care to assigned patients

Weeks 10 to 12 and Thereafter

The orientee will be responsible for enlisting the assistance of the preceptor and all other nursing resources as needed in the ongoing process of planning for and delivering quality patient care.

SUGGESTIONS FOR FURTHER READING

American Society of Anesthesiologists: Practice advisory for recovery room, ASA Newsletter, May 2, 1978.

Drain CB and Shipley S: The recovery room, Philadelphia, 1979, WB Saunders Co.

Fraulini KE: After anesthesia: a guide for PACU, ICU, and medical-surgical nursing, Los Altos, Calif, 1987, Appleton & Lange.

Israel JS and DeKornfeld TJ: Recovery room care, Springfield Ill, 1982, Charles C Thomas, Publisher.

Luczun ME: Postanesthesia nursing, a comprehensive guide, Rockville, Md, 1984, Aspen Publications, Inc.

Plasse NJ and Lederer JR: Preceptors: a resource for new nurses, J Nurs Leadership Management, June, 1981.

Post Anesthesia Care Unit Clinical Preceptor Program, Memorial Sloan Kettering Cancer Center, Department of Nursing, New York, 1987.

Smith CE: Planning, implementing and evaluating learning experiences for adults. Nurse Educ, Nov-Dec, 1978.

CHAPTER 20

A Role for the PACU Nurse on the Nursing Unit

Ann Marie Terra
Elizabeth A. M. Frost

HOLISTIC NURSING

The involvment and interaction of the PACU nurse on the unit is a primary facet in a multidisciplinary approach complementing holistic care. Modern technology has influenced and necessitated the expansion of PACU nursing practice to incorporate critical care expertise. This evolutionary factor is essential to ensure the patient's safe and smooth passage through the crisis of surgical intervention. Juxtaposed is the increased scope of knowledge and skills required in the formulation of nursing diagnoses and use of the nursing process assuring effective, efficient, quality care.

Terminology

Health, defined epidemiologically, is the state of complete well-being of the physical, mental, and social processes, not merely the absence of disease. *Disease* results from an imbalance in equilibrium as governed by the environment and is a state of unwellness, a manifestation of a pathological condition. *Holistic* is termed more than the sum total of parts. *Holistic medicine* includes the metaphysical or spiritual approach and deals with the well individual who becomes unwell (Figure 20-1).

In our efforts to maintain equilibrium, various coping mechanisms attempt to compensate for stress, strain, and the unwellness of the disease state (Figure 20-2). Holistic nursing may be defined as the concept involving total care of the patient in an integrated manner encompassing all patient systems in the well/ill continuum. The goals are based on the standards of care.

Holistic Approach

1. Emphasis on the interrelatedness of all systems subject to vascillation, affected by the exogenous and endogenous environment
2. Structure and application of the nursing process as a tool with the patient as the framework
3. Identification of patient needs and coping mechanisms, such as fear, anxiety, loss of control over self—which will affect learning and recovery (return to wellness); physiological and emotional support then required
4. Use of a perioperative role (Figure 20-3)

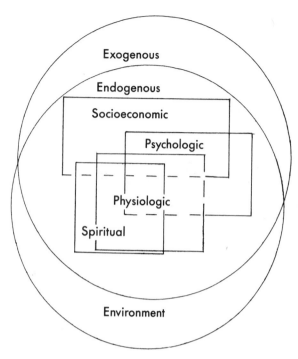

FIGURE 20-1
Holistic concept of man and environment.

Methodology

1. Collect data from the chart and unit nurses
2. Preoperative visit: establish rapport with patient and family; observe all systems; listen and obtain history; initiate or reinforce patient teaching; discuss expectations
3. Postoperative visit and phone calls: evaluate care delivered; reinforce teaching

Communication

Effective communication with the unit nurses fosters teamwork, which is vital for quality care and an holistic approach. In addition, it promotes a safe environment and effective and efficient nursing care.

The nursing diagnosis originating on the unit can be transferred to the operating room and PACU with appropriate reassessment. Previously identified problems in other settings can become the basis

of a nursing care plan and assist in determining a baseline (Figure 20-4).

Age, sex, value systems, and beliefs, as well as life experience, are influential factors in determining the patient's accommodation to the proposed surgical experience.

Preparation for preoperative teaching should include review of chart, identification of previous surgery and type, and a brief discussion with the unit RN.

PREOPERATIVE TEACHING

Preoperative teaching and counseling are recognized not only as the patient's right but as important determinants of good outcome. In many centers these tasks have been assigned to operating room nurses. However, rather than the nurse spending time describing and explaining the operative situation—a time when the patient may well be unaware of his surroundings—it may be more important to emphasize the postoperative period. During the preanesthetic interview, anesthesiologists stress not simply "you are going to sleep," but rather "you will wake up." Thus preoperative teaching should describe the environment and functioning of the PACU, as well as the sensations the patient may experience when recovering from anesthesia. Ideally, the nurse who performs the preoperative interview should be assigned to the postanesthetic care.

A blind study, designed to test the hypothesis that preoperative instruction of the patient by a PACU nurse has a positive effect on the patient's immediate postoperative adaptation to the recovery environment, had positive results. Patients in the instructed group require 14% fewer analgesics than the control group, and the average length of stay in the PACU was reduced by 15 minutes. Also, 93% of those who received preoperative teaching cooperated easily with instruction compared with 85% of those who received only routine preoperative instruction from a member of the floor staff. Other benefits of the preoperative interview included a decreased incidence of vomiting and obvious discomfort, and fewer "surprises."

The instruction time of 8 minutes per patients

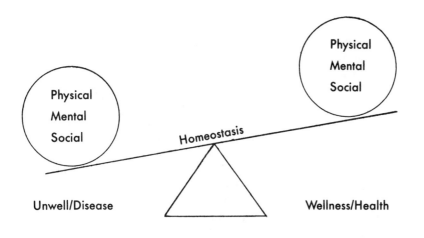

FIGURE 20-2
Maintenance of homeostasis.

Physical
Mental
Social

Physical
Mental
Social

Homeostasis

Unwell/Disease

Wellness/Health

Surgical experience

Preoperative	Assessment	Preoperative visits Patient teaching
Intraoperative	Planning	Identification of patient problems (anesthesia, positioning, surgical complications)
Postoperative	Implementation Intervention	of goals formulated (nursing care plan, patient teaching)
	Evaluation	and surveillance of post- anesthetic care, requires continuous reassessment

FIGURE 20-3
The nursing process:
perioperative role of
the PACU nurse.

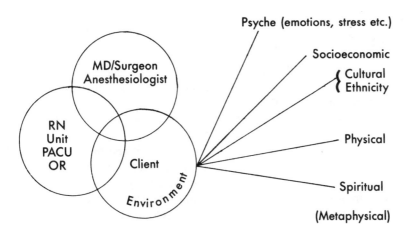

Psyche (emotions, stress etc.)

Socioeconomic

{ Cultural
  Ethnicity

MD/Surgeon
Anesthesiologist

RN
Unit
PACU
OR

Client

Physical

Environment

Spiritual

(Metaphysical)

FIGURE 20-4
Interrelatedness of team
(holistic) approach.

was more than offset by the 15 minutes deducted from PACU time. Thus such a program can prove cost effective, as well as provide improved patient care and better public relations. Also, PACU nurses who have participated in preoperative teaching have appreciated the ability to communicate with an awake patient and to develop greater awareness of individual patient needs that could be incorporated in the PACU care plan.

During preoperative teaching, the PACU nurse can help the patient in the following ways:

1. Understand proposed surgery and outcome (this validates informed consent). Appropriate explanation and discussion in laymen terminology can be positive reinforcement.
2. Discuss routine preoperative preparation (that is, shave, antiseptic shower, premedication, transfer to the operating room, family waiting area).
3. Describe the environment: holding area; operating room (narrow bed, surgical lights, personnel dress); and PACU (recovery from anesthesia until stable for transfer to unit or intensive care). Although patients may hear noise on awakening, every effort is made to keep this to a minimum.
4. When applicable, explain spinal anesthesia block and its effect on the patient in the immediate recovery period.
5. Explain nature and type of equipment attached to the patient (that is, ECG, pulse oximeter, Foley catheter, nasogastric tube, airway, endotracheal tube, intravenous cannulae).
6. Explain general nature of discomfort upon emerging from anesthesia; reassurance of availability of pain-relief medication. Mention the dry, scratchy throat after endotracheal intubation and why water is not generally given in the PACU but that ice chips are usually allowable in very small quantities.
7. When applicable, mention the use of restraints and that these will be removed when the patient is in control of his actions.
8. Discuss the use of warm blankets to improve patient comfort.

9. Reinforce patient teaching on deep breathing, coughing, leg exercises, changing position.
10. Review incision and type of dressing.
11. Assist in coping with feelings of anxiety, fear, and depression by encouraging verbalization on such matters as body image, loneliness, and powerlessness. This is of prime importance, since learning and retention are related to the level of stress and coping adaptability.
12. Set achievable goals in dealing with illness and surgery, and reinforce, whenever possible, information given by the anesthesiologist and surgeon.

Instruction should also be given to family members as follows:

- An approximate length of time that the patient will be in the operating room and PACU
- An explanation as to why relatives are not allowed in the operating room or PACU
- Directions to the family room or waiting room

TYPES OF LEARNING

Knowledge and assessment of the type of learning the patient requires are necessary to determine the manner of presentation:

- Cognitive learning: need for information
- Affective learning: need to learn (or change) attitudes, behavior
- Psychomotor learning: need to acquire new skills

Teaching Aids

Recommended teaching aids that can be adapted according to availability of financial resources and staffing patterns are as follows:

I. Preoperative interview
   A. Objectives
      1. Instruct patient and family.
      2. Identify patient needs and assist with problem solving.
      3. Document patient needs (ensures continuity of care).

4. Establish rapport and trust.
5. Collect data: obtain history and perform physiological assessment (physical impairment, handicaps, limitations) and psychological assessment (mental status, orientation, fears, apprehension).
6. Develop and implement individualized nursing care plan.
7. Coordinate care plan with other members of health team.
8. Increase job satisfaction.
9. Reduce postoperative level of stress and complications.
10. Minimize hospital stay.

B. Methodology
1. Observe patient's color, respiration, muscle activity, circulation.
2. Listen and encourage client verbalization.
3. Question and obtain a history; elicit patient participation.

C. Types of interviewing techniques
1. Direct: assertive, direct questioning, uses confrontation and interpretive methods.
2. Nondirect: Rogerian, less assertive approach, encourages patient to initiate communication regarding perceptions and concerns without blocking him or assuming what his fears are.
3. Transactional analysis employing the three defined levels (child, parent, mature adult) requires cognizance regarding role interchanges.

D. Recommendation: Conduction of the preoperative interview should occur sitting at the patient's level and initiated by self-introduction. Specific questions concerning surgery or anesthesia can be referred to the appropriate physician. Application of effective communication skills, both verbal and nonverbal (body language), contribute to the accomplishment of established goals.

II. Group classes: Planned, regularly scheduled classes for prospective surgical patients and families can be arranged preoperatively or before admission. Coordination of classes with presurgical testing may be convenient. Patient education and staff development departments can assist in conjunction with OR and PACU inservice personnel in the development and implementation of informative classes. Staff participation should be encouraged and used to promote efficacy of the program and self-actualization. Suggested modalities for adaptation and presentation of classes are the following:
1. Self-teaching instructional modules
2. Lectures
3. Role playing
4. Pictures, posters
5. Booklets and/or pamphlets

III. Audiovisual aids: Presentations recorded or filmed on site or obtained commercially range from simple to elaborate, depending on institutional resources available. Ingenuity and adaptability are primary ingredients in initiating an effective and rewarding program. Considerations include the following:
1. Slide presentation (with or without documentary, taped or lecture)
2. Video tapes
3. Movies, films
4. Closed-circuit television

IV. Tours: Recommended times are geared toward personnel availability and traffic hours. Obvious areas to include are the following:
1. Presurgical testing (laboratory, diagnostic imagining department)
2. Ambulatory surgery unit
3. Surgical units
4. Holding area
5. Operating room
6. PACU
7. Family waiting area
8. Intensive care areas (optional)

Classes or tours can be held at predetermined intervals compatible with patient and staff scheduling and arranged via the admitting office.

V. Recommended sources of assistance for initiation and implementation of proposed programs are the following:
   1. Patient education department
   2. Audiovisual department
   3. Volunteer department
   4. Surgical specialty department
   5. Social service department
   6. Public relations department
   7. Multidisciplinary committees
   8. Nursing committees
   9. Community relations committees
   10. Specialty committees (such as OR and PACU committee)

PEDIATRIC PATIENTS

Elective surgery for the pediatric patient involves consideration and focus on (1) stages of growth and development and (2) the family unit. Education of child and parents allays fear and anxiety and accelerates the child's return to homeostasis with minimal negative incidence. Public awareness through creative avenues of education satisfies attainment of goals.

Class participation can be elicited via contact with the local school's health education departments. Initially a brief presentation to the class can include the following:
   1. Dress in "scrubs"
   2. Discussion and visual aids integrated with the human body system currently being studied
   3. Discussion regarding surgery and role of the OR and PACU nurse
   4. Introduction of poster contest illustrating these discussions
   Prize awards for most outstanding, etc. (such as, T-shirts, ribbons)
   Prearranged poster display at school or at local mall in conjunction with Health Education Week or health fair
   Publicity through school and newspaper coverage

Preoperative preparation ideally begins in the surgeon's office, where the child and parents should have specific needs identified and addressed. A preparatory hospital tour is highly indicated, and a "show and tell" is also beneficial.

Recommendations

During the preoperative visit, the child should be addressed directly. At this time, determination of language and comprehensive skills can be assessed. Nickname, age, height, and weight are ascertained to formulate an individualized teaching care plan (Table 20-1).

Availability of medical equipment for handling is suggested, such as anesthesia masks, blood pressure apparatus, stethoscope. Based on indications and the preference of the anesthesiologist, premedication for pediatric patients may not be ordered. If ordered however, preferable administration is one hour before transport to the holding room to allow

TABLE 20-1	
Assessment and implementation for the teaching plan	
Development level	**Consideration**
Preschool children (4-6 years)	
Have limited time concept	Demonstrate with dolls or drawings
Short attention span	Note any comfort object, i.e., blanket, animal, doll
Ritualistic	
School age (6-12 years)	
Higher cognitive level	Demonstrate equipment
Ability to focus on several sequential concepts	Encourage play sessions (to act out fears and fantasies)
Greater attention span	Provide simple explanation
Adolescent (12-18 years)	
Increased complexity of understanding	Increase complexity of explanation
Fear of body exposure	Use visual aids
	Assure protection of privacy

for full effect. The holding area should be quiet and screened; parents should be encouraged to remain with the child. Research regarding parental presence in the PACU has demonstrated stress reduction in the postanesthetic phase. Alleviation of the child's fear of separation appears to be of consequence.

AMBULATORY PATIENTS

Patients benefit significantly when seen ahead of time by the anesthesiologist, the surgeon, and the nurse from the ambulatory unit or PACU. Although there may be some duplication of effort and information, the interviews allow positive reinforcement and encourage interaction. Patients have more opportunities to verbalize and to understand the instructions and explanations. Although telephone interviews are an often-used option, the personal interview before the day of surgery is preferred.

Arranging a time for interview may be difficult because the ambulatory patient is not the ''captive audience'' that the inpatient becomes. Preoperative teaching and preparation can be coordinated with preadmission testing. If possible, evening hours may be preferable to avoid the necessity of the patient taking time from work. Coordination must be made also through the department of anesthesiology to ensure availability of an anesthesiologist. One of the benefits of arranging a meeting before the day of surgery is a rather practical one—the patient learns the location of the parking lot and the ambulatory unit!

Focus on the short-term aspects of hospital stay requires definitive instructions regarding the admission procedure and preoperative instructions (see Chapter 13.) General, stand-by, or local anesthesia is of considerable importance to the disposition of the patient and length of stay. Discharge instructions are essential. Standard admission and specific preoperative protocol regarding preparation and instructions should be documented. Communication by telephone postoperatively provides the following:

1. Reinforcement of instructions
2. Clarification of information
3. Reassurance
4. Improved public relations

Nursing involvement in the ambulatory process has been capsulated by Burden:

The preoperative evaluation and interviews are probably the most important parts of the entire outpatient surgery process. No financial savings or administrative efficiency is worth compromising a patient's safety: proper evaluation of the patient is the key to success. Any complication is undesirable, but one resulting from poor evaluation and selection is a tragedy because it is easily prevented.

SUMMARY

A holistic approach using the nursing process can enhance the postanesthetic recovery of adult and pediatric patients. Adaptation is dictated by need, institutional size, and budgetary allowance. The key is innovativeness and creativity of those involved to devise, coordinate, and implement from available effective programs and techniques.

SUGGESTIONS FOR FURTHER READING

Ayers C and Walton L: A guide for the preoperative visit, AORN J 19:413, 1974.

Bille DA: Preoperative teaching: rights and responsibilities, Today's OR Nurse, p. 9, Oct 1979.

Boegli EH and Boegli RG: Can preop learning be improved? AORN J 16:43, 1972.

Burden N: Preoperative assessment of the ambulatory surgery patient, J Post Anesth Nurs 1:1, 48, 1986.

Cote CJ: Management of induction and emergence in pediatrics, 39th Annual Refresher Course Lectures, no. 211, Amer Soc Anes, San Francisco, 1988.

Crain WC: Theories of development: concepts and applications, Englewood Cliffs, NJ, 1980, Prentice Hall.

Crawford FJ: Ambulatory surgery: the elderly patient, AORN J 41:357, 1985.

Diniaio MJ and Ingoldsbry B: Parental presence in the recovery room, AORN J 38:685, 1983.

Dunn R and Dunn K: Practical approaches to individualized instruction, West Nyack, NY, 1972, Parker Publishing Co.

Feeley TW: Assessments and management of patients in the recovery room, 39th Annual Refresher Course Lectures, no. 175, Amer Soc Anes, San Francisco, 1988.

Gewolb J, Hanes R, and Barash PG: A survey of 3244 consecutive admissions to the post anesthesia recovery room at a university teaching hospital, Anesthesiology 67:3A A471 1987

Hercules PR: Nursing in the postoperative care unit, AORN J 28:047, 1978.

Hercules PR: O.R. experience teaches continuity of care, AORN J 32:299, 1983.

Kanda NL: Staff development for R.R. nurses, Aorn J 26:664, 1977.

Kempe A and Gelozis R: Patient anxiety levels: an ambulatory surgery study, AORN J 41:391, 1985.

Lockhart CH: Practical consideration in the preoperative psychological preparation of the pediatric patient. In Guerra F and Aldrete JA, editors: Emotional and psychological responses to anesthesia and surgery, New York, 1980, Grune & Stratton, Inc.

Lorig K: An overview of needs assessment tools for continuing education, Nurse Educ, p. 12, Mar/Apr 1977. McClintoc J: Preoperative care of the pediatric patient, Today's OR Nurse 2(5):7, 1980.

McClurg E: Developing an effective patient teaching program, AORN J 3:474, 1981.

Milazzo V: A study of the differences in health knowledge gained through formal and informal teaching. Heart Lung 9:1079, 1980.

Quinn MJC: Another dimension of PACU nursing, J Post Anesth Nurs 1:1, 26, 1986.

Ridgway M: Preop interviews assure quality care, AORN J 2:1083, 1976.

Rozman F: Nursing process in the recovery room, AORN J 2:1069, 1976.

Schmidt FE and Woolridge PJ: Psychological preparation of surgical patients, Nurs Res, p. 108, Mar/Apr 1973.

CHAPTER 21

Risk Management and Liabilities of the Post Anesthesia Care Team

Richard B. Patt
Estelle White

THE ROLE OF THE NURSE

The evolving role of the medical/surgical nurse has introduced additional obligations and responsibilities to members of the nursing profession (see Appendix 9). As a consequence, increased awareness of risk management issues and participation in the process of risk management are essential. The role of the nurse continues to include the traditional tasks of administering medications and carrying out physicians' orders. In addition, contemporary nursing includes independent assessment and planning, as well as the recognition of alterations in the clinical status of patients and determination of the need for appropriate intervention.

MEDICAL MALPRACTICE

Medical malpractice is a form of negligence that exists when, in the course of treatment, a health care professional has not practiced with reasonable skill. For malpractice to exist, there must be a professional relationship between the care giver and

the patient, a departure from the accepted standard of care must occur, and that departure must be the proximate cause of injury to the patient. Although each of these elements must be proven to establish malpractice, in the current legal environment, the simple presence of an injury or allegation of injury may be sufficient cause for the initiation of a malpractice suit, which, regardless of outcome, can be professionally and personally devastating.

Persons Involved in a Lawsuit

The *plaintiff* is the person who brings on the complaint and initiates the lawsuit. Generally, it is the patient who is the plaintiff. However, in the case of a deceased patient, the plaintiff is often a spouse or other family member and is referred to as the *executor* of the decedent plaintiff's estate. In the case of an infant (any person who has not reached majority is considered an infant under the law), it is usually the parent who, as the *guardian,* brings about the lawsuit on behalf of the infant plaintiff.

The *defendant* is the person or hospital against whom the lawsuit is brought. This is the *party* to the suit who must be defended in the courtroom. Usually, the decision as to which hospital personnel are to be named as defendants is made by the plaintiff's attorney, not by the plaintiff. It is common for a plaintiff to sue physicians and nurses with whom he has a good relationship because his attorney convinces him that it is necessary for the prosecution of a case. Some attorneys will name only those people who had a direct role in an alleged injury, whereas others will name everyone who cared for the patient and whose name appears in the medical record. Either way, a defense must be prepared for each of the defendants.

STANDARDS OF CARE

The term *standard of care* refers to the level of skill, knowledge, and care to which a professional is expected to adhere, and describes what a reasonable person acting under similar circumstances might do. Increasingly, the courts have tended to recognize national standards of care rather than accepting varied standards in different local communities. In any given case, the standard of care to which a nurse or physician is expected to adhere may not be inherently obvious, and the testimony of expert witnesses is generally relied on to establish the standard of care that is pertinent. A judgment of what actually constitutes appropriate care is often reached only with difficulty, since testimony from multiple specialists for the defense and plaintiff may be in conflict.

STATUTE OF LIMITATIONS

The statute of limitations is the period of time during which a plaintiff can institute a lawsuit. The statutory period begins when an injury occurs, although in some cases (usually involving foreign objects left in the body) the statutory period begins when the injured person discovers the injury.

The statute of limitations is a great concern to both defendants and plaintiffs because, depending on the nature of the particular malpractice case, several years may elapse before institution of the suit. This can be beneficial for the plaintiff but extremely problematic for the defendant. The difficulty is that with the passage of time memories fade and hospital witnesses move away. It is crucial for the hospital staff to report any unusual incidents or probable future lawsuits to the hospital's risk management department. Careful, factual documentation is essential.

The statute of limitations varies from state to state. In New York, for example, an adult patient may sue up to $2\frac{1}{2}$ years from the time that the alleged malpractice took place. If a patient dies as a result of medical or nursing treatment, the executor of the estate can bring about a suit up until 2 years from the date of death. If a patient undergoes a surgical procedure, continues to complain of discomfort for several years, and then learns through surgery or an x-ray that a sponge was left behind, another full year may elapse before the statute of limitations has run out. In the case of an infant, the statute is either 10 years or until the infant has reached majority plus $2\frac{1}{2}$ years.

Obviously, the statute of limitations need not be memorized at this juncture, but suffice it to say, the plaintiff can sometimes wait several years. The importance of early reporting by the hospital staff cannot be overemphasized, so that witnesses can recount the occurrence while memories are fresh.

NURSING LIABILITY

Historically, most malpractice actions are directed against physicians and hospitals. Allegations against hospitals can involve claims arising from nursing care. If a nurse has acted within the scope of her employment, the employer or hospital is held vicariously liable.

Although the nurse may be held primarily liable, the hospital employer generally pays any damages under theories of vicarious liability and the contractual obligation to provide insurance for nurses.

Nurses' individual responsibility should not be

minimized. Involvement in a claim can be a difficult experience, and loss of licensure or professional actions can result from cases in which patients are harmed.

POST ANESTHESIA NURSING AND RISK MANAGEMENT

Post anesthesia care is an area of particularly high medical risk and potential liability. A study on malpractice claims conducted by the National Association of Insurance Commissioners in 1978 rated the PACU as the area in the hospital with the highest percentage of injuries and claims. The postsurgical patient is subject to acute stresses related to surgical intervention and recovery from anesthetic drugs. With advances in medical technology, surgery and anesthesia have become more sophisticated and sicker patients are subjected to more complex and invasive surgery. The post anesthesia nurse is responsible for interpreting data from increased numbers of complex monitors and at the same time is expected not to be distracted from keen observation of clinical parameters. Nurses are expected to be familiar with a myriad of medications (and their interactions), many of which are administered intravenously to produce rapid changes in physiology. New drugs are rapidly introduced into perioperative therapeutics, and old drugs are administered for new indications and by new routes.

The most common sources of problems resulting in malpractice action against nurses include allegations of the following:

- Failure to follow nursing protocols
- Failure to adequately monitor or observe the patient
- Failure to administer medications properly and promptly
- Failure to follow physician orders properly and promptly
- Failure to properly record and execute verbal orders
- Failure to promptly detect and report changes in a patient's condition
- Failure to intervene appropriately

- Failure to protect the patient from falls or burns

In no setting is exposure to risk greater than in the large teaching hospital where medical students and residents with varying degrees of training, experience, and supervision write orders and are involved in patient care. The post anesthesia nurse often has more experience than the treating physicians and is expected to exercise independent judgment in the patient's interest. Further, in the case of an inconsistency between nurse and physician perception, the nurse is charged with resolving the conflict in a professional manner in accordance with existing protocol. This can include going beyond the initial physician contacted to resolve a problem where the response is deemed unsatisfactory. The hospital and its clinical departments (nursing, medicine, surgery, risk management) are responsible for creating an environment that supports the delivery of quality care and for developing systems that facilitate and demand that deviations from the standard be reported and corrected.

Some representative cases follow.

1. Failure to Follow Physician's Orders Promptly and Properly. The nurse is responsible for reviewing the medical record to ascertain whether the doctor's orders have been modified. In the case of *Toth* v. *Community Hospital at Glen Cove,* twin girls born prematurely were placed under oxygen. One baby suffered total blindness, and the other suffered severe damage to one eye. The physician ordered 6 L of oxygen per minute for the first 12 hours, then 4 L per minute thereafter. The nurses continued to give 6 L of oxygen for several weeks. The jury found the nurses guilty of malpractice for not following the doctor's orders correctly. Nurses can also be found negligent if they carry out an order that is unsafe or erroneous. If the order appears questionable, it is incumbent upon the nurse to have the order clarified *by the physician who wrote it*. If the nurse is not familiar with the medication ordered, the dosage, or manner of administration, it is her responsibility to check with her supervisor or the physician who wrote the order.

2. Failure to Take Correct Telephone Orders. Because the physician, unlike the nurse, usually does not maintain a vigil by the patient's bedside, telephone orders often become a necessity. Because it is incumbent upon the nurse to transcribe the orders, every effort must be made to be careful and accurate. Orders should be repeated, once transcribed, for verification purposes. Verification of an order by another nurse on a second phone is helpful

3. Failure to Report Significant Changes. In the case of *Goff* v. *Doctor's Hospital,* a patient in the PACU was seriously bleeding because the doctor failed to suture properly. Although the attending physician was no longer present in the hospital once the bleeding was recognized by the nurses, he was the only physician who was contacted. The patient died. The court held that the nurses were negligent in their failure to report the condition in a way that could be handled promptly.

4. Failure to monitor. An 18-year-old boy with a history of sleep apnea was admitted to the PACU, arousable but sleepy. Staffing was reduced by illness and lunch break, and vital signs were not monitored for about 25 minutes. Flat line on the ECG monitor was noted by an anesthesiologist accompanying another patient. All resuscitative attempts were futile. The nurses and hospital communicated immediately with the family and admitted liability, and the case was settled out of court.

RISK MANAGEMENT

Risk management, once practiced informally and extemporaneously, has become an integral part of hospital-based medical practice. Most individual departments within a hospital are required to have active quality assurance programs that address risk management, and increasing numbers of hospitals staff an independent department for this purpose.

The basis for risk management lies jointly in the reduction of liability, claims, and financial loss, and the prevention of injury to patients and employees. The concepts and the practice of reducing financial loss and reducing personal injury are closely related and are complementary goals of risk management programs. Risk management and quality assurance programs have closely related missions, but they are not identical. Risk management focuses more acutely on patients and how they are affected by policies and events, with an eye toward avoiding claims. Quality assurance focuses closely on the providers of health care and patterns of practice to ascertain that the best quality of care possible is delivered to patients. Both processes serve the patient, institution, and providers by elevating the standard of care. Risk management focuses on standards mandated by law and emphasizes the provision of care that meets at least those minimal requirements, whereas quality assurance may apply higher standards.

The process of risk management involves identification, analysis, and modification. Identification may take place through incident reporting or quality assurance activity. The concept of an "incident" has broadened to include not just an injury, but any event that might have resulted in an injury. For example, a pharmacy error resulting in the delivery of an incorrect dosage of medication is an incident and must be reported, regardless of whether the drug was actually administered.

Evaluation involves investigation and assessment of both the incident and the system within which the incident occurred, to detect any pattern of system breakdown that is potentially remedial. Evaluation is carried out through interviews, chart review, and consultation.

Modification depends on the nature and seriousness of the event. In the case of an incident involving patient well-being, a patient representative may work with family members to resolve their concerns or anger, and a portion or the entire patient's bill is often absorbed by the institution. In the case of a serious injury, the insurer is notified and funds may be set aside to offset potential liability. The risk management department works closely with the involved department to determine whether protocols need to be revised or entire systems need reorganization. Education of hospital staff is an important component of this phase of risk management. The analysis of the event becomes part of the risk management data base, and further monitoring is planned to ascertain that efforts at remediation are successful.

Recognition of situations that could potentially result in medicolegal action is an important aspect of risk management. By informing nursing supervisors and the central risk management office early, damage can often be averted or minimized. Misguided efforts to shift blame or alter the medical record can produce disastrous results. In consultation with the hospital's legal department, the risk management department often encourages and supervises frank, early disclosure of problems to patients and family members. Some patient charges may be deferred. The patient's chart may be reviewed, and interviews with staff may take place to record the details of events while they are still fresh.

One of the greatest values of a proactive risk management program is that potential injuries, including disability and death, are prevented, based on the observation of events that have not yet resulted in injury. Although key hospital personnel are typically identified as expert risk managers, the system functions effectively only when all staff regard risk management as a part of their job description and practice it on a daily basis.

RISK MANAGEMENT STRATEGIES: DOCUMENTATION

Although a detailed description of good nursing practice is beyond the scope of this chapter, documentation is discussed in some depth because even if nursing care has been impeccable, it is difficult or impossible to prove in the absence of careful documentation. Unfortunately, in the care of critically ill patients, it is a common but serious error to take documentation shortcuts.

Standards of care, quality assurance activities, and nursing regulations require thorough and complete documentation at administrative levels. In addition, documentation in the patient's medical record is of paramount importance, since entries may be scrutinized as potential or actual evidence in legal proceedings. The information in the record, as well as the style in which it is presented, can pro-

vide support for the actions of health care providers or alternatively can furnish a ''prepackaged'' line of attack to a plaintiff's attorney. Requisition and review of pertinent medical records are essential preliminary steps undertaken by the legitimate malpractice attorney before deciding whether to bring suit on a client's behalf. Instances of averted malpractice claims based on impeccable charting are well documented in the literature.

In general, the administration of health care requires that a record be maintained by its provider. Documentation is especially critical in the perioperative period because of the rapid pace and the necessity for frequent intervention. Because modern medicine involves interaction among numerous specialists and providers of care, one of the primary purposes of the medical record is to serve as a means of communication to ensure continuity and quality of care. To be effective, the record must be written legibly, its style should reflect professionalism, and its content must be concise without sacrificing accuracy and detail. At the most basic level, proper charting is the responsibility of each individual involved in the care of a patient. In addition, maintaining quality in charting also represents an important goal for nursing leadership, nursing educators, and quality assurance and risk management programs. Proactive remediation is infinitely more desirable than lessons learned from destructive malpractice events.

Ideally, nursing notes are thoughtful records of patients care activities, events, and observations. Nursing notes are intended to record the details of a medical scenario in such a way that, whether mundane or dramatic, it is readily reconstructed and understood retrospectively. Proper notes do not raise questions without outlining a plan for action nor do they assign responsibility to other care providers or lay blame, but rather they relay a dispassionate account of medically pertinent events and information.

For example, it is not enough merely to report a changing condition to the appropriate personnel. The nurse must also document all observations and nursing actions taken while awaiting the physician's arrival. Many lawsuits have been lost simply because of a lack of documentation in this area. In the case of a patient who, for example, is suddenly showing signs of respiratory distress, writing "Patient dyspneic. Dr. Smith paged stat," is not adequate. A note regarding a patient whose condition is significantly changing should be as specific and detailed as possible. A good nursing note would read as follows:

9:00 PM   Patient complaining of difficulty in "catching his breath." BP, 120/80; P, 90; R, 30. Dr. Smith, anesthesia, paged stat. Head of bed raised. O_2 at 5 L via face mask. Color good.

9:03 PM   BP 100/70; P, 90; R, 30.

9:05 PM   Complaining of chest pain. Pale. Diaphoretic. BP 90/60; P, irregular, 90; R, 30. Dr. Smith not arrived. Paged again stat. Emergency cart at bedside. ECG being done now. Mrs. Chu, nursing supervisor, paged stat.

9:07 PM   BP, 90/60; P, ?60; R, shallow.

9:10 PM   Dr. Smith here. BP palpable at 80. Pulse-? Cardiology called stat.

9:12 PM   Intubated by Dr. Smith. Dr. Jones, cardiology, arrived.

This sample note not only illustrates the detail involved, but also shows how to document when a physician does not respond to an emergency page. The nurse must note what she is doing for the patient while awaiting the doctor, and who else she has paged. In this case, a full 10 minutes elapsed before the doctor arrived, and this must be factually documented. However, as the anesthesiologist on call may be involved in other emergencies elsewhere in the hospital, the nursing supervisor should be called simply to offer assistance in locating other physicians.

An entry in a patient's chart reading "I.V. infusing well" is of negligible value, both because it transmits no objective information and because easily obtainable data are omitted. The omission represents poor charting, which in and of itself suggests the possibility of poor care and also reflects the likelihood that the intravenous site was not thoroughly examined. An appropriate entry might read, "I.V.: 18-gauge Intracath in dorsum of right hand infusing D_5LR at 100 ml/hr. Insertion site without redness or swelling and nontender." If some information is documented on a flow sheet, such as the type of I.V. solution and catheter hardware, an appropriate note would address all aspects not indicated on the flow sheet. By considering the medical record as one entity rather than a collection of isolated parts, completeness can be met without needless repetition.

An entry reading, "Patient appears to be in pain," is likewise inadequate because it conveys judgment but does not provide information. The entry documents that a significant event has occurred, but the subjective quality of the note raises questions rather than providing data. An appropriate entry might read, "Patient is restless and moaning. Heart rate and blood pressure are elevated. Appears to be in pain. House officer called." The amended entry provides facts and observations that lead to the assessment that the patient is probably in pain.

Documenting clinical patterns creates an obligation for action, which also must be documented. Further entries in the patient's medical record should include the planned intervention and, finally, its effectiveness.

Improper alteration or disposition of the medical record is absolutely contraindicated. Sophisticated methods of verification of the legitimacy of records have been used in the courts, and evidence of altered records historically has resulted in the award of huge sums to the plaintiff, almost without regard to the case's other merits. An acceptable means of acknowledging an error is to draw a single line through the error without obliterating it, and write "error" nearby, followed by the date, the clinician's initials, and the corrected entry.

Thus to minimize legal exposure, the professional nurse can take certain general measures when documenting. They are as follows:

Be objective. Do not label your patient (or the physician) as being "obnoxious" or "demanding." Even though this might be the case, remarks like this will infuriate a jury and cause them to look upon the author of the note in a disfavorable light. Brief, factual notes are essential.

Do not obliterate. If an error in charting has been made, simply draw a line through the sentence. It should be initialed by the person who both wrote the note and made the correction. Any attempts to obliterate or white out a note will be viewed in the courtroom as an attempt to falsify the record.

Avoid discrepancies. Read the previous entry. If the information is contrary to your findings, document that you are aware of the discrepancy and that the doctor will be made aware.

Use addendums when necessary. If the nurse wishes to add to a previously written note, it must be done in a separate note, dated and timed when the additional note is written. The addendum should never be written in the margin or between lines, because this will be viewed by a jury as an attempt to ''doctor'' the record.

CONCLUSION

This chapter has emphasized the importance of both the concept and daily practice of risk management as a foundation for the administration of optimal health care. Adherence to principles of risk management ensures that the hospital is a safe place both for patients to receive health care and for nurses and physicians to provide health care.

Medical malpractice litigation is a sad but true reality, reflecting modern society and the changing trends in the public mind. It can never be completely avoided, because as long as there are human beings involved, human error will exist. Meticulous record keeping, prudent judgment, and early reporting of cases will help to minimize exposure.

SUGGESTIONS FOR FURTHER READING

Brooten KE Jr and Chapman S: Malpractice: a guide to avoidance and treatment, Orlando, 1987, Grune & Stratton, Inc.

Curtin L and Flaherty MJ: Nursing ethics: theories and pragmatics, Bowie, Md, 1982, Robert J. Brady Co.

Duran GS: On the scene: risk management in health care, NAQ: Legal Aspects and Legislation 5:19, 1980.

Fiesta J: The law and liability: a guide for nurses, New York, 1988, John Wiley & Sons, Inc.

Northrop CE and Kelly ME: Legal issues in nursing, St. Louis, 1987, The CV Mosby Co.

Pierce EC: The medical liability crisis: where are we going? Curr Rev Recov Room Nurses 8:91, 1986.

APPENDIXES

APPENDIX I

NURSING CARE STANDARD: CARE OF THE PATIENT IN THE PACU

Patients recovering from anesthesia will receive short-term intensive nursing care. Through continuous observation, monitoring, assessment, and nursing care, postanesthetic complications will be prevented or be recognized and treated promptly.

Assessment	Plan	Intervention
1. Adequacy of airway	1. On admission to PACU and q 15 minutes.	1. If airway not patent, suction (oral, nasal, pharyngeal) or insert nasal/oral airway.
2. Adequacy of ventilation a. Strength of voluntary muscles b. Use of accessory muscles c. Respirations, rate, and rhythm	2. On admission and q 15 minutes; administer oxygen as ordered by physician; encourage coughing and deep breathing.	2. Notify anesthesiologist if patient in respiratory distress and requires mechanical assistance or medications.
3. Presence of protective reflexes a. Gag b. Cough	3. On admission.	3. Stay at patient's bedside until present.
4. Cardiovascular status a. Pulse, rate, and rhythm b. Blood pressure	4. On admission and q 15 minutes; apply warm blankets.	4. With any pulse dysrhythmias, place on ECG monitor. Notify anesthesiologist and surgeon of significant deviations in vital signs or ECG.
5. Fluid status	5. Monitor intake and output; administer fluids and blood products as ordered.	5. Notify surgeon of signs and symptoms of dehydration or fluid overload.

6. Allergic reactions
7. Pain
   a. Type
   b. Location
   c. Severity
   d. Effects of nursing care
8. Neuromuscular status
   A. Nerve blocks: Assess sensation, spontaneous or reflex movement, color, warmth, edema of area around and distal to operative site.
   B. Spinals, epidurals: Assess upper level of anesthesia, respiratory function, sensations, spontaneous or reflex movements, color, warmth of lower extremities.
9. Level of consciousness
   a. Response to noxious stimuli
   b. Response to verbal stimuli
   c. Orientation to person, place, and time
10. Condition of operative site
    a. Type of dressing or suture line
    b. Drainage tubes
    c. Drainage
    d. Edema

6. On admission and continuously.
7. On admission and continuously; proper positioning and support for operative reassurance, psychological support; medicate as ordered.
   A. On admission and q 15 minutes; elevate limb/area as indicated.
   B. Have patient attempt to move lower extremities on admission and q 15 minutes until movement is restored; reassure patient of temporary nature of anesthetic effects.
9. On admission and q 15 minutes.
10. On admission and q 15 minutes.

6. Notify surgeon or anesthesiologist of any signs or symptoms.
7. Notify surgeon if plan ineffective or if pain unexplained.
9. Notify anesthesiologist if decreasing level of consciousness.
10. Notify surgeon of any abnormal finding.

APPENDIX II

POSTANESTHETIC RECOVERY SCORE

J. A. Aldrete

A. PURPOSE

1. To be used as a guideline for the evaluation of the postanesthetic patient.
2. To provide set criteria that the postanesthetic patient should meet before discharge from the PACU
3. To provide objective information of the physical condition of patients arriving in the PACU after anesthesia

B. SCORING SYSTEM

1. *Activity.* The muscular activity is assessed by observing the ability of the patient to move his limbs either spontaneously or on command.
   a. Ability to move all four extremities scores 2.
   b. Ability to move two extremities scores 1.
   c. Unable to move any extremity scores 0.
2. *Respiration.* No complicated apparatus or sophisticated physical tests are used.
   a. Ability to deep breathe and cough scores 2.
   b. Limited respiratory effort (i.e., splinting) or dyspnea scores 1.
   c. No evident spontaneous respiratory effort scores 0.
3. *Circulation.* This is the most difficult sign to evaluate by a simple method. Changes in the arterial blood pressure from the preanesthetic level were chosen because it is reliable, it is monitored throughout the anesthetic period, and it is one of the first signs taken on arrival in the PACU.
   a. Systolic arterial blood pressure 20% ± preanesthetic level scores 2.

b. Systolic arterial blood pressure 20% to 50% ± preanesthetic level scores 1.
   c. Systolic arterial blood pressure 50% ± preanesthetic level scores 0.
   (Note: Great differences in diastolic blood pressure should be noted.)
4. *Consciousness.* Ability of patients to answer simple questions and follow verbal commands. Only verbal stimuli are to be used.
   a. Full alertness with ability to answer question scores 2.
   b. Patient arousable by calling his name scores 1.
   c. Auditory stimuli fail to elicit any response scores 0.
5. *Color.* Patients are to be scored on their color in the PACU, whether this skin color was present before surgery or not (example: jaundiced preoperatively and postoperatively).
   a. Obviously normal or pink skin color scores 2.
   b. Any alteration from the normal pink, but not cyanotic; for example: pale, dusky, blotchy, jaundiced scores 1.
   c. Cyanotic nailbed, lips, and skin scores 0.
   (Note: Check patient oral mucosa if any questions.)

C. RESULTS OF POSTANESTHETIC RECOVERY SCORE

1. Optimum score is 10. Patient may be discharged from the PACU with scores of 8, 9, or 10. Nursing judgment must be used, since this scoring system is not infallible.
2. Patients who had scores of 10 preoperatively

but received scores less than 8 during the postoperative state require more constant observation and may need a specialized nursing care area, such as the intensive care unit.

3. Chronically debilitated, senile, or paralyzed patients may never receive an optimum score. Each patient must be treated individually and discharged from the PACU at the discretion of the attending anesthesiologist.

4. There are variables that may influence patient's emergence from anesthesia and thus his score. These include the following:
   a. Type of anesthetic agent used
   b. Use of paralyzing drugs and narcotics during surgery
   c. Type of surgery performed
   d. Duration of surgery and anesthesia

APPENDIX III

ABBREVIATIONS, NORMAL VALUES, CONVERSION FACTORS, AND BLOOD GAS AND ACID-BASE ANALYSES

Abbreviations

a	Artery
ac	Before meals
ad lib	As needed
amt	Amount
ant	Anterior
approx	Approximately (about)
bid or bd	Twice a day
BP	Blood pressure
C	Centigrade
c̄	With
cc	Cubic centimeters
DC	Discontinue
ECG (EKG)	Electrocardiogram (tracing of heart function)
EEG	Electroencephalogram (brain wave tracing)
ER	Emergency room
F	Fahrenheit
f	Frequency
fld	Fluid
GI	Gastrointestinal (stomach and intestine)
g	Gram
gr	Grain
gtt	Drop
h	Hour
Hgb	Hemoglobin
H_2O	Water
hs	Bedtime
I and O	Intake and output
IV	Intravenous
kg	Kilogram
lab	Laboratory
lat	Lateral
lb	Pound
med	Medial
min	Minute
mg	Milligram
no.	Number
noc	Night
NPO	Nothing by mouth (nihil per os)
O_2	Oxygen
OB	Obstetrics
OR	Operating room
p	Pulse
Ped, or Peds, Pedi	Pediatrics
po	Per os or by mouth
postop	Postoperative
prn	When necessary
preop	Preoperative
pt	Patient
PT	Physical therapy
qd	Every day
qh	Every hour
qid	Four times a day
qod	Every other day
qs	Quantity sufficient
r or resp	Respirations
sol	Solution
stat	At once
sup	Superior
tab	Tablet
TPR	Temperature, pulse, respiration
via	By way of
wt	Weight

Abbreviations for Respiratory Patterns

SR	Spontaneous respiration
AR	Assisted respiration
CV	Controlled respiration
IPPB(V)	Intermittent positive-pressure breathing (Ventilation)

IMV	Intermittent mandatory ventilation
CPAP	Continuous positive airway pressure
PEEP	Positive end-expiratory pressure
HFJV	High-frequency jet ventilation

Conversion Factors
Measurement conversion

centimeter $=$ inches $\times$ 2.54

inches $= \dfrac{\text{centimeter}}{2.54}$

kilogram $=$ pound $\times$ 2.2

pound $= \dfrac{\text{kilogram}}{2.2}$

1 meter $=$ 39.37 inches

Temperature conversion

Centigrade $=$ Fahrenheit $(0.555) - 32$
Fahrenheit $=$ Centigrade $(1.8) + 32$

Pressure unit conversions

To convert from	To	Multiply by
cm H_2O	mm Hg	0.735
	inches Hg	0.0290
	psi	0.0142
mm Hg	cm H_2O	1.36
	inches Hg	0.0394
	psi	0.0193
inches Hg	mm Hg	25.4
	cm H_2O	34.5
	psi	0.491
psi	mm Hg	51.7
	cm H_2O	70.4
	inches Hg	2.04

Respiration abbreviations

Abbreviation	Example	
A alveolar gas	PAO_2	Partial pressure of oxygen in the alveolus
B barometric	PB	Barometric pressure
D dead space gas	VD	Volume of the dead space
E expired gas	$PECO_2$	Partial pressure of expired carbon dioxide
i inspired gas	FiO_2	Fraction of oxygen inspired
a arterial blood	PaO_2	Partial pressure of arterial oxygen
b blood	Qb	Rate of blood flow
c capillary blood	PcO_2	Pressure of oxygen in the capillaries
v venous blood	$PvCO_2$	Venous pressure of carbon dioxide
$\bar{v}$ mixed venous blood	$P\bar{v}CO_2$	Central venous pressure of carbon dioxide
C concentration of gas	CaO_2	Arterial concentration of oxygen
F fractional concentration of gas	$FECO_2$	Fraction of expired carbon dioxide
P pressure of gas		
Q blood volume	Qb	Rate of blood flow
V gas volume		
S saturation	SaO_2	Arterial saturation of oxygen
TV	tidal volume	
f	frequency	
MV	minute ventilation	

Arterial Blood Gases

pH	7.35-7.45
$PaCO_2$	35-45 mm Hg
PaO_2	95-100 mm Hg
CO_2 content	26-28 mEq/L
Bicarbonate (HCO_3)	22-28 mEq/L
O_2 saturation	
Arterial	94%-100%
Venous	60%-85%
O_2 content	
Arterial	15-23 vol %
Venous	10-16 vol %

Arterial Blood Gas Analyses

I. Reason

To determine if the patient is well oxygenated

To determine the acid-base status of the patient

II. Obtained from an artery because

Arterial blood is a good way to sample a mixture of blood. (There is incomplete mixing of blood in a venous sample.)

Normal values

Test	Normal range	Test	Normal range
Blood		**CSF**	
Hematocrit	45% ± 7% males	Albumin	10-30 mg/dl
	40% ± 6% females	Cell count	0.8 cells/ml
Hemoglobin	14-18 g/dL males	Glucose	45-75 mg/dl
	12-16 g/dL females	Protein total	15-45 mg/dl
	12-15 g/dL children	**Urine**	
	14.5-24.5 g/dL newborns		
Platelet count	150,000-400,000/mm^3	pH	4.6-8.0
Erythrocytes	5×10^6/mm^3 males	SG	1.012-1.024
	4.5×10^6/mm^3 females	Glucose	negative
Leukocytes	5000-10,000/mm^3	Acetone	negative
Blood volume	69 ml/kg males		
	65 ml/kg females	**Vital Signs**	
Bleeding time	1-6 minutes	Pulse	
Prothrombin time	12-14 seconds	Infants	112-130 beats/min
Alcohol levels		Adult	70-80 beats/min
Intoxication	0.3-0.4%	Elderly	56-62 beats/min
Stupor	0.4-0.5%	Respiration rate	
Coma	Above 0.5%	Infants	30-50 breaths/min
Serum barbiturates		Adults	12-20 breaths/min
Coma	1.5 mg/100 ml	Blood pressure	
Serum electrolytes		Infants	80/58-50/40
Potassium	3.5-5 mEq/L	Adults	110/60-148/90
Sodium	136-145 mEq/L		
Chlorides	100-106 mEq/L	**Respiration**	
Bicarbonate	21-28 mEq/L	Rate	12-35 min
Phosphate	2-4 mEq/L	Rhythm	regular
Sulfate	1 mEq/L	Tidal volume	4-8 ml/kg (250 $\rightarrow$ 500 ml)
Organic acids	6 mEq/L	Vital capacity	20-50 ml/kg (1.5 $\rightarrow$ 4L)
Calcium	5 mEq/L	Negative inspiratory pressure	$-40 \rightarrow -80$ cm H_2O
Magnesium	2 mEq/L	Dead space/tidal volume (VD/VT)	<0.3

Arterial blood determines how well the lungs are oxygenating the blood.

III. Performing arterial puncture

  A. Equipment

    1. 20- or 22-gauge needle.

      a. There is less potential for a hematoma with a smaller needle.

      b. Causes less pain for the patient.

    2. Syringe

      a. A glass syringe with a Luer-Lok is preferred to prevent disconnection of the needle from the syringe. A glass syringe is preferred because the gases may diffuse out from some types of plastic.

      b. The syringe should be a larger capacity than the volume required for analysis (usually 2 to 3 ml suffices).

      c. The plunger should slide freely the entire length of the barrel.

    3. Heparin

    The syringe should be coated with heparin (1000 unit/ml). Excess heparin should be discarded. (Too much in the syringe will alter the pH of the blood, but heparin should be left in the needle and hub of syringe.)

    4. Rubber tip cap

    Both can be used to seal off the sample from air, but the rubber stopper is preferred.

    5. Rubber stopper

    6. Prep pads

    Although alcohol pads are supplied, a betadine prep is preferred.

Disorders of Acid-Base Balance

Respiratory acidosis: pH ↓ ; Pco_2 ↑ ; HCO_3 normal or ↑

  1. Obstructive lung disease

  2. Oversedation and other causes of compromised function of the respiratory center (even with healthy lungs)

  3. Other causes of hypoventilation

Respiratory alkalosis: pH ↑ ; Pco_2 ↓ ; HCO_3 normal or ↓

  1. Hypoxia

  2. Anxiety

  3. Pulmonary embolus

  4. Pregnancy

Metabolic acidosis: pH ↓ ; Pco_2 normal or ↓ ; HCO_3 ↓

  1. Diabetic acidosis

  2. Poisonings; salicylate, methyl alcohol, paraldehyde

  3. Renal failure

  4. Lactic acidosis

  5. Diarrhea

  6. Treatment with Diamox

Metabolis alkalosis: pH ↑ ; Pco_2 normal or ↑ ; HCO_3 ↑

  1. Diuretic therapy, Edecrin, furosemide, and the thiazides

  2. Steroid therapy

  3. Cushing's disease

  4. Fluid losses from the upper gastrointestinal tract—vomiting, nasogastric suction resulting in loss of acid

APPENDIX IV

GUIDELINES FOR BLOOD COMPONENT THERAPY

Product	Content	Indications	Volume	Shelf life	Comments
Whole blood	Red cells, leukocytes, platelets, plasma	Acute massive blood loss; neonatal exchange transfusion	500 ml	35 days in CPDA-1 at 106° C	~$50 per unit; not available in all hospital blood banks
Red blood cells	Red cells, leukocytes, some plasma	Anemia	200-350 ml	35 days in CPDA-1 at 106° C	~$50 per unit
Red blood cells frozen-thawed	Red cells, very few leukocytes, platelets, plasma	Anemia; prevent reactions to white blood cells, platelets, plasma proteins; storage of rare bloods	170-190 ml	Frozen, 3 yr; thawed, 24 hr	Rare bloods are frozen in large reference centers; expensive (~$90 per unit)
Red blood cells (leukocyte-poor)	Red cells, few leukocytes, some plasma	Prevent febrile reactions caused by white blood cell antibodies; anemia	200-250 ml	35 days in CPDA-1 at 106° C	Try before using frozen-thawed red blood cells in patients with febrile transfusion reaction.
Platelet concentrate	Platelets, few leukocytes, some plasma	Bleeding caused by low platelet count or poor platelet function	20-50 ml	72 hr	Red blood cells contaminate most units of platelets; (Use Rh-negative units for Rh-negative recipients)
Leukocyte concentrate	Leukocytes, platelets, few red cells	Serious infections in leukopenic patients	30-50 ml	24 hr	Patients may experience febrile reaction to transfused leukocytes

Product	Composition	Indication	Volume	Storage/Expiration	Comments
Fresh frozen plasma	Clotting factors, no platelets	Clotting disorders	220-250 ml	Frozen, 1 yr; thawed, 6 hr	Discouraged for simple volume expansion
Cryoprecipitated AHF (antihemophiliac factor)	Factors VIII and XIII, fibrinogen, von Willebrand's factor, fibronectin	Deficiencies in factors VIII and XIII and von Willebrand's factor	10-25 ml	Frozen, 1 yr; thawed, 6 hr	
Purified AHF concentrate	Factor VIII	Factor VIII deficiency	Lyophilized powder	Determined by manufacturer	300-1600 units/vial $30-$150/vial
Autoplex	Activated procoagulants	Inhibitor to factor VIII	30 ml sterile water; lyophilized powder	2 yr	Prohibitively expensive; hepatitis and DIC risk; use only with consultation of hematologist
Factor IX	Factors II, VII, IX, X; 500 or 1000 units Factor IX	Factor IX deficiency (Christmas disease); factors II, VII, IX, X deficiency	20-40 ml sterile water; lyophilized powder	Determined by manufacturer; store at 2.8° C	Hepatitis risk great; cost, $60 or $140/vial
Albumin	5% albumin or 25% albumin	Plasma volume expansion required	250 or 500 ml	3 yr	Product of choice for volume expansion; risk of hepatitis minimal
Plasma protein fraction	Albumin α- and β-globulins	Plasma volume expansion required	5% 250 or 500 ml	3 yr	Minimal risk of hepatitis
Rh(D) immune globulin	γ-globulin rich in anti-D immunized donors	Prevention Rh(D) sensitization in Rh-negative patients	1-2 ml	3 yr	To be used in Rh-negative patients without anti-Rh(D) antibody
Immune serum	γ-globulin	hypo-γ-globulinemia or disease prophylaxis	2 ml / 10 ml	3 yr	IV preparation recently available

APPENDIX V

CARDIOPULMONARY RESUSCITATION (CPR)
SUMMARY PERFORMANCE SHEET

Objectives	Actions		
	Adult (over 8 yrs)	**Child (1 to 8 yrs)**	**Infant (under 1 yr)**
A. Airway			
1. Assessment: Determine unresponsiveness.	Tap or gently shake shoulder.		
	Say, "Are you okay?"		Observe.
2. Get help.	Call out "Help!"		
3. Position the victim.	Turn on back as a unit, supporting head and neck if necessary (4-10 seconds).		
4. Open the airway.	Head-tilt/chin-lift		
B. Breathing			
5. Assessment: Determine breathlessness.	Maintain open airway. Place ear over mouth, observing chest. Look, listen, feel for breathing (3-5 seconds).		
6. Give 2 rescue breaths.	Maintain open airway.		
	Seal mouth to mouth.		Mouth to nose/mouth.
	Give 2 rescue breaths, 1 to 1½ seconds each. Observe chest rise. Allow lung deflation between breaths.		
7. Option for obstructed airway.	a. Reposition victim's head. Try again to give rescue breaths.		
	b. Activate the EMS system.		
	c. Give 6-10 subdiaphragmatic abdominal thrusts (the Heimlich maneuver).		Give 4 back blows.
			Give 4 chest thrusts.
	d. Tongue-jaw lift and finger sweep.	Tongue-jaw lift, but finger sweep only if you see a foreign object.	
	If unsuccessful, repeat a, c, and d until successful.		

Section	Step			
C. Circulation	8. Assessment: Determine pulselessness.	Feel for carotid pulse with one hand; maintain head-tilt with the other (5-10 seconds).		Feel for brachial pulse; keep head-tilt.
	9. Activate EMS system.	If someone responded to call for help, send them to activate the EMS system.		
	Begin chest compressions: 10. Landmark check.	Run middle finger along bottom edge of rib cage to notch at center (tip of sternum).		Imagine a line drawn between the nipples.
	11. Hand position.	Place index finger next to finger on notch:		Place 2-3 fingers on sternum, 1 finger's width below line. Depress ½-1 in.
		Two hands next to index finger. Depress 1½-2 in.	Heel of one hand next to index finger. Depress 1-1½ in.	
	12. Compression rate.	80-100 per minute.		At least 100 per minute.
CPR Cycles	13. Compressions to breaths.	2 breaths to every 15 compressions.	1 breath to every 5 compressions.	
	14. Number of cycles.	4 (52-73 seconds).	10 (60-87 seconds).	10 (45 seconds or less).
	15. Reassessment.	Feel for carotid pulse (5 seconds).		Feel for brachial pulse.
		If no pulse, resume CPR, starting with 2 breaths.		If no pulse, resume CPR, starting with 1 breath.
Option for entrance of 2nd rescuer: "I know CPR. Can I help?"	1st rescuer ends CPR.	End cycle with 2 rescue breaths.	End cycle with 1 rescue breath.	
	2nd rescuer checks pulse (5 seconds).	Feel for carotid pulse.		Feel for brachial pulse.
	If no pulse, 2nd rescuer begins CPR.	Begin one-rescuer CPR, starting with 2 breaths.		Begin one-rescuer CPR, starting with 1 breath.
	1st rescuer monitors 2nd rescuer.	Watch for chest rise and fall during rescue breathing; check pulse during chest compressions.		
Option for pulse return	If no breathing, give rescue breaths.	1 breath every 5 seconds.	1 breath every 4 seconds.	1 breath every 3 seconds.

APPENDIX VI

PERFORMANCE GUIDELINES
ONE-RESCUER CPR: ADULT

	Objectives	Critical Performance	Reason
	Airway		
	Assessment: Determine unresponsiveness. Get help if possible.	Tap or gently shake shoulder. Shout "Are you OK?" Call out "help!"	One concern about teaching people CPR is the risk of possible damage from unnecessarily resuscitating sleepers, fainters, etc. Call for help will summon nearby bystanders.
	Position the victim (4-10 seconds).	Turn on back as a unit, if necessary, supporting head and neck.	Frequently the victim will be facedown. Effective CPR can be provided only with the victim flat on back. The head cannot be above the level of the heart or CPR is ineffective.
	Open the airway (head-tilt/chin-lift).	Kneel beside victim's shoulder; lift the chin up gently with one hand while pushing down on the forehead with the other to tilt the head back. The chin should be lifted so that the teeth are brought almost together. Avoid completely closing the mouth.	Airway must be opened to establish breathlessness. Many victims may be making efforts at breathing that are ineffective because of obstruction by the tongue.
	Breathing		
	Assessment: Determine breathlessness (3-5 seconds).	Maintain open airway. Turn your head toward victim's chest with your ear directly over and close to victim's mouth. *Look* at the chest for movement. *Listen* for the sounds of breathing. *Feel* for breath on your cheek.	Hearing and feeling are the only true ways of determining the presence of breathing. If there is chest movement but you cannot feel or hear air, the airway is still obstructed. Accurate diagnosis is important; rescue breathing should not be performed on someone who is breathing.

Give 2 full breaths (1 to 1½ seconds per breath).	Pinch nostrils closed with thumb and forefinger of upper hand while maintaining pressure on victim's forehead to keep the head tilted. Open your mouth wide, take a deep breath, and make a tight seal. Breathe into victim's mouth 2 times with complete refilling of your lungs after each breath. Watch for victim's chest to rise. Rescue breaths are given at the rate of 1 to 1½ seconds each, allowing the lungs to deflate between breaths. [If you cannot give rescue breaths to a victim, start the obstructed airway sequence (see Step 7, p. 242).]	When you are beginning rescue breathing, it is important to get as much oxygen as possible to the victim. If your rescue breathing is effective, you will: • feel air going in as you blow • feel the resistance of the victim's lungs • feel your own lungs emptying • see the rise and fall of the victim's chest and belly
Circulation Assessment: Determine pulselessness (5-10 seconds).	Place 2-3 fingers on the Adam's apple (voice box) just below chin. Slide fingers into the groove between Adam's apple and muscle, on the side nearest you. Maintain head-tilt with the other hand. Feel for the carotid pulse.	This activity should take 5 to 10 seconds because it takes time to find the right place, and the pulse itself may be slow or very weak and rapid. The victim's condition must be properly assessed.
Activate the EMS system.	Know your local EMS or rescue unit telephone number. Send second rescuer to call.	Notification of the EMS system at this time allows the caller to give complete information about the victim's condition.

Reproduced with permission, *Heartsaver Manual: A Student Handbook for Cardiopulmonary Resuscitation and First Aid for Choking.* 1987. American Heart Association.   *Continued.*

PERFORMANCE GUIDELINES
ONE-RESCUER CPR: ADULT—cont'd

Objectives	Critical performance	Reason
Begin first cycle of rescue breathing *with* chest compressions:	To begin first cycle: Move your hands to the victim's chest. Run the index and middle fingers up the lower margin of the rib cage and locate the sternal notch with your middle finger. With index finger on sternum, place heel of the hand closest to the head on the sternum next to, but not covering, the index finger. Place second hand on top of first. Position body. Compress with weight transmitted vertically downward, elbows straight and locked, and shoulders over hands. Between compressions the pressure must be released and the chest allowed to return to its normal position, but the hands should not be lifted off the chest. Say mnemonic at proper rate and ratio. (Count aloud to establish rhythm: "one-and-two-and-three-and-four-and . . .") Compress smoothly and evenly, keeping fingers off victim's ribs. The rescuer must apply enough force to depress the sternum 1½-2 inches (4-5 cm), at a rate of 80-100 compressions per minute.	Precise hand placement is essential to avoid serious injury. 50% of compression/relaxation is downward to empty the heart; 50% of compression/relaxation is upward to fill the heart. With each compression, you want to squeeze the heart or increase pressure within the chest so that blood moves to the vital organs.

15 compressions (9 to 11 seconds) and 2 ventilations.	Ventilate properly: After every 15 compressions, deliver 2 rescue breaths.	Adequate oxygenation must be maintained.
At the end of 4 cycles (52-73 seconds), check for return of pulse for 5 seconds.	Check pulse. If no pulse, resume CPR. If there is a pulse but no breathing, give 1 rescue breath every 5 seconds (12 per minute).	To establish whether there is a spontaneous return of pulse or breathing.
	Entrance of a 2nd rescuer to replace the 1st rescuer	1st rescuer ends cycle with 2 breaths. Second rescuer appears and 1. identifies self: "I know CPR: can I help?" 2. checks pulse for 5 seconds. If no pulse, second rescuer starts one-rescuer CPR with two breaths. 1st rescuer assesses the adequacy of 2nd rescuer by • watching for chest to rise during rescue breaths • checking the pulse during chest compressions.

APPENDIX VII

AMERICAN HEART ASSOCIATION CARDIOPULMONARY RESUSCITATION AND EMERGENCY CARDIAC CARE RATIONALE FOR ONE- AND TWO-RESCUER CPR

Activity and time (seconds)	Critical performance	Rationale
1st rescuer resumes CPR. 2nd rescuer identifies himself and checks pulse for effective compressions.	Technique for single rescuer. 2nd rescuer says, "I know how to do CPR." Fingers palpate for carotid pulse.	To locate the carotid pulse.
2nd rescuer calls out "Stop compressions" and checks for spontaneous pulse and breathing. (5 sec.)	Five seconds pause to check for spontaneous pulse and breathing. 2nd rescuer should inform the 1st rescuer of the status of the victim and the need for either ventilations, compressions, or both. Says, "No pulse, continue CPR."	Provides a second assessment of pulse and breathing and the need for CPR.
2nd rescuer ventilates once.	Ventilates properly and observes chest rise.	

1st rescuer resumes compressions.	Two-rescuer rate and ratio.	2nd rescuer ventilation triggers change of rate and ratio.
Minimum of two cycles of 5 compressions and 1 ventilation. (8-10 sec.) Switch and repeat until examiner is satisfied.	Correct rate of compressions.	
	Says mnemonic.	Necessary to establish rhythm.
	Interposes breath.	
	No pause for ventilation.	
	Calls for switch.	Signal for change must be clear.
	Switches.	
	Switches back.	
	Checks pulse (by ventilator).	
	Technique as above.	

TWO RESCUERS ....

(....)

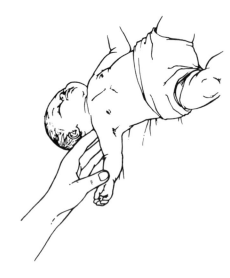

APPENDIX VIII

ONE-RESCUER CPR: INFANT (LESS THAN 1 YEAR)

When a victim is at this very early stage of physical development, CPR must be managed with special considerations for size and vulnerabilities. For this reason there are several differences in technique in CPR, and in first aid for choking, in infants.

A. AIRWAY

1. *Assessment: Determine unresponsiveness.* Tap or gently shake the shoulder.
2. *Call out "Help!"*
3. *Position the infant* on his or her back, on a firm surface, supporting the head and neck if you have to turn him or her.
4. *Open the airway,* using head-tilt/chin-lift. Take care not to tilt the head too far back.

Continued.

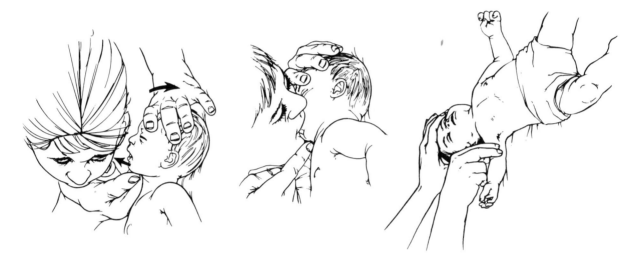

B. BREATHING

5. *Assessment: Determine breathlessness.* While maintaining an open airway, place your ear over the infant's mouth, and *look* at the chest for movement, *listen* for breathing, and *feel* for breaths on your ear.

6. *Give two gentle rescue breaths,* with your mouth covering the mouth and nose of the infant, while maintaining an open airway. Observe the rise and fall of the chest. Breaths should be 1 to 1½ seconds per breath.

C. CIRCULATION

7. *Assessment: Determine pulselessness.* Feel for the brachial pulse on the inside of the upper arm with one hand while maintaining head-tilt with the other hand.

Reproduced with permission, *Heartsaver Manual: A Student Handbook for Cardiopulmonary Resuscitation and First Aid for Choking,* 1987, American Heart Association.

ONE-RESCUER CPR: INFANT (LESS THAN 1 YEAR)—cont'd

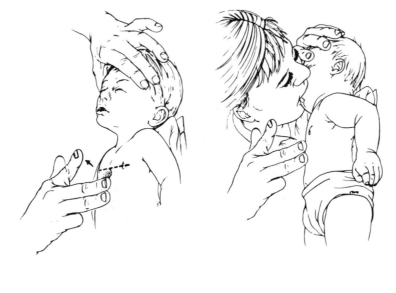

8. *Activate the EMS system.* If someone else is now present, that person should activate the EMS system.

9. *Begin chest compressions.* Imagine a line drawn between the nipples. Place 2 fingers 1 finger's width below that line. Because of wide variations in the relative sizes of rescuers' hands and infants' chests, these instructions are only guidelines; after finding the position for compressions, make sure that you are not on the xiphoid process. Compress chest ½ to 1 inch (1.25-2.5 cm) at least 100 times per minute, giving 1 rescue breath for every 5 compressions.

10. Do 10 cycles of compressions and rescue breaths.

11. Check brachial pulse.

12. If no pulse, give 1 rescue breath and continue compressions with rescue breaths.

13. Feel for the pulse every few minutes.

14. If the pulse returns, check for spontaneous breathing. If there is no breathing, give 1 rescue breath every 3 seconds (20 rescue breaths per minute) and monitor the pulse. If there is breathing, maintain an open airway and monitor breathing and pulse.

APPENDIX IX

PERFORMANCE GUIDELINES
OBSTRUCTED AIRWAY: CONSCIOUS ADULT

	Objectives	Critical performance	Reason
	Rescuer must identify complete airway obstruction by determining if victim is able to speak or cough. Victim may be using the "Universal Distress Signal" of choking: clutching the neck between thumb and index finger.	Rescuer asks, "Are you choking?"	In the conscious victim it is essential to recognize the signs of an airway obstruction and take action immediately. If the victim is able to speak or cough effectively, do not interfere with his or her attempts to expel the foreign body. Continually check for success.
Abdominal Thrust	Perform the Heimlich maneuver (subdiaphragmatic abdominal thrusts) until the foreign body is expelled or the victim becomes unconscious.	SUBDIAPHRAGMATIC ABDOMINAL THRUSTS (the Heimlich maneuver): Stand behind victim and wrap your arms around victim's waist. Grasp one fist with your other hand and place thumb side of your fist in the midline slightly above the navel. Press fist into abdomen with quick inward and upward thrusts. Each abdominal thrust should be delivered decisively, with the intent of relieving the obstruction.	Such thrusts can force air upward into the airway from the lungs with enough pressure to expel the foreign body.
For victims in late pregnancy or who are obese: **Chest Thrust**		CHEST THRUSTS: Stand behind victim and place your arms under victim's armpits to encircle the chest. Grasp one fist with other hand and place thumb side on the middle of the breastbone. Press with quick backward thrusts.	Chest thrusts are more easily done than abdominal thrusts when the abdominal girth is large, as in gross obesity or in advanced pregnancy.

Reproduced with permission, *Heartsaver Manual: A Student Handbook for Cardiopulmonary Resuscitation and First Aid for Choking,* 1987, American Heart Association.

Continued.

PERFORMANCE GUIDELINES
OBSTRUCTED AIRWAY: CONSCIOUS ADULT WHO BECOMES UNCONSCIOUS

	Objectives	Critical performance	Reason
	Position the victim and get help. Activate the EMS system.	Turn victim on back as a unit, if necessary, supporting head and neck. Call out "Help!" Activate EMS; or if someone responds to call for help, send them.	The victim must be properly positioned on his or her back in case CPR becomes necessary. It is vitally important to gain access to advanced life support.
	Foreign body check.	Perform tongue-jaw lift. Sweep deeply into mouth to remove foreign body.	This can be done only in the unconscious victim.
	Open airway and give rescue breaths.	Use head-tilt/chin-lift. Attempt rescue breathing.	Complete airway obstruction by a foreign body is assumed present, but at this point an attempt must be made to get some air into the lungs just in case the victim's fall has dislodged the foreign body.

	Airway remains obstructed? Give 6-10 abdominal thrusts.	SUBDIAPHRAGMATIC AB-DOMINAL THRUSTS (the Heimlich maneuver): Straddle the victim's thighs. Place heel of one hand on the abdomen in the midline slightly above the navel and well below the tip of the xiphoid. Place the second hand directly on top of the first hand. Press into the abdomen with quick upward thrusts. Perform 6-10 thrusts. Continually check for success. Each abdominal thrust should be delivered with the intent of relieving the obstruction. (CHEST THRUSTS: Same hand position as that for applying external chest compression. Exert quick downward thrust.)	Such thrusts can force air upward into the airway from the lungs with enough pressure to expel the foreign body. Chest thrusts are preferred in the presence of large abdominal girth (advanced pregnancy or obesity). Downward thrusts generate effective airway pressure.
	Check for foreign body using finger sweep.	Turn head up, open mouth with tongue-jaw lift technique and sweep deeply into mouth along cheek with hooked finger.	A dislodged foreign body may now be manually accessible if it has not been expelled. Dentures may need to be removed to improve finger sweep.
	Open airway and give rescue breaths. Repeat sequence until successful.	Open airway by the head-tilt/chin-lift maneuver, and attempt rescue breathing. Alternate the above maneuvers in rapid sequence: • abdominal thrusts • finger sweep • attempt rescue breathing	By this time another attempt must be made to get some air into the lungs. Persistent attempts are rapidly made in sequence in order to relieve the obstruction. As the victim becomes more deprived of oxygen, the muscles will relax and maneuvers that were previously ineffective may become effective.

Continued.

PERFORMANCE GUIDELINES
OBSTRUCTED AIRWAY: UNCONSCIOUS ADULT

	Objectives	Critical performance	Reason
	Airway remains obstructed? Open airway and give rescue breaths.	Reposition head; attempt again to give rescue breaths.	Improper head-tilt is the most common cause of airway obstruction.
	Activate the EMS system.	If unsuccessful, and a second person is available, he or she should activate EMS system. Know your local EMS or rescue unit number.	Advanced life support capability may be required.
	Give 6-10 subdiaphragmatic abdominal thrusts.	SUBDIAPHRAGMATIC ABDOMINAL THRUSTS (the Heimlich maneuver): Straddle the victim's thighs. Place heel of one hand on the abdomen midline slightly above the navel and well below the tip of the xiphoid. Place the second hand directly on top of the first hand. Press into the abdomen with quick upward thrusts. (CHEST THRUSTS: Same hand position as that for applying chest compression. Exert quick downward thrusts.)	Such thrusts can force air upward into the airway from the lungs with enough pressure to expel the foreign body. Chest thrusts are preferred in the presence of large abdominal girth (advanced pregnancy or obesity). Downward thrusts generate effective airway pressure.

APPENDIX X

COMPLETE OBSTRUCTION IN A CONSCIOUS CHOKING INFANT

Elapsed time (seconds) min.	max.	Activity and time (seconds)	Critical performance	Rationale
2	3	Rescuer checks for airway obstruction. (2-3 sec.)	Rescuer must identify complete obstruction by looking, listening, and feeling for ventilation and for blueness of the lips.	The presence of complete airway obstruction must be properly diagnosed before proceeding with treatment.
5	8	4 Back blows (3-5 sec.)	The infant is straddled over the rescuer's arm with the head lower than the trunk. The 4 back blows are delivered rapidly and forcefully between the shoulder blades.	Back blows when used alone may relieve the obstruction.
9	13	4 Chest thrusts (4-5 sec.)	The infant is supported between 2 hands, turned onto the back, and the thrusts are delivered in the midsternal region in the same manner as external chest compression. The head is lower than the trunk.	The combination of back blows and chest thrusts is superior to one technique when used alone. Abdominal thrusts are not recommended in infants because of the potential injury to the abdominal organs.
		Verbally indicate repeat of above sequence until effective.	Verbalize alternating the above maneuvers in rapid sequence.	Time is of the essence. The two techniques are rapidly repeated alternatively until obstruction is relieved or unconsciousness occurs.

APPENDIX XI

AIRWAY OBSTRUCTION MANAGEMENT

SUMMARY PERFORMANCE SHEET

	Objectives	Actions		
		Adult (over 8 yrs.)	Child (1 to 8 yrs.)	Infant (under 1 yr.)
Conscious victim	1. Assessment: Determine airway obstruction.	Ask, "Are you choking?" Determine if victim can cough or speak.		Observe breathing difficulty.
	2. Act to relieve obstruction.	Perform subdiaphragmatic abdominal thrusts (Heimlich maneuver).		Give 4 back blows. Give 4 chest thrusts.
	Be persistent.	Repeat Step 2 until obstruction is relieved or victim becomes unconscious.		
Victim who becomes unconscious	3. Position the victim; call for help.	Turn on back as a unit, supporting head and neck, face up, arms by sides. Call out, "Help!" If others come, activate EMS.		
	4. Check for foreign body.	Perform tongue-jaw lift and finger sweep.	Perform tongue-jaw lift. Remove foreign object only if you actually see it.	
	5. Give rescue breaths.	Open the airway with head-tilt/chin-lift. Try to give rescue breaths.		
	6. Act to relieve obstruction.	Perform subdiaphragmatic abdominal thrusts (Heimlich maneuver).		Give 4 back blows. Give 4 chest thrusts.
	7. Check for foreign body.	Perform tongue-jaw lift and finger sweep.	Perform tongue-jaw lift. Remove foreign object only if you actually see it.	
	8. Try again to give rescue breaths.	Open the airway with head-tilt/chin-lift. Try to give rescue breaths.		
	9. Be persistent.	Repeat Steps 6-8 until obstruction is relieved.		

Unconscious victim			
1. Assessment: Determine unresponsiveness.	Tap or gently shake shoulder. Shout, "Are you okay?"	Tape or gently shake shoulder.	
2. Call for help; position the victim.	Turn on back as a unit, supporting head and neck, face up, arms by sides. Call out, "Help!" If others come, activate EMS.		
3. Open the airway.	Head-tilt/chin-lift.	Head-tilt/chin-lift, but do not tilt too far.	
4. Assessment: Determine breathlessness.	Maintain an open airway. Ear over mouth; observe chest. Look, listen, feel for breathing (3-5 seconds).		
5. Give rescue breaths.	Make mouth-to-mouth seal.	Make mouth-to-nose-and-mouth seal.	
	Try to give rescue breaths.		
6. Try again to give rescue breaths.	Reposition head. Try rescue breaths again.		
7. Activate the EMS system.	If someone responded to the call for help, that person should activate the EMS system.		
8. Act to relieve obstruction.	Perform subdiaphragmatic abdominal thrusts (Heimlich maneuver).	Give 4 back blows.	
		Give 4 chest thrusts.	
9. Check for foreign body.	Perform tongue-jaw lift and finger sweep.	Perform tongue-jaw lift. Remove foreign object only if you actually see it.	
10. Rescue breaths.	Open the airway with head-tilt/chin-lift. Try again to give rescue breaths.		
11. Be persistent.	Repeat Steps 8-10 until obstruction is relieved.		

Reproduced with permission, *Heartsaver Manual: A Student Handbook for Cardiopulmonary Resuscitation and First Aid for Choking*, 1987.

APPENDIX XII

AMERICAN SOCIETY OF ANESTHESIOLOGISTS
STANDARDS FOR POSTANESTHESIA CARE

(Approved by House of Delegates on October 12, 1988)

These Standards apply to postanesthesia care in all locations. These Standards may be exceeded based on the judgment of the responsible anesthesiologist. They are intended to encourage high quality patient care, but cannot guarantee any specific patient outcome. They are subject to revision from time to time as warranted by the evolution of technology and practice.

STANDARD I

ALL PATIENTS WHO HAVE RECEIVED GENERAL ANESTHESIA, REGIONAL ANESTHESIA, OR MONITORED ANESTHESIA CARE SHALL RECEIVE APPROPRIATE POSTANESTHESIA MANAGEMENT.

1. A Postanesthesia Care Unit (PACU) or an area which provides equivalent postanesthesia care shall be availabe to receive patients after surgery and anesthesia. All patients who receive anesthesia shall be admitted to the PACU except by specific order of the anesthesiologist responsible for the patient's care.

2. The medical aspects of care in the PACU shall be governed by policies and procedures which have been reviewed and approved by the Department of Anesthesiology.

3. The design, equipment and staffing of the PACU shall meet requirements of the facility's accrediting and licensing bodies.

4. The nursing standards of practice shall be consistent with those approved in 1986 by the American Society of Post Anesthesia Nurses (ASPAN).

STANDARD II

A PATIENT TRANSPORTED TO THE PACU SHALL BE ACCOMPANIED BY A MEMBER OF THE ANESTHESIA CARE TEAM WHO IS KNOWLEDGEABLE ABOUT THE PATIENT'S CONDITION. THE PATIENT SHALL BE CONTINUALLY EVALUATED AND TREATED DURING TRANSPORT WITH MONITORING AND SUPPORT APPROPRIATE TO THE PATIENT'S CONDITION.

STANDARD III

UPON ARRIVAL IN THE PACU, THE PATIENT SHALL BE RE-EVALUATED AND A VERBAL REPORT PROVIDED TO THE RESPONSIBLE PACU NURSE BY THE MEMBER OF THE ANESTHESIA CARE TEAM WHO ACCOMPANIES THE PATIENT.

1. The Patient's status on arrival in the PACU shall be documented.
2. Information concerning the preoperative condition and the surgical/anesthetic course shall be transmitted to the PACU nurse.
3. The member of the Anesthesia Care Team shall remain in the PACU until the PACU nurse accepts responsibility for the nursing care of the patient.

STANDARD IV

THE PATIENT'S CONDITION SHALL BE EVALUATED CONTINUALLY IN THE PACU.

1. The patient shall be observed and monitored by methods appropriate to the patient's medical condition. Particular attention should be given to monitoring oxygenation, ventilation and circulation. While qualitative clinical signs may be adequate, quantitative methods are encouraged.
2. An accurate written report of the PACU period shall be maintained. Use of an appropriate PACU scoring system is encouraged for each patient on admission, at appropriate intervals prior to discharge, and at the time of discharge.
3. General medical supervision and coordination of patient care in the PACU should be the responsibility of the anesthesiologist.
4. There shall be a policy to assure the availability in the facility of a physician capable of managing complications and providing cardiopulmonary resuscitation for patients in the PACU.

STANDARD V

A PHYSICIAN IS RESPONSIBLE FOR THE DISCHARGE OF THE PATIENT FROM THE POSTANESTHESIA CARE UNIT.

1. When discharge criteria are used, they must be approved by the Department of Anesthesiology and the medical staff. They may vary depending upon whether the patient is discharged to a hospital room, to the ICU, to a short stay unit, or home.
2. In the absence of the physician responsible for the discharge, the PACU nurse shall determine that the patient meets the discharge criteria. The name of the physician accepting responsibility for discharge shall be noted on the record.

From American Society of Anesthesiologists, Park Ridge, Illinois; Copyright © 1988.

APPENDIX XIII

MULTIPLE-CHOICE QUESTIONS AND ANSWERS

Questions

Select the single best answer.

CHAPTER 1

1. The main functions of the PACU nurse include all the following except:
   a. Recognition and initial treatment of respiratory problems
   b. Measuring oxygen saturation
   c. Maintaining accurate records
   d. Monitoring the cardiovascular system
   e. Determining which patients should be admitted to the PACU

2. During transport of the patient from the operating room to the PACU:
   a. Adequate monitoring should be maintained
   b. Resuscitative equipment should be readily available
   c. Two people should be in attendance
   d. No more than 5 minutes should elapse
   e. All of the above

3. The initial report from the anesthesiologist to the PACU nurse need not include:
   a. Patient's name
   b. Operation performed
   c. Past medical history
   d. Name of insurance carrier
   e. Physical impairments

4. All of the following are important in the initial respiratory observation of the patient coming to the PACU except:
   a. Lip and fingernail color
   b. Ability to talk or cry
   c. Respiratory rate
   d. Chest excursion
   e. Adequate arterial blood gases at the beginning of surgery

5. Assessment of recovery from anesthesia may be simply made by:
   a. The Aldrete score
   b. Electroencephalographic recording
   c. Observation
   d. Blood pressure recording
   e. All of the above

6. Each of the instructions evaluate the ability to comprehend and perform a motor function except:
   a. "Lift your head"
   b. "Open your eyes"
   c. "Put out your tongue"
   d. "Are you having pain?"
   e. "Can you move your toes?"

7. In using the postanesthetic recovery score, which of the following does not score 1 point?
   a. Ability to move only the lower extremities
   b. Dyspnea
   c. Arousable on calling
   d. Dusky color
   e. Blood pressure 15% below preanesthetic level

8. Negative inspiratory pressure:
   a. Cannot be easily measured at the bedside
   b. Should be measured only by the respiratory therapist
   c. Must be at least -40 cm H_2O to allow adequate coughing
   d. Can be measured only if the patient has an endotracheal tube in place
   e. Is of little value

9. Phase 2 neuromuscular blockade:
   a. Develops after prolonged succinylcholine administration
   b. May be a residual effect of pancuronium administration
   c. Is associated with posttetanic facilitation
   d. Is not increased by administration of penicillin
   e. All of the above
10. A flow-directed, balloon-tipped pulmonary artery catheter (Swan-Ganz) is used to measure all of the following except:
    a. Cardiac output
    b. Pulmonary capillary wedge pressure
    c. Central venous pressure
    d. Right ventricular pressure
    e. Left ventricular pressure

CHAPTER 2

1. Pain impulses to the spinal cord are transmitted through:
   a. β fibers
   b. φ fibers
   c. Unmyelinated C fibers
   d. Myelinated B fibers
   e. Nodes of Ranvier
2. Which of the following are endogenous peptides exhibiting opioid properties?
   a. Somatostatin
   b. Diamorphine
   c. β-lipoprotein
   d. Met-enkephalin
   e. α-endorphin
3. Opioid receptors are found in which of the following parts of the central nervous system?
   a. Baroreceptor trigger zone
   b. Anterior horn cells
   c. Substantia gelatinosa of the dorsal horn
   d. Basal ganglia
   e. Reticulospinal tract
4. Which of the following opioids have agonist effects primarily at μ receptors?
   a. Pentazocine
   b. Heroin
   c. Fentanyl
   d. Nalbuphine
   e. Naloxone

5. Morphine:
   a. Is highly lipophilic
   b. Is a $\varkappa$ receptor antagonist
   c. Is an agonist at μ receptors
   d. Antagonizes labyrinthine vomiting
   e. Is highly suitable for epidural analgesia
6. Methadone:
   a. Is a naturally occurring opioid
   b. Has a very long elimination half-life
   c. Is unsuitable for intravenous administration
   d. Has a fast clearance
   e. Is metabolized to a highly active metabolite
7. Bupivacaine:
   a. Is an aminoester local anesthetic
   b. Is poorly lipid soluble
   c. Should never be repeated until the effects of a previous block have worn off.
   d. Produces intense motor nerve blockade
   e. Has a longer onset of action than lidocaine
8. Opioids suitable for intravenous infusion analgesia:
   a. Should have a slow hepatic clearance
   b. Are usually partial agonists at μ receptors
   c. Should have a short elimination half-life
   d. Do not cause ventilatory depression
   e. Are not suitable for patient-controlled demand analgesia
9. Narcotic (morphine) overdose:
   a. Is associated with dilation of the pupil
   b. May be treated with naloxone
   c. Is characterized by rapid shallow breathing
   d. Should be treated with metoclopramide
   e. May be completely reversed by buprenorphine
10. Midthoracic segmental (T4-12) epidural block in the postoperative period:
    a. Cannot be achieved by the use of opioids
    b. Is best achieved by repeated lidocaine injection
    c. Is associated with weakness of leg movements
    d. Can be produced by 15 ml 0.5% bupivacaine injected at T8 interspace
    e. Blocks the sympathetic nerve supply to the adrenal gland.

CHAPTER 3

1. Postoperatively, the trachea may be extubated safely:
   a. Even if the respiratory pattern is irregular
   b. As long as the patient is kept in a lateral position
   c. When the patient is responsive to commands
   d. Only when the surgeon has given the order
   e. As soon as the temperature reads 35° C

2. The simplest initial indication of adequate oxygenation is:
   a. Awake patient
   b. Pink lips
   c. Respiratory rate of 16 per minute
   d. Oxygen saturation by oximetry of 98%
   e. PaO_2 90 mm Hg

3. Respiratory insufficiency is least likely to develop after 1 hour in the PACU if:
   a. The initial temperature was 30° C
   b. Morphine 10 mg is given intravenously
   c. 1.5 L of normal saline has been infused over 1 hour
   d. Trendelenburg position is employed to correct hypotension
   e. Meperidine 12.5 mg is given intravenously

4. Signs of inadequate ventilation include all of the following except:
   a. Cyanosis
   b. Sternal retraction
   c. Respiratory rate of 38 per minute in an adult
   d. PaO_2 of 60 mm Hg with an FiO_2 of 0.35
   e. $PaCO_2$ 32 mm Hg

5. Immediate postoperative hypoxia may be caused by all of the following except:
   a. Intraoperative hyperventilation
   b. Intraoperative hypoventilation
   c. 2 L normal saline intraoperatively
   d. Epidural anesthesia to T10 level
   e. Meperidine 150 mg in the previous hour

6. The alveolar-arterial oxygen tension gradient:
   a. Indicates no pulmonary damage as long as it is < 200 mm Hg
   b. Bears no relationship to the barometric pressure
   c. Is a conveniently calculated number used to assess the ability of pulmonary oxygen transfer
   d. Increases as pulmonary function improves
   e. Has an ideal value of 100 mm Hg

7. Respiratory criteria that should be met before the patient may be safely discharged include all of the following except:
   a. A vital capacity of > 1.5 L
   b. Respiratory rate stability for 15 minutes
   c. Ability to cough
   d. $PaCO_2$ 35 mm Hg
   e. PaO_2 120 mm Hg at FiO_2 of 0.25

8. The vital capacity is:
   a. The amount of air moved in or out during normal respiration
   b. Measured by a Wright respirometer
   c. Not affected after upper abdominal surgery
   d. An inspiratory measurement
   e. Part of the dead space to tidal volume ratio

9. Negative inspiratory force:
   a. Cannot be suitably measured at the bedside
   b. Should be at least 15 mm Hg if ventilation is to be considered adequate
   c. Must be at least -25 cm H_2O to allow effective gas exchange
   d. Can be measured only if the patient has a tracheostomy tube in place
   e. Is of little value

10. All the following drugs are likely to result in significant ventilatory depression in the recovery period except:
   a. Meperidine 25 mg IV 15 minutes after discontinuing general anesthesia
   b. Diazepam 10 mg orally, given 30 minutes before cystoscopy in an 85-year-old man.
   c. Succinylcholine 550 mg given intraoperatively over a 90-minute period
   d. Curare 3 mg given before intubation
   e. Meperidine 25 mg IM after an anesthetic technique that employed droperidol 12.5 mg (5 ml)

CHAPTER 4

1. The treatment of choice for a patient with hypotension complicating sinus bradycardia is:
   a. Methoxamine 2 mg IV
   b. Digoxin 0.25 mg IV
   c. Glycopyrrolate 0.2 mg IV
   d. Phentolamine
   e. Epinephrine infusion 1 μg/kg per minute
2. A characteristic sign of pulmonary edema arising in the postoperative period is:
   a. Bradypnea
   b. ST segment depression
   c. Basal crepitations
   d. Sinus bradycardia
   e. Prolonged P-R interval
3. Which of the following is a complication of postoperative hypertension?
   a. Pulmonary embolism
   b. Cerebral thrombosis
   c. Atrial fibrillation
   d. Cor pulmonale
   e. Pulmonary edema
4. A high systolic pressure with a wide pulse pressure but normal diastolic pressure is compatible with:
   a. Pheochromocytoma
   b. Renovascular hypertension
   c. Coronary artery disease
   d. Coarctation of the aorta
   e. Arteriosclerosis

5. The rate of change of arterial pressure (dP/dt) is a measure of:
   a. Cardiac conduction
   b. Systemic vascular resistance
   c. Stroke volume
   d. Myocardial contractility
   e. Venodilation
6. Propranolol (1-2 mg) IV is indicated for which of the following circumstances?
   a. Junctional bradycardia
   b. Sinus tachycardia
   c. Möbitz Type II block
   d. First-degree heart block
   e. R on T extrasystoles
7. Lidocaine (1 mg/kg) IV is indicated in which of the following?
   a. R on T phenomenon
   b. Junctional tachycardia
   c. Sinus bradycardia
   d. First-degree heart block
   e. Atrial fibrillation
8. In which of these conditions should postoperative hypertension *not* be treated?
   a. After carotid endarterectomy
   b. In the presence of elevated intracranial pressure
   c. When CVP is low
   d. When the urinary bladder is distended
   e. After administration of methylprednisolone
9. Septicemia should be suspected when:
   a. Tachycardia is associated with hypertension
   b. Low cardiac output is associated with elevated left atrial pressure
   c. Hypotension is associated with high cardiac output
   d. Paroxysmal tachycardia will not respond to propranolol
   e. Bradycardia will not respond to atropine
10. Subendocardial ischemia is manifest in the ECG as:
   a. Raised, coved ST segments
   b. Widening of the QT interval
   c. Depressed ST segments
   d. Widened QRS complexes in precordial leads
   e. μ waves

CHAPTER 5

1. Who are candidates for platelet transfusion?
   a. Patients who are actively bleeding
   b. Patients who are to undergo surgery and have platelet counts less than 50,000 per cu mm
   c. Persons with platelet counts less than 20,000 per cu mm
   d. Patients who have had massive transfusions or open heart surgery
   e. All of the above

2. How much colloid would a 70 kg man with 10% burn require over 24 hours?
   a. None, he should receive blood
   b. 5 ml/kg
   c. 10 ml/kg
   d. 20 ml/kg
   e. Depends on his age

3. In the postoperative patient:
   a. Ringer's lactate should never be used
   b. Salt retention is a dreaded complication
   c. Normal saline is preferable to Ringer's lactate
   d. A certain degree of fluid retention is expected
   e. D_5W is complete replacement

4. Use of colloid solutions:
   a. Are indicated in the burn patient
   b. Are controversial for resuscitation of patients other than those with burns
   c. May impair organ function
   d. All of the above
   e. None of the above

5. Whole blood:
   a. Should be used instead of packed red cells at every opportunity
   b. Is useful for 3 years if frozen
   c. Is rich in clotting factors
   d. Is useful for acute massive blood loss
   e. Rarely causes allergic reactions

6. Platelet concentrates:
   a. Should be used for patients with an elevated prothrombin time
   b. Are useful for bleeding caused by a low platelet count
   c. Have a long shelf life (longer than 1 year)
   d. Can last at room temperature for 2 to 4 days
   e. Can be obtained immediately from the blood bank

7. After a TURP, a patient should be observed for:
   a. Water overload
   b. Hyponatremia
   c. Changes in mental function
   d. Congestive heart failure
   e. All of the above

8. Patients receiving chronic diuretic therapy:
   a. Are often salt depleted and have increased fluid requirements
   b. Should be run "dry"
   c. May have increased body stores of potassium
   d. Should be maintained with a blood pressure over 150 mm Hg at all times
   e. Are usually tachycardic

9. Total body water:
   a. Is the largest single component of body weight
   b. Is least in young, muscular males
   c. Is greatest in elderly, obese females
   d. Is made up at least 50% by rate of oxidation
   e. Is replenished daily

10. Extracellular fluid:
    a. Is increased during shock
    b. Decreases with resuscitation
    c. Is altered by permeability of cell membranes
    d. Is independent of ion exchange
    e. Averages about 15% of normal weight

CHAPTER 6

1. Immediate postoperative hypoxia may be caused by all of the following except:
   a. Intraoperative hyperventilation
   b. Intraoperative hypoventilation
   c. 2 L normal saline intraoperatively
   d. Epidural anesthesia to T10 level
   e. 300 μg fentanyl in the previous hour

2. Rapid emergence from anesthesia is usually seen after:
   a. Droperidol and fentanyl
   b. Methoxyflurane
   c. Continuous pentothal infusion
   d. Isoflurane 0.5% for 4 hours
   e. Fentanyl 25 μg/kg—muscle relaxant technique for 2 hours

3. Therapy of a patient in whom there has been only partial reversal of muscle relaxant action should include all of the following except:
   a. Ventilatory support
   b. Supportive verbal communication
   c. Neostigmine and atropine
   d. Sodium bicarbonate
   e. Naloxone

4. Demerol 25 mg in the postoperative period will cause hypoventilation:
   a. In old patients only
   b. In 25% of all patients
   c. Especially in a patient who has just had a gastrectomy
   d. In 80% of patients
   e. Only if the surgical dressing is too tight

5. Prolonged effects of muscle relaxants are least likely to occur:
   a. In patients who received 0.4 mg atropine and 2.0 mg neostigmine at the end of the operation
   b. In patients who have an arterial pH of 7.28
   c. In incipient myasthenia gravis
   d. If the patient has received curare 75 mg over 3½ hours
   e. If a single dose of succinylcholine 200 mg was used for intubation 30 minutes previously

6. A patient who is admitted to the PACU with a temperature of 31° C:
   a. Must have continuous cardiac monitoring
   b. Must be rewarmed with hot blankets immediately
   c. Can be safely moved for diagnostic x-rays within 15 minutes
   d. Should be catheterized to monitor urinary output
   e. Should be given large doses of diazepam to prevent shivering

7. The least common cause of postoperative coma is:
   a. Blood sugar level of 1200 mg%
   b. Regional epidural anesthesia at T5 level
   c. Intraoperative intracranial aneurysm rupture
   d. Incision and drainage of a fascial abscess of thigh
   e. Temperature of 30° C

8. Respiratory insufficiency exists if:
   a. Respiratory rate is 12 per minute
   b. Tidal volume is 350 ml
   c. Vital capacity is <1L
   d. Oxygen saturation by pulse oximetry is 98.5%
   e. $PaCO_2$ is 37 mm Hg

9. Therapy of postoperative hypoventilation does not include:
   a. Assisted ventilation
   b. Naloxone
   c. Continuous ECG monitoring
   d. Diazepam to decrease confusion
   e. Increased FiO_2

10. Which of the following is not commonly observed in allergic drug response?
    a. Skin wheal
    b. Bronchospasm
    c. PaO_2 65 mm Hg
    d. Blood pressure 80/50
    e. Bradycardia 50 per minute

CHAPTER 7

1. According to JCAHO, the person responsible for the decision to discharge a patient from PACU is:
   a. The PACU nurse manager or staff nurse
   b. The patient's surgeon or anesthesiologist
   c. The hospital administrator or OR supervisor
   d. The patient or family
   e. Any physician

2. Written discharge criteria should include:
   a. The physiological parameters of the patient to be evaluated
   b. The length of time a patient may remain in PACU
   c. The time a patient is discharged from PACU
   d. The destination of the patient
   e. All of the above

3. A post anesthesia scoring system provides:
   a. Long-term evaluation of the patient's recovery
   b. More paperwork for the nurse.
   c. An objective measurement of the patient's recovery from anesthesia
   d. A standard for discharge criteria
   e. An essential part of the patient's record

4. Which of the following classifications of patients *do not* require specific discharge criteria?
   a. Pediatric patients
   b. Ambulatory surgery patients
   c. Critical care patients
   d. Abdominal surgery patients
   e. Postcraniotomy patients

5. Established discharge criteria provide:
   a. A tool for evaluating discharge eligibility
   b. Professional accountability for the nurse
   c. A means to comply with JCAHO guidelines
   d. Improved patient care
   e. All of the above

6. Standards identified for written discharge criteria should include all of the following except:
   a. A definition of acceptable temperature range
   b. A definition of stability for vital signs
   c. The patient's ability to drive himself home
   d. Documentation requirements
   e. Discharge to the care of a responsible adult

7. The Aldrete postanesthetic recovery score is most similar in concept to the:
   a. Glasgow coma scale
   b. Carignan scoring system
   c. Apgar score
   d. Graphic score
   e. None—it is a new concept

8. An anesthesiologist's discharge signature is required:
   a. In 32 states and 6 countries
   b. By JCAHO
   c. When that is the policy in a particular institution
   d. When the patient is ready to leave the PACU
   e. Throughout the United States

9. The pediatric patient in PACU, on discharge, should be able to:
   a. Cry or talk
   b. Retain fluids
   c. Focus his eyes
   d. Maintain stable vital signs
   e. All of the above

10. A verbal report from the PACU nurse to the next nurse who will be caring for the patient is important for all of the following reasons except:
    a. Alerts the nurse to the patient's imminent arrival
    b. Provides continuity in the patient's care
    c. Enables the PACU nurse to use nursing assistants for transport
    d. Assists the next nurse to plan for the patient's continuing care needs
    e. Summarizes patient care in the postanesthetic period

CHAPTER 8

1. The estimated blood volume of a 3 kg neonate is:
   a. 90 ml
   b. 120 ml
   c. 195 ml
   d. 240 ml
   e. 300 ml

2. The minimum systolic blood pressure (mm Hg) considered normal in a healthy 6-hour-old, full-term infant is:
   a. 70
   b. 60
   c. 50
   d. 40
   e. 30

3. Heat loss in the newborn infant is enhanced by each of the following except:
   a. Large surface area to body weight ratio
   b. Environmental temperature of 21°C (70° F)
   c. Presence of only small amounts of subcutaneous tissue
   d. Heat loss from brown fat deposits
   e. Radiation to surrounding surfaces (for example, incubator walls)

4. True statements about the infant airway include all the following except:
   a. The larynx is more cephalad than in the adult
   b. The widest part is just below the cords
   c. Edema after intubation may critically compromise the airway
   d. An appropriately sized endotracheal tube allows a leak
   e. Humidified oxygen is appropriate therapy to treat early edema

5. A 2-year-old, 15 kg child, after an uneventful endotracheal general anesthetic, becomes restless in the PACU, with a ''croupy'' cough, mild retractions, and a respiratory rate of 45 per minute. Appropriate initial therapy is:
   a. Epinephrine 0.2 mg subcutaneously
   b. Endotracheal intubation
   c. Nebulized racemic epinephrine and cool mist
   d. Dexamethasone 15 mg intravenously

6. In addition to 5% dextrose in 0.2% saline solution, a 3-day-old infant undergoing surgery for bowel resection should be given:
   a. An electrolyte-containing solution at a rate of 4 to 6 ml/kg per hour
   b. D_5W at a rate of 4 to 6 ml/kg per hour
   c. No additional fluids
   d. Whole blood as replacement for third-space loss
   e. Plasmanate 5 ml/kg per hour

7. One hour after tonsillectomy, a 4-year-old, 20 kg child vomits approximately 300 ml of fresh blood. He is restless, blood pressure is 60/40 mm Hg, and the pulse is 160 per minute. The best approach is to:
   a. Draw blood for hemoglobin and hematocrit determination
   b. Administer lactated Ringer's solution
   c. Await fully cross-matched blood before operative intervention
   d. Alert the surgeon immediately, and administer partially cross-matched blood

8. Appropriate doses of agents used in pediatric cardiopulmonary resuscitation include all the following except:
   a. Atropine, 0.02 mg/kg
   b. Epinephrine, 1:10,000 solution, 0.01 ml/kg
   c. Calcium chloride, 10 mg/kg
   d. Sodium bicarbonate, 2 mEq/kg
   e. 100% O_2

9. When using an inflatable cuff to measure blood pressure:
   a. The width of the cuff should equal two thirds the length of the upper arm
   b. Use of a narrower cuff leads to pressure measurements lower than actual pressures
   c. The width of the cuff should be related to age
   d. Pressures are measured in the arm
   e. All of the above

10. Drugs and techniques to relieve postoperative pain include all the following except:
    a. Narcotics
    b. Regional analgesia
    c. Acetaminophen
    d. Diazepam
    e. Parental visit

CHAPTER 9

1. The normal intracranial pressure is:
   a. 22 mm Hg
   b. 10 mm Hg
   c. 32 mm Hg
   d. 40 mm Hg
   e. 5 cm H_2O
2. The following physiological variable will increase ICP:
   a. Hypocarbia
   b. Hypercarbia
   c. Hypothermia
   d. Hypotension
   e. Hypoxia to 70 mm PaO_2
3. The factor that will decrease the ICP is:
   a. Tachycardia
   b. Hypertension
   c. Nitroprusside
   d. Mannitol
   e. Nitroglycerin
4. Persistent poor neurological function in the PACU may be the result of all of the following except:
   a. Intracranial bleeding
   b. Spasm of cerebral vessels
   c. Pneumocephalus
   d. Shivering
   e. Hypoxia
5. The ideal position for a patient after craniotomy is:
   a. Head low
   b. Feet up
   c. Head turned to the left
   d. Head up
   e. Flat
6. Patients after cervical cord injury are liable to manifest all of the following except:
   a. Pulmonary edema
   b. Hypotension
   c. Respiratory disease
   d. Increased ICP
   e. Hallucinations

7. Increasing intracranial pressure is detected by:
   a. Monitoring ICP
   b. Diuresis
   c. Low arterial $PaCO_2$
   d. Hypothermia
   e. Falling blood pressure
8. Clinical deterioration in the neurological function can be detected by all except:
   a. Pupillary reaction to light
   b. Unequal size of pupils
   c. Shivering (nonconvulsive)
   d. Deteriorating mental status
   e. Decreasing handgrip
9. All of the following are true features in direct intraventricular ICP monitoring except:
   a. Early detection of neurological deterioration
   b. Withdrawal of CSF to decrease ICP
   c. Sterile heparinized saline in a highly pressurized system is used
   d. Intracranial hemorrhage and infection can result
   e. Requires making a burr hole
10. Glasgow coma scale uses all of the following parameters except:
    a. Motor response
    b. Verbal response
    c. Eye opening ability
    d. Pupillary reaction to light
    e. Response to commands

CHAPTER 10

1. Which of the following patient is most likely to have a local anesthetic reaction when he arrives in the PACU?
   a. A man who had a spinal anesthetic an hour ago for hernia repair
   b. A patient who had multiple intercostal blocks 20 minutes ago and was brought to the PACU before surgery
   c. A patient who had a digital nerve block with 5 ml of 1% xylocaine 10 minutes ago
   d. Any patient who received bupivacaine 0.25%
   e. Any case in which epinephrine was added to the solution

2. Which of the following procedures is least likely to result in a pneumothorax?
   a. Supraclavicular brachial plexus block
   b. Multiple intercostal block for gallbladder surgery
   c. Lumbar epidural for varicose vein surgery
   d. Subclavian placement of CVP catheter
   e. Internal jugular placement of a Swan-Ganz catheter

3. A T6–level spinal anesthetic may result in all except which of the following?
   a. Make most vascular beds below the waist vasodilate
   b. Block all nerve supply to the bladder
   c. Generally increase the blood pressure
   d. Relax the lower abdominal muscles
   e. Cause a decrease in blood pressure

4. Which of the following is not appropriate treatment for significant hypotension from spinal anesthesia?
   a. Place patient in 90-degree head-up position to keep spinal from going higher
   b. Give 5 L/min nasal oxygen
   c. Infuse 200 ml of Ringer's lactate solution quickly
   d. Place patient in slight head-down position
   e. Give ephedrine 12.5 mg

5. The adverse reaction to spinal anesthesia most likely to be seen in the PACU is:
   a. Pneumothorax
   b. Local anesthetic toxicity
   c. Sympathetic nerve block causing hypotension
   d. Headache
   e. Backache

6. Possible adverse reactions after topical anesthesia for bronchoscopy include all the following except:
   a. Seizures
   b. Hypotension
   c. Aspiration
   d. Pneumothorax
   e. Tachycardia

7. Which statement about epidural morphine is not true?
   a. It has been used for surgical anesthesia
   b. It is used most for postoperative pain relief
   c. Because small doses are used, it is safer than morphine administered intramuscularly
   d. It may cause itching
   e. Its use is still controversial

8. Which statement about the respiratory effects of spinal anesthesia is true?
   a. Spinal anesthesia rarely paralyzes the diaphragm
   b. Hypotension from a spinal anesthesia may cause respiratory arrest
   c. Spinal anesthesia can have a significant effect on respiration
   d. Narcotics given to supplement spinal anesthesia may cause respiratory depression
   e. All of the above

9. Which statement about spinal headaches is not true?
   a. There is evidence that lying flat after a spinal anesthetic does not help prevent a headache
   b. It is unlikely that a patient would get a headache after epidural anesthesia
   c. If a patient is going to get a spinal headache, it will be starting in the PACU
   d. Increasing fluid administration helps to prevent and treat spinal headache
   e. Severity of headache is related to the gauge of the spinal needle

10. Heat loss in the PACU is:
    a. More of a problem with a high spinal anesthetic
    b. More of a problem after general anesthesia
    c. No different after spinal or general anesthesia for similar operations
    d. Increased by shivering
    e. Decreased by narcotic administration

CHAPTER 11

1. The most useful indicator of renal function is:
   a. Urine output
   b. Serum creatinine
   c. Urine specific gravity
   d. U/P creatinine
   e. Blood urea nitrogen

2. Which of the following statements about the patient with chronic renal disease is true?
   a. Congestive heart failure is rare
   b. Should never receive Na^+-containing solutions because Na^+ cannot be excreted
   c. Alteration of dosages of all drugs is required
   d. Anemia is caused by decreased red blood cell synthesis
   e. None of the above

3. All of the following are ECG signs of hyperkalemia except:
   a. Presence of U waves
   b. Tall, peaked T waves
   c. Loss of P waves
   d. Wide QRS complexes
   e. ST segment changes

4. The anephric adult at rest requires:
   a. ~1200 ml H_2O per day to replace insensible loss
   b. ~ 500 ml H_2O per day to replace insensible loss
   c. ~2500 ml H_2O and electrolytes per day to replace gastrointestinal and respiratory loss
   d. ~ 500 ml H_2O and electrolytes per day to replace gastrointestinal and respiratory loss
   e. ~1000 ml colloid daily

5. Which of the following parameters will give the least information about the patient with chronic renal disease during the perioperative period?
   a. ECG
   b. Urine specific gravity
   c. Central venous pressure
   d. Blood pressure
   e. Serum electrolytes

6. All of the following statements about acute renal failure are true except:
   a. Acute renal failure may be the result of administration of aminoglycoside antibiotics
   b. Perioperative acute renal failure carries a poor prognosis
   c. Acute renal failure may occur secondary to sepsis
   d. Perioperative oliguria is always an indication of acute renal failure
   e. None of the above

7. The correct treatment of established acute renal failure includes all of the following except:
   a. "Flushing" the kidneys to remove pigments
   b. Hemodialysis
   c. Fluid restriction
   d. Peritoneal dialysis
   e. Precise fluid balance charting

8. Hyperkalemia may be treated by administration of all of the following except:
   a. Sodium bicarbonate
   b. Diuretics
   c. Insulin and glucose
   d. Exchange resins
   e. Normal saline infusion

9. Each of the following tests may be useful in distinguishing prerenal from renal oliguria except:
   a. Urine specific gravity
   b. Fractional excretion of Na^+
   c. U/P potassium
   d. U/P creatinine
   e. None of the above

10. Which of the following statements about the patient with chronic renal failure is true:
    a. Insensible loss is greater than in the patient with normal renal function
    b. Urine output, when present, should be replaced with infusion of 0.5% or 0.33% saline solution
    c. Colloid solutions should never be administered
    d. Perioperative Na^+ requirements are less than in the patient with normal renal function
    e. Low hemoglobin concentrations are poorly tolerated

CHAPTER 12

1. To avoid pain after thoracotomy, patients may:
   a. Reflexly contract their expiratory muscles (splint)
   b. Actively exhale
   c. Avoid coughing
   d. All of the above
   e. None of the above
2. The decrease in vital capacity that follows thoracotomy is:
   a. Minimal
   b. 10%
   c. 40%
   d. 75%
   e. 90%
3. Postoperative hypoxemia is most commonly caused by;
   a. Worsening relationship between FRC and closing capacity
   b. Hypoxic vasoconstriction
   c. Posthyperventilation apnea
   d. Atelectasis
   e. Pneumonia

4. Chest tube drainage systems:
   a. Employ four chambers
   b. Allow air from the drainage system to enter the lung during inspiration
   c. Develop a negative pressure that is determined solely by the amount of suction applied
   d. Have an underwater seal, which should fluctuate with respirations
   e. Are always placed on suction even during patient transport
5. A patient being mechanically ventilated who has a bronchopleural fistula is optimally managed with:
   a. Double-lumen endotracheal tube
   b. A standard endotracheal tube
   c. An uncuffed endotracheal tube
   d. The chest tube attached to suction
   e. Removal of the chest tube
6. Life-threatening complications after pneumonectomy include:
   a. Pulmonary vascular hemorrhage
   b. Herniation of the heart through a pericardial defect
   c. Tension pneumothorax
   d. Right-to-left shunting through a patent foramen ovale
   e. All of the above
7. Which of the following will not improve pulmonary function after thoracotomy?
   a. Incentive spirometry
   b. Supplemental humidified oxygen
   c. Keeping the diseased lung dependent as much as possible
   d. Chest percussion and postural drainage
   e. Adequate analgesia
8. Patients with myasthenia gravis:
   a. Rarely need postoperative mechanical ventilation
   b. Can have weakness of respiratory and pharyngeal muscles
   c. Have antibodies to acetylcholine
   d. Should automatically be started on their full dose of anticholinesterase postoperatively
   e. Show resistance to muscle relaxants

9. Epidural morphine can cause all of the following except:
   a. Hypotension
   b. Early respiratory depression
   c. Late respiratory depression
   d. Nausea and vomiting
   e. Pruritus

10. Which technique when used alone cannot provide adequate postoperative analgesia after thoracotomy?
    a. Epidural narcotics
    b. Administration of local anesthetics through an intrapleural catheter
    c. Patient-controlled analgesia (PCA)
    d. Transcutaneous electrical nerve stimulation (TENS)
    e. Cryoanalgesia

CHAPTER 13

1. The advantages of using the PACU as a special procedures unit include all the following except:
   a. Proximity to the operating room
   b. Improvement in PACU efficiency
   c. Accessibility of sterile precautions
   d. Ready availability of an anesthesiologist
   e. No need to wear operating room garb

2. Special procedures that may conveniently be performed in the PACU include all of the following except:
   a. Electroconvulsive therapy
   b. Celiac plexus block
   c. Swan-Ganz catheter insertion
   d. Administration of last rites
   e. Blood patch for spinal headache

3. The nursing role in special procedures in the PACU includes all of the following except:
   a. Verification of signed consent forms
   b. Careful monitoring of vital signs
   c. Application of the current during cardioversion
   d. Emotional support
   e. Completion of the customary preanesthetic checklist if anesthesia is to be administered

4. Cardiovascular complications after electroconvulsive therapy:
   a. Are mainly the result of excess vagal tone
   b. Usually resolve in 10 to 15 minutes
   c. Are exaggerated if there is preexistent vascular disease
   d. Are characterized by hypertension and tachycardia after 5 minutes
   e. All of the above

5. In considering cardioversion, which of the following is not true?
   a. It is an effective means of converting cardiac dysrhythmias to sinus rhythm
   b. It is indicated mainly for atrial flutter and atrial fibrillation
   c. Fairly deep general anesthesia is required because of burn pain
   d. On rare occasions, pulmonary edema may be a severe complication
   e. It is less likely to be successful if the patient is receiving large doses of propranolol

6. Epidural anesthesia:
   a. Provides patchy pain relief
   b. Has a sympatholytic effect
   c. Does not increase blood supply to the legs
   d. Is performed through a 22- or 25-gauge needle
   e. None of the above

7. A brachial plexus block:
   a. Takes about 20 to 30 minutes for total blockade
   b. Involves placement of a small-gauge needle close to the brachial plexus sheath
   c. Requires 5-10 ml local anesthetic solution
   d. Can be completely successful only if a supraclavicular route is used
   e. Is the first line of treatment for angina pectoris

8. The most common severe complication of nerve block is:
   a. Allergic response
   b. Peripheral rash
   c. Cardiovascular collapse
   d. Tachycardia
   e. Hemiplegia

9. After hemolytic transfusion reaction, all of the following steps should be taken except:
   a. Blood administration should be immediately discontinued
   b. The patient's blood and urine should be checked for free hemoglobin
   c. No diuretics should be given because the patient is already hypovolemic
   d. Steroids should be given to modify the antigen-antibody reaction
   e. Step-by-step documentation on the hospital record is essential

10. The least common complication of blood transfusion is:
    a. Hemolytic transfusion reaction
    b. Shivering caused by hypothermia
    c. Septicemia caused by pyrogens
    d. Transmission of serum hepatitis
    e. Congestive cardiac failure if the blood is given over 2 hours

CHAPTER 14

1. Hypotension in burn patients occurs because of:
   a. Increased vascular permeability leading to decreased intravascular volume
   b. Release of histamine and prostaglandins
   c. Loss of skin barrier leading to hypoproteinemia
   d. Hypoxia
   e. All of the above

2. Volume replacement:
   a. Should be given as rapidly as possible for the first 24 hours of hospitalization after thermal injury
   b. Should contain 10% dextrose
   c. May result in generalized edema because of increased vascular permeability
   d. Can cause edema that is limited to the burn site
   e. Should be with blood.

3. Routine therapy for burn patients includes all of the following *except:*
   a. Tetanus prophylaxis
   b. Full-thickness wound biopsy to identify organisms before clinical evidence of infection
   c. Prophylactic intravenous antibiotics
   d. Monitoring of antibiotic level after intravenous antibiotics are started
   e. Frequent electrolyte analyses

4. Mortality in burn patients is most directly affected by:
   a. Age
   b. Percent of body surface area affected
   c. Inhalation injury
   d. Depth of burn
   e. Causative agent

5. A difference between pediatric and adult patients is that:
   a. Adults require more glucose during resuscitation
   b. Adults are more likely to have airway obstruction after inhalation injury
   c. Adults have higher baseline relative O_2 and metabolic demands, which are increased with large surface burns
   d. Adults have more respiratory reserve, and fatigue less rapidly with the increased work associated with respiratory tract injury
   e. Inability to communicate with children increases morbidity

6. Carbon monoxide:
   a. Is a foul-smelling gas with a high affinity for hemoglobin
   b. Inhalation causes a fall in PaO_2
   c. In the blood may cause nausea, dizziness, and headache
   d. Can result in coma at concentrations of 5% carboxyhemoglobin
   e. Rarely causes fatality

7. Intraoperative management of the burn victim should include all of the following *except:*
   a. Warmed intravenous fluids to avoid hypothermia
   b. Ready use of surgical placement of intravenous cannulae if there are extensive skin burns
   c. Central venous pressure measurements
   d. Urinary catheter
   e. Pulse oximetry

8. Anesthetic management of the burn victim should include:
   a. Heavy sedation before examination of possibly injured airways
   b. Avoidance of narcotics because of patient's altered metabolism
   c. Avoidance of positive end-expiratory pressure (PEEP) in the presence of airway injury
   d. Inflation of endotracheal cuff just enough to prevent a leak
   e. Immediate blood transfusion

9. In burn patients:
   a. Use of succinylcholine should be completely avoided because of risk of hyperkalemia
   b. Use of all muscle relaxants should be avoided because of their prolonged action
   c. Nondepolarizing muscle relaxants can be safely used up to 25% of the usual dose
   d. Reversal of muscle relaxants requires the usual dose
   e. Any muscle relaxant may be safely used

10. All of the following regarding topical antibiotics in burn patients are true *except:*
   a. Topical antibiotics have been found to increase bacterial superinfection
   b. Mafenide can cause a metabolic acidosis and pain on application
   c. Silver nitrate often stains skin and clothing
   d. Silver sulfadiazine has less toxicity and intermediate absorption when compared with other topical agents
   e. Systemic complications may occur

CHAPTER 15

1. Basic life support includes:
   a. Use of ECG
   b. Endotracheal intubation
   c. Cannulation of vein
   d. Cardiac compression rate of 80 to 100 per minute
   e. Protective measures against corneal abrasions

2. Endotracheal intubation:
   a. Should aways be performed as a first step in CPR
   b. Should be preceded by oxygenation of the lungs by other methods
   c. Should be done with an EOA or EGTA tube
   d. Makes it difficult to compress chest at a rate of 80/minute
   e. Should best be done through the nose

3. Aspiration of gastric contents has these characteristics:
   a. May follow removal of an esophageal airway
   c. May follow removal of an endotracheal tube
   d. Is particularly hazardous if the pH of the aspirate is less than 2.5
   e. All of the above

4. Lidocaine is an antidysrhythmic drug that:
   a. Can cause seizures
   b. Is usually given as a 2% infusion
   c. Is given as 1 mg/kg bolus
   d. Increases ventricular contractility
   e. Is no longer used as a first-line drug

5. Atropine sulfate is:
   a. of no value in ventricular tachycardia
   b. always required if the heart rate is less than 60/minute
   c. usually given in 2 mg boluses up to a total of 10 mg
   d. not indicated in high-degree atrioventricular block
   e. not given to children because it causes fever

6. Epinephrine is given in cardiac arrest to:
   a. Increase myocardial contractility
   b. Increase myocardial blood flow
   c. Coarsen ventricular fibrillation
   d. Convert asystole to ventricular fibrillation
   e. All of the above
7. Defibrillation requires:
   a. Initial energy of 50 joules
   b. Reduction in transthoracic impedance
   c. Synchronized switching
   d. Two paddles on the lateral chest walls
   e. Lidocaine be given first
8. Ventricular tachycardia presents:
   a. As three or more sequential ventricular complexes at a rate greater than 100 per minute
   b. With a regular or irregular rate
   c. With or without a pulse
   d. No fixed relationship between P waves and QRS complexes
   e. All of the above
9. $NaCHO_3$ is no longer a first-line drug because:
   a. It crosses rapidly into cells
   b. Each mEg yields 10 mm Hg CO_2
   c. It causes a paradoxical worsening of hypercarbia and acidosis
   d. The initial dose of 1 mEq/kg is too large a volume
   e. It causes CSF alkalosis
10. Which of the following drugs is indicated in recurrent ventricular fibrillation?
    a. Amrinone
    b. Verapamil
    c. Calcium chloride
    d. Epinephrine
    e. Bretylium

CHAPTER 16

1. Which of the following organizations has mandated criteria for determining brain death?
   a. The Presidents' Cabinet
   b. Congress
   c. Individual states
   d. The American Medical Association
   e. Hospital boards

2. According to the President's Commission guidelines for determining brain death, which region of the brain must be shown to be completely and irreversibly lost?
   a. Cerebral cortex
   b. Cerebral hemispheres
   c. Brainstem
   d. Entire central nervous system
   e. None; heart must stop spontaneously
3. Which statement concerning spinal reflexes is *false*?
   a. They consist of withdrawal of the legs in response to noxious stimulation
   b. They indicate that the spinal cord, which is part of the central nervous system, and afferent and efferent nerve tracts are intact
   c. Cephalic reflexes, unlike spinal reflexes, rely on the brainstem and cranial nerves
   d. When absent, indicate brain death
   e. When spinal reflexes are present, the President's Commission guidelines preclude a determination of brain death.
4. In testing for apnea, according to most criteria, at which level must the $PaCO_2$ rise before it is considered an adequate stimulus to breathing?
   a. 20 to 30 mm Hg
   b. 30 to 40 mm Hg
   c. 40 to 50 mm Hg
   d. $\geq$ 50 mm Hg
   e. It does not necessarily rise at all because the patient is not breathing
5. In which condition is an isoelectric EEG a valid indicator of brain death?
   a. Hypothermia
   b. Barbiturate intoxication
   c. Presence of cardiac rhythms or ventilator artifacts
   d. Prematurity of an infant
   e. All of the above
6. If an EEG cannot be performed, which test is the most readily available, reliable alternative confirmatory test in the United States?
   a. Four-vessel angiography
   b. Radioisotope angiography
   c. Evoked responses
   d. Observation for 24 hours
   e. CT scan

7. In children and full-term infants older than 7 days, which is the recommended confirmatory test?
   a. EEG
   b. Apnea test
   c. Four-vessel angiography
   d. Concomitant radionuclide angiography
   e. CT scan

8. In which condition might a patient be apneic, mute, and quadriplegic, but have normal mentation?
   a. Persistent vegetative state
   b. Carbon monoxide poisoning
   c. Hysteria
   d. Locked-in syndrome
   e. Aspirin overdose

9. In which case cannot criteria for brain death be applied?
   a. Premature infant
   b. Pregnant woman
   c. Attempted murder victim
   d. Neurosurgical patient
   e. Any intraoperative death

10. Of the following guidelines from the President's Commission, which is treated with the most flexibility?
    a. Exclusion of barbiturate intoxication
    b. Exclusion of hypothermia
    c. Requirement for a confirmatory test
    d. Period of observation being at least 6 hours
    e. All are flexible

CHAPTER 17

1. The structural configuration of the PACU that is capable of accommodating a large bed capacity (more than 15 beds) is the:
   a. Rectangle
   b. Circle
   c. Square
   d. Semicircle
   e. Oval

2. Dividing walls between individual patient units in the PACU provide:
   a. Complete visual surveillance of all patients
   b. Patient privacy
   c. Cost-efficient staff requirements
   d. Complete auditory observation of the patient
   e. Structural improvement

3. The intubation cart or tray (adult and pediatric) provides:
   a. All necessary emergency medications
   b. ECG monitoring capabilities
   c. All equipment necessary to manage a respiratory emergency
   d. Cardiac pacing equipment
   e. Defibrillator

4. The ambient temperature in the PACU should be maintained at:
   a. 18.5° C (70° F)
   b. 24.0° C (80° F)
   c. 20.75° C (75° F)
   d. 26.25° C (85° F)
   e. Temperature is not important if humidity is high enough

5. The relative humidity in the PACU should be maintained at:
   a. 50% to 60%
   b. 60% to 70%
   c. 40% to 50%
   d. 80% to 90%
   e. Depends on temperature

6. To reduce sensory stimulation in the PACU:
   a. Lighting should be bright and direct
   b. Colors of walls, wallpaper, and draperies should be pastels or beige
   c. Ceiling tiles should be of an intricate design involving twisting shapes and patterns
   d. Discussion should occur at the patient's bedside
   e. Auditory signal on the ECG should be turned off

7. For every OR surgical suite there should be at least the following number of available patient care units in the PACU:
   a. ½ to 1
   b. 1½ to 2
   c. 2½ to 3
   d. 3½ to 4
   e. Varies from day to day

8. An alternative location if a PACU isolation room is not available for recovering a patient who is on strict or respiratory isolation is:
   a. The patient's private room
   b. A semiprivate room on the patient's unit
   c. An open design PACU
   d. An open design SICU
   e. The OR until recovered

9. Fire extinguishers (regardless of type) must be located in the PACU every:
   a. 300 square meters (3300 square feet)
   b. 200 square meters (2200 square feet)
   c. 100 square meters (1100 square feet)
   d. 400 square meters (4400 square feet)
   e. 50 square meters (500 square feet)

10. It is highly recommended that these mandatory items—sphygmomanometer, oxygen therapy, suction, ECG monitor—be:
    a. Ceiling suspended
    b. Wall mounted
    c. Portable
    d. Retrieved from a central location within the PACU
    e. Easily and quickly borrowed from the department of anesthesiology

CHAPTER 18

1. Elements of the nursing process include:
   a. Assessment
   b. Plan
   c. Intervention
   d. Evaluation
   e. All of the above

2. Assessment skills include all the following except:
   a. Observation
   b. Evaluation
   c. Percussion
   d. Auscultation
   e. Palpation

3. Criteria to be considered when designing a classification system would not include:
   a. Size of patient
   b. Admission score
   c. Length of stay
   d. Degree of nursing intervention required
   e. Monitoring requirements

4. When determining staffing patterns, the following statistics are vital:
   a. Census
   b. Hours of operation
   c. Peak activity levels
   d. Acuity levels
   e. All of the above

5. The use of flowsheets and checklists is advisable in the PACU for all the following except:
   a. Time element
   b. Ease of documentation
   c. Eliminates need for direct observation
   d. Data retrieval
   e. Objective versus subjective

6. Before writing nursing care standards, it is essential to have preestablished:
   a. Policies
   b. Procedures
   c. Standing orders
   d. Role delineations
   e. All of the above

7. Components of a good quality assurance program would not include:
   a. Established criteria
   b. Method of monitoring
   c. Unlimited time elements
   d. Problem-solving techniques
   e. Isolating problems

8. Resources to be used when establishing standards of care include all the following except:
   a. Accreditation manual for hospitals
   b. State guidelines for care
   c. ASPAN guidelines
   d. ASA guidelines
   e. AORN standards

9. Responsibilities that can be delegated to ancillary personnel include all the following except:
   a. Transportation
   b. Stocking
   c. Charting
   d. Requisitions
   e. Maintenance of equipment

10. The role of the LPN in the PACU is limited to all but which of the following?
    a. Monitoring
    b. Direct patient care
    c. Assessment
    d. Reporting to RN
    e. Charting

CHAPTER 19

1. One of the major premises of adult learning principles is that the adult learner wants to learn.
   True/False

2. Programmed instruction is the least time-consuming and therefore has become the most widely used teaching method.
   True/False

3. No matter what method of evaluation is used, the greater the frequency of feedback, the greater the possibility of performance consistent with a standard.
   True/False

4. How long should a typical PACU orientation program be for a new nurse?
   a. 1 day
   b. 1 week
   c. 6 weeks
   d. 8 to 12 weeks
   e. More than 3 months

5. Which method do orientees prefer when learning a PACU skill?
   a. Dynamic lecture
   b. Hands-on experience
   c. Reading policy and procedure manuals
   d. Involvement in paper work and charting
   e. Acting as ward liaison

6. Nursing personnel policies should be written by:
   a. Head nurse
   b. Assistant director
   c. Director of the unit
   d. Staff nurses
   e. All of the above

7. The PACU nurse should have training in:
   a. Anesthetic drugs
   b. Cardiopulmonary resuscitation
   c. ECG interpretation
   d. Basic anesthetic techniques
   e. All of the above

8. Planning for staff development includes:
   a. Assessment
   b. Planning
   c. Implementation
   d. Evaluation
   e. All of the above

9. A preceptor should be:
   a. The head nurse
   b. The clinical instructor
   c. The senior staff nurse
   d. A collaboration of all three
   e. Separate from the day-to-day PACU nurse

10. Orientation to any new work environment is a time of adjustment and stress.
    True/False

CHAPTER 20

1. Health may be defined as:
   a. Absence of disease
   b. Balance of equilibrium
   c. Complete state of well-being
   d. Maintenance of homeostasis
   e. All of the above

2. A holistic concept of human beings includes:
   a. Endogenous and exogenous environment
   b. Physiological, psychological, socioeconomical processes
   c. Metaphysical/spiritual process
   d. Homeostasis of all systems
   e. All of the above

3. The preoperative visit:
   a. Contributes to client apprehension and fear
   b. Has a definite effect on length of stay
   c. May cause tension between surgeon and patient
   d. Is a methodology in a holistic approach for increased communication and patient teaching
   e. Is not necessary

4. Recommended preparation for preoperative teaching should include the following:
   a. Discussion with surgeon regarding patient
   b. Discussion with unit RN, review of chart, identification of previous surgery and type
   c. Discussion with surgeon and unit RN
   d. Review of chart and identification of previous surgery and type
   e. Knowledge of patient's value systems and life experience

5. Recommended teaching aids are structured:
   a. According to patient's age and financial status
   b. To include staff participation
   c. To accommodate consumer and staff schedules
   d. According to availability of institutional financial resources and staffing patterns
   e. For adaptation in certain surgical specialties only

6. Interviewing techniques may be classified as:
   a. Direct, nondirect, communicative
   b. Nondirect, communicative, transactional analysis (child, parent, mature adult)
   c. Direct, Rogerian, transactional analysis (child, parent, mature adult)
   d. Direct, assertive, Rogerian
   e. Direct, assertive, transactional analysis (child, parent, mature adult)

7. The nursing process applied to the perioperative role of the PACU nurse involves:
   a. Preoperative interviews and patient teaching
   b. Identification of patient problems and potential problems
   c. Individualized nursing care plan
   d. Evaluation of postanesthetic care
   e. All of the above

8. The pediatric patient:
   a. Requires no special preoperative preparation or treatment
   b. Should never be spoken to directly
   c. Cannot be identified by an individual teaching care plan
   d. Is assessed depending on developmental level and determination of language and comprehensive skills
   e. Is difficult to handle when the parents are present

9. Recommendations regarding pediatric patients:
   a. Preoperative teaching need not include both child and parents
   b. Medical equipment for handling is not significant (show and tell)
   c. Preoperative class or tour is not meaningful to children or parents
   d. Presence of parents in the holding area and PACU alleviates the child's fear of separation (from parents)
   e. All of the above

10. Ambulatory patients:
    a. Do not require preoperative teaching, since length of stay is short
    b. Require no reenforcement of instructions
    c. Cannot be included in preoperative classes, tours, or interviews because of scheduling difficulties
    d. Should not be communicated with via phone, preoperatively and postoperatively because it causes unnecessary anxiety
    e. Should have specific preoperative instructions, as well as discharge instructions

CHAPTER 21

1. Medical malpractice:
   a. Is a form of negligence
   b. Involves imprudent acts
   c. Shows a lack of conformance with the standards of the medical community
   d. Is not a criminal act
   e. All of the above

2. A plaintiff is:
   a. The person who institutes the lawsuit
   b. The person to be defended in a lawsuit
   c. Often the godparents, in the case of an infant
   d. Often a spouse, in the case of a paralyzed adult
   e. The lawyer's friend

3. The standard of care:
   a. Cannot be explained in a courtroom
   b. Is presented by expert witnesses
   c. Is an imaginary concept that holds no weight in a lawsuit
   d. Is determined by what a reasonably prudent nonmedical person would do
   e. All of the above

4. The statute of limitations:
   a. Varies from state to state
   b. Is the period during which a lawsuit may be instituted
   c. Sometimes begins when the patient discovers the injury
   d. Is of extreme importance when a lawsuit is initiated
   e. All of the above

5. The doctor's order is for digoxin 5.0 mg. You believe this is an excessive dose. You:
   a. Give the medication because you trust and respect the doctor
   b. Question the anesthesia resident on call for the PACU
   c. Contact the physician who wrote the order to clarify it
   d. Do not give it and forget about it
   e. None of the above

6. A medication you are unfamiliar with is ordered by the physician. You:
   a. Ask other staff members about it
   b. Look it up in the *Physician's Desk Reference*
   c. Give it because you trust and respect the doctor
   d. Give it, and hope for the best
   e. Give something you know and believe the patient needs

7. The physician calls and gives a telephone order. You:
   a. Have another staff nurse verify the order
   b. Write it as it is being said
   c. Repeat what you have written back to the doctor
   d. All of the above
   e. None of the above

8. Your patient's condition suddenly starts to deteriorate. You:
   a. Page the doctor stat
   b. Take the necessary nursing actions
   c. Document everything that is done while awaiting the doctor
   d. Continue to call for help until there is a response
   e. All of the above

9. Your patient suffers complications in the PACU and needs to be brought back to surgery. You:
   a. Call the risk management department to report the complication
   b. Refuse to sign your nursing note because you do not want to be implicated
   c. Tell the patient's family that they should sue
   d. Do not follow up on the patient's condition
   e. All of the above

10. Exposure on a case can be minimized by:
    a. Reporting fewer cases to the risk management department
    b. Extremely careful record keeping
    c. Signing your note illegibly
    d. Refusing to care for more than one patient
    e. All of the above

Answers

CHAPTER 1

1. e
2. e
3. d
4. e
5. a
6. d
7. e
8. c
9. e
10. e

CHAPTER 2

1. c
2. d
3. c
4. c
5. c
6. b
7. e
8. c
9. b
10. e

CHAPTER 3

1. c
2. d
3. e
4. e
5. d
6. c
7. e
8. b
9. c
10. d

CHAPTER 4

1. c
2. c
3. e
4. e
5. d
6. b
7. a
8. b
9. c
10. c

CHAPTER 5

1. e
2. b
3. d
4. d
5. d
6. b
7. e
8. a
9. a
10. c

CHAPTER 6

1. d
2. d
3. e
4. d
5. a
6. a
7. b
8. c
9. d
10. e

CHAPTER 7

1. b
2. e
3. c
4. d
5. e
6. c
7. c
8. c
9. e
10. c

CHAPTER 8

1. d
2. b
3. d
4. b
5. c
6. a
7. d
8. b
9. a
10. d

CHAPTER 9

1. b
2. b
3. d
4. d
5. d
6. d
7. a
8. c
9. c
10. d

CHAPTER 10

1. b
2. c
3. c
4. a
5. c
6. d
7. c
8. e
9. c
10. a

CHAPTER 11

1. b
2. d
3. a
4. b
5. b
6. d
7. a
8. b
9. c
10. b

CHAPTER 12

1. a
2. c
3. a
4. d
5. a
6. e
7. c
8. b
9. a
10. d

CHAPTER 13

1. e
2. d
3. c
4. e
5. c
6. b
7. a
8. b
9. c
10. e

CHAPTER 14

1. d
2. c
3. c
4. c
5. d
6. c
7. b
8. d
9. d
10. a

CHAPTER 15

1. d
2. b
3. e
4. c
5. a
6. e
7. b
8. e
9. c
10. e

CHAPTER 16

1. c
2. c
3. d
4. d
5. c
6. a
7. d
8. d
9. a
10. d

CHAPTER 17

1. a
2. b
3. c
4. c
5. a
6. b
7. b
8. b
9. b
10. b

CHAPTER 18

1. e.
2. b
3. a
4. e
5. c
6. e
7. c
8. e
9. c
10. c

CHAPTER 19

1. True
2. False
3. True
4. d
5. b
6. e
7. d
8. e
9. d
10. True

CHAPTER 20

1. e
2. e
3. d
4. b
5. d
6. c
7. e
8. d
9. d

CHAPTER 21

1. e
2. a
3. b
4. d
5. c
6. b
7. d
8. d
9. a
10. b

INDEX